Antiviral Methods and Protocols

METHODS IN MOLECULAR MEDICINE™

John M. Walker, SERIES EDITOR

42. **Vaccine Adjuvants: *Preparation Methods and Research Protocols***, edited by *Derek T. O'Hagan*, 2000
41. **Celiac Disease: *Methods and Protocols***, edited by *Michael N. Marsh*, 2000
40. **Diagnostic and Therapeutic Antibodies**, edited by *Andrew J. T. George and Catherine E. Urch*, 2000
39. **Ovarian Cancer: *Methods and Protocols***, edited by *John M. S. Bartlett*, 2000
38. **Aging Methods and Protocols**, edited by *Yvonne A. Barnett and Christopher P. Barnett*, 2000
37. **Electrically Mediated Delivery of Molecules to Cells**, edited by *Mark J. Jaroszeski, Richard Heller, and Richard Gilbert*, 2000
36. **Septic Shock Methods and Protocols**, edited by *Thomas J. Evans*, 2000
35. **Gene Therapy of Cancer: *Methods and Protocols***, edited by *Wolfgang Walther and Ulrike Stein*, 2000
34. **Rotavirus Methods and Protocols**, edited by *James Gray and Ulrich Desselberger*, 2000
33. **Cytomegalovirus Protocols**, edited by *John Sinclair*, 2000
32. **Alzheimer's Disease: *Methods and Protocols***, edited by *Nigel M. Hooper*, 1999
31. **Hemostasis and Thrombosis Protocols: *Methods in Molecular Medicine***, edited by *David J. Perry and K. John Pasi*, 1999
30. **Vascular Disease: *Molecular Biology and Gene Therapy Protocols***, edited by *Andrew H. Baker*, 1999
29. **DNA Vaccines: *Methods and Protocols***, edited by *Douglas B. Lowrie and Robert Whalen*, 1999
28. **Cytotoxic Drug Resistance Mechanisms**, edited by *Robert Brown and Uta Böger-Brown*, 1999
27. **Clinical Applications of Capillary Electrophoresis**, edited by *Stephen M. Palfrey*, 1999
26. **Quantitative PCR Protocols**, edited by *Bernd Kochanowski and Udo Reischl*, 1999
25. **Drug Targeting**, edited by *G. E. Francis and Cristina Delgado*, 1999
24. **Antiviral Methods and Protocols**, edited by *Derek Kinchington and Raymond F. Schinazi*, 2000
23. **Peptidomimetics Protocols**, edited by *Wieslaw M. Kazmierski*, 1999
22. **Neurodegeneration Methods and Protocols**, edited by *Jean Harry and Hugh A. Tilson*, 1999
21. **Adenovirus Methods and Protocols**, edited by *William S. M. Wold*, 1998
20. **Sexually Transmitted Diseases: *Methods and Protocols***, edited by *Rosanna Peeling and P. Frederick Sparling*, 1999
19. **Hepatitis C Protocols**, edited by *Johnson Yiu-Nam Lau*, 1998
18. **Tissue Engineering**, edited by *Jeffrey R. Morgan and Martin L. Yarmush*, 1999
17. **HIV Protocols**, edited by *Nelson Michael and Jerome H. Kim*, 1999
16. **Clinical Applications of PCR**, edited by *Y. M. Dennis Lo*, 1998
15. **Molecular Bacteriology: *Protocols and Clinical Applications***, edited by *Neil Woodford and Alan Johnson*, 1998
14. **Tumor Marker Protocols**, edited by *Margaret Hanausek and Zbigniew Walaszek*, 1998
13. **Molecular Diagnosis of Infectious Diseases**, edited by *Udo Reischl*, 1998
12. **Diagnostic Virology Protocols**, edited by *John R. Stephenson and Alan Warnes*, 1998
11. **Therapeutic Application of Ribozymes**, edited by *Kevin J. Scanlon*, 1998
10. **Herpes Simplex Virus Protocols**, edited by *S. Moira Brown and Alasdair MacLean*, 1998
9. **Lectin Methods and Protocols**, edited by *Jonathan M. Rhodes and Jeremy D. Milton*, 1998
8. ***Helicobacter pylori* Protocols**, edited by *Christopher L. Clayton and Harry L. T. Mobley*, 1997
7. **Gene Therapy Protocols**, edited by *Paul D. Robbins*, 1997
6. **Molecular Diagnosis of Cancer**, edited by *Finbarr Cotter*, 1996
5. **Molecular Diagnosis of Genetic Diseases**, edited by *Rob Elles*, 1996

METHODS IN MOLECULAR MEDICINE™

Antiviral Methods and Protocols

Edited by

Derek Kinchington

St. Bartholomew's and the Royal London School of Medicine and Dentistry, London, UK

and

Raymond F. Schinazi

Emory University, Decatur, GA

Humana Press **Totowa, New Jersey**

999 Riverview Drive, Suite 208
Totowa, New Jersey 07512

This publication is printed on acid-free paper. ∞
ANSI Z39.48-1984 (American Standards Institute)
Permanence of Paper for Printed Library Materials.

Cover illustration: Figure 1 from Chapter 11, "Antiviral Screening Assays for Human Herpesviruses 6 and 7," by Jodi B. Black and Philip E. Pellett.

Cover design by Patricia F. Cleary.

For additional copies, pricing for bulk purchases, and/or information about other Humana titles, contact Humana at the above address or at any of the following numbers: Tel.: 973-256-1699; Fax: 973-256-8341; E-mail: humana@humanapr.com, or visit our Website: http://humanapress.com

Printed in the United States of America. 10 9 8 7 6 5 4 3 2 1

Library of Congress Cataloging in Publication Data

Main entry under title:

Methods in molecular medicine™.

Antiviral methods and protocols/edited by Derek Kinchington and Raymond F. Schinazi.
p. cm.—(methods in molecular medicine; vol. 24)
Includes index.
ISBN 0-89603-561-1 (alk. paper)
1. Antiviral agents—Laboratory manuals. I. Kinchington, Derek. II. Schinazi, Raymond F. III. Series: Methods in molecular medicine; 24.
[DNLM: 1. Hepatitis, Viral, Human—drug therapy. 2. Antiviral Agents—therapeutic use. 3. DNA Virus Infections—drug therapy. 4. RNA Virus Infections—drug therapy. WC 536 A633 1999]
RM411.A575 2000
616.9'25061—dc21
DNLM/DLC
for Library of Congress 99-25099
CIP

Preface

This latest addition to the *Methods in Molecular Medicine* series, *Antiviral Methods and Protocols*, is opportune because there is an increasing interest in discovering compounds that are effective against both chronic and acute viral infections. A number of the methods described in the volume are unpublished and their inclusion indicates the speed at which this field is moving. This volume is not a review but each chapter contains methods validated by the experts who have spent time in developing the protocols.

The hallmark of this series is the comprehensive way in which the methods are described, which includes a list of all the reagents needed for each protocol. Of importance is the section on tips and pitfalls that the authors have discovered while developing their protocols. The manual itself is designed to be used by researchers in universities and industry who are familiar with a range of biological techniques but who want to set up quickly a novel assay system. We encourage a dialog between readers and authors, which may also result in useful collaborations.

The first chapter gives an overview of the change in methodologies that have been used for discovering active compounds. Safety considerations have also been reviewed because there are some significant differences in containment requirements between the United States and the United Kingdom, for example. Routine quality testing of cell cultures has also been highlighted because there are many stories of results being invalidated when target cells have been contaminated by microorganisms, which, even at low levels, may significantly alter antiviral endpoints.

For each virus group the chapters that describe the assays start with cell-based systems and progress through to those of biochemical and molecular design. Those associated with hepatitis viruses predominantly describe protocols for HBV, but a relatively new method is described for a high throughput screen for compounds against HVC. In the herpesvirus section, cell-based assays are described for HSV 1 and 2, CMV, VZV, and EBV. A chapter details the methodology for monitoring drug resistance in clinical herpesviruses, which is now mandatory in immunocompromised patients. The section on HIV methods contains a wide variety of methods ranging from those evaluating the activity of topical virucidal agents, an area that may prove to be important in reducing the rates of infection, through cell-based assays and molecular techniques used in identifying agents active against reverse transcriptase, protease, and integrase. Of importance is the chapter describing the methods that identify the phenotypic and genotypic properties of resistant clinical isolates. This methodology undoubtedly will become more automated, but in nondiagnostic settings it will be necessary to carry out such studies on a small scale. The two assays on human papillomaviruses describe a relatively simple method for identifying E6 and E7 proteins, responsible for cellular immortalization, in cell lysates and a molecular approach for identifying the E1 and E2 proteins by in vitro translation. Finally, some chapters describe the virological and biochemical assays that measure the resistance of viruses against one of the new generations of neuraminidase inhibitors.

Production of volumes such as this are always flawed by the passage of time. However, we hope that it will provide a snapshot of the valuable and exciting work that continues in this area of science and be a significant aid to those involved in discovering new compounds.

Derek Kinchington
Raymond F. Schinazi

Contents

Contributors

GRACIELA ANDREI • *Rega Institute for Medical Research, Katholieke Universiteit, Leuven, Belgium*
JANE ANGIER • *Glaxo-Wellcome Medicines Research Centre, Stevenage, UK*
JAN BALZARINI • *Rega Institute for Medical Research, Katholieke Universiteit, Leuven, Belgium*
RICHARD C. BETHELL • *Discovery Biology Unit, Pfizer Ltd., Kent, UK*
JODI B. BLACK • *Centers for Disease Control and Prevention, Atlanta, GA*
TONY J. BLICK • *Biomolecular Research Institute, Parkville, Australia*
JÜRG BÖNI • *Swiss National Center for Retroviruses, Zurich, Switzerland*
SALVATORE T. BUTERA • *Retrovirus Disease Branch, Centers for Disease Control and Prevention, Atlanta, GA*
GILDA M. CIVITICO • *Victorian Infectious Diseases Reference Laboratory, Fairfield Hospital, Fairfield, UK*
MARIE-PIERRE DE BÉTHUNE • *Tobotec, Mechelen, Belgium*
ERIC DE CLERQ • *Rega Institute for Medical Research, Katholieke Universiteit, Leuven, Belgium*
JAN DESMYTER • *Rega Institute for Medical Research, Katholieke Universiteit, Leuven, Belgium*
DONNA DEVINE • *Celltech, Slough, UK*
PETER ERTL • *Glaxo-Wellcome Medicines Research Centre, Stevenage, UK*
PAUL M. FEORINO • *Department of Medical Microbiology, Section of Virology and Cell Biology, Imperial College of Science, Technology, and Medicine, London, UK*
MAUREEN C. FERRAN • *Laboratory of Viral Diseases, NAIAID, National Institutes of Health, Bethesda, MD*
PIERRE FITEN • *Rega Institute for Medical Research, Katholieke Universiteit, Leuven, Belgium*
ERIC S. FURFINE • *Molecular Biochemistry Department, Glaxo-Wellcome, Inc., Research Triangle Park, NC*
J. DAVID GANGEMI • *Department of Microbiology and Molecular Medicine, Clemson University, Clemson, SC*
J. GERARDO GARCIA LERMA • *Retrovirus Disease Branch, Centers for Disease Control, Atlanta, GA*

DAVID R. HARPER • *Department of Virology, St. Bartholomew's and the Royal London School of Medicine and Dentistry, London, UK*
GRAHAM J. HART • *Enzyme Pharmacology Unit, Glaxo-Wellcome Research and Development, Stevenage, UK*
WALID HENEINE • *Retrovirus Diseases Branch, Centers for Disease Control and Prevention, Atlanta, GA*
KURT HERTOGS • *Tibotec, Mechelen, Belgium*
JEFFERY A. JOHNSON • *Department of Microbiology and Molecular Medicine, Clemson University, Clemson, SC*
PHILIP S. JONES • *Roche Research Centre, Welwyn Garden City, UK*
AMANDA J. JOWETT • *Respiratory Diseases Unit, Glaxo-Wellcome Research and Development, Stevenage, UK*
DEREK KINCHINGTON • *Department of Medical Microbiology and Virology, St. Bartholomew's and the Royal London School of Medicine and Dentistry, University of London, UK*
ROBERT W. KING • *The DuPont Merck Co., Wilmington, DE*
BRENT KORBA • *Division of Molecular Virology and Immunology, Georgetown University, Rockville, MD*
ANN D. KWONG • *Vertex Pharmaceuticals, Cambridge, MA*
STEPHANIE K. LADNER • *The DuPont Merck Co., Wilmington, DE*
JUNG-CHUNG LIN • *Department of Microbiology, Tzu Chi College of Medicine, Hualien, Taiwan*
STEPHEN A. LOCARNINI • *Research and Molecular Development, Victorian Infectious Diseases Reference Laboratory, North Melbourne, Australia*
NAOMI MATHEWS • *Celltech, Slough, UK*
ABHIJIT MAZUMDER • *Laboratory of Molecular Pharmacology, National Institutes of Health, Bethesda, MD*
ALISON A. MCBRIDE • *Laboratory of Viral Diseases, NAIAID, National Institutes of Health, Bethesda, MD*
JENNIFER L. MCKIMM-BRESCHKIN • *Biomolecular Research Institute, Parkville, Australia*
NOURI NEAMATI • *Laboratory of Molecular Pharmacology, National Institutes of Health, Bethesda, MD*
TIMOTHY O'CONNOR • *Department of Virology, St. Bartholomew's and the Royal London School of Medicine, University of London, UK*
GHISLAIN OPDENAKKER • *Rega Institute for Medical Research, Katholieke Universiteit, Leuven, Belgium*
MICHAEL J. OTTO • *Department of Clinical Research, Rhone-Poulenc Rorer, Collegeville, PA*

JOSHUA OWEN • *Laboratory of Molecular Pharmacology, National Institutes of Health, Bethesda, MD*
CHRISTOPHE PANNECOUQUE • *Rega Institute for Medical Research, Katholieke Universiteit, Leuven, Belgium*
PHILIP E. PELLETT • *Centers for Disease Control and Prevention, Atlanta, GA*
YVES POMMIER • *Laboratory of Molecular Pharmacology, National Institutes of Health, Bethesda, MD*
SHARON RANDALL • *Clinical Virology and Surrogates Unit, Glaxo Wellcome Research and Development, Stevenage, UK*
CHRISTINE RISANO • *Vertex Pharmaceuticals, Cambridge, MA*
RUDI ROSSAU • *Innogenetics NV, Gent, Belgium*
LINDA RUSSELL • *Glaxo-Wellcome Medicines Research Centre, Stevenage, UK*
ANJALI SAHASRABUDHE • *Biomolecular Research Institute, Parkville, Australia*
JÖRG SCHÜPBACH • *Swiss National Center for Retroviruses, University of Zurich, Switzerland*
RAYMOND F. SCHINAZI • *Veterans Affairs Medical Center and Emory University, Decatur, GA*
KAREN SCHMIDT • *Division of Molecular Virology and Immunology, Georgetown University, Rockville, MD*
JEAN-CLAUDE SCHMIT • *Rega Institute for Medical Research, Katholieke Universiteit, Leuven, Belgium*
TIMOTHY SHAW • *Victorian Infectious Diseases Reference Laboratory, Carlton, Australia*
ROBERT SNOECK • *Rega Institute for Medical Research, Katholieke Universiteit, Leuven, Belgium*
ALISON STACEY • *Centre for Applied Microbiology and Research, Porton Down, UK*
GLYN STACEY • *Centre for Applied Microbiology and Research, Porton Down, UK*
LIEVEN STUYVER • *Innogenetics NV, Gent, Belgium*
SANJAY SUNDER • *Laboratory of Molecular Pharmacology, National Institutes of Health, Bethesda, MD*
ANNE-MIEKE VANDAMME • *AIDS Reference Center, Rega Institute for Medical Research and University Hospital, Katholieke Universiteit, Leuven, Belgium*
KRISTEL VAN LAETHEM • *Rega Institute for Medical Research, Katholieke Universiteit, Leuven, Belgium*

Gonda Verpooten • *Innogenetics NV, Gent, Belgium*
Richard A. Whitaker • *Rhone-Poulenc Rorer, Collegeville, PA*
John D. Williamson • *Department of Medical Microbiology, Section of Virology and Cell Biology, Imperial College of Science, Technology, and Medicine, London, UK*
Myriam Witvrouw • *Rega Institute for Medical Research, Katholieke Universiteit, Leuven, Belgium*
Ann Wyseur • *Innogenetics NV, Gent, Belgium*

1

Changing Methods for Discovering Antiviral Drugs

Philip S. Jones

1. Introduction

Viral diseases were largely untreatable 40 yr ago. Now effective and safe therapies are available. This has led to significant improvements in the quality of life for large numbers of patients. New viral diseases are, however, continuing to emerge and established viruses have been shown to develop resistance to available therapies making this a fertile area for continued drug discovery. The processes used to discover drugs have also changed enormously over the past 40 yr. Nowhere have these changes been more apparent than in the field of antiviral therapy. Therefore, the development of antiviral drugs makes an excellent example for documenting the changes in approaches used to discover active agents. This brief chapter describes some of these changes—from the broad screening in animals and tissue culture first used to the mechanism–based approaches using computer assisted techniques and biostructural information.

2. Beginnings

The origins of antiviral therapies can be traced to the early 1950s, when sulfonamide antibiotics were tested for activity against poxviruses using mice infected with vaccinia *(1)*. A decade of work at the Wellcome laboratories culminated in the development of methisazone, which was introduced in 1960 for the prophylaxis of smallpox (*see* **Scheme 1**). Notable success in the smallpox epidemic in Madras in 1963 demonstrated the value of this compound, but vaccines introduced soon after led to eradication of the disease and made the compound redundant. However, the principle that chemotherapy was effective for treating antiviral diseases had been demonstrated.

Influenza was another viral disease where chemotherapeutics were available in this early period. Once again this can be ascribed in part to appropriate

From: *Methods in Molecular Medicine, vol. 24: Antiviral Methods and Protocols*
Edited by: D. Kinchington and R. F. Schinazi © Humana Press Inc., Totowa, NJ

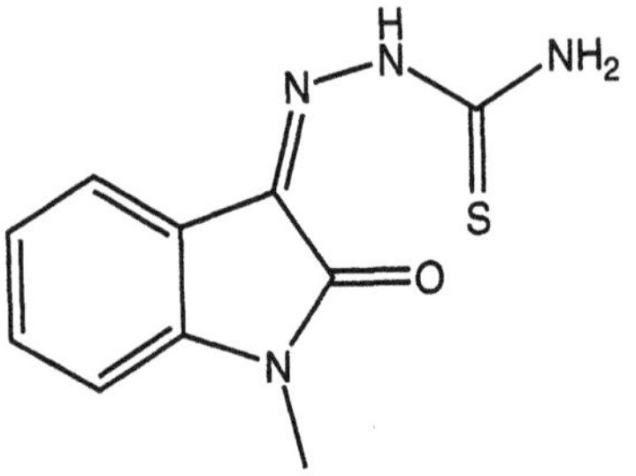

Scheme 1. Methisazone.

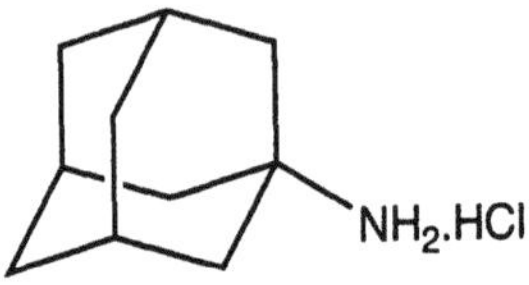

Scheme 2. Amantidine.

animal models being available for the testing of compounds. Antiviral activity against influenza A was observed for amantidine (licensed in 1966) and the related rimantidine (*see* **Scheme 2**). The mechanism of action of these compounds was elucidated much later. Analysis of nucleotide sequences of drug-resistant mutants revealed that the proton channel M2 protein had changed. Blockade of this channel leads to interference of virus uncoating *(2)*.

3. Nucleoside Analogs

In the mid-1960s, screening of natural product nucleosides, isolated for anticancer programs, revealed activity vs some DNA viruses. However, the development of acyclovir for the treatment of herpes infections in the late 1970s marked the "coming of age" of antiviral therapy as it was the first example of a highly selective, efficacious antiviral drug. The discovery of acyclovir also preceded a detailed knowledge of its mechanism of action. Studies subsequently showed that the active entity is acyclovir triphosphate, which can be incorporated into a nascent DNA chain preventing further extension (*see* **Scheme 3**) *(3)*. The triphosphate also inhibits the DNA polymerase directly. The administered drug is initially converted to its monophosphate by a viral enzyme and then to triphosphate by host kinases. The viral enzyme carries out the initial phosphorylation approx 200 times faster than host cell enzymes. This leads to higher concentrations of the active inhibitor in infected cells than in healthy ones and, therefore, to a high degree of selectivity *(4)*. A second facet of selectivity is derived from the fact that the viral polymerase incorporates acyclovir triphosphate more readily than natural nucleoside phosphates.

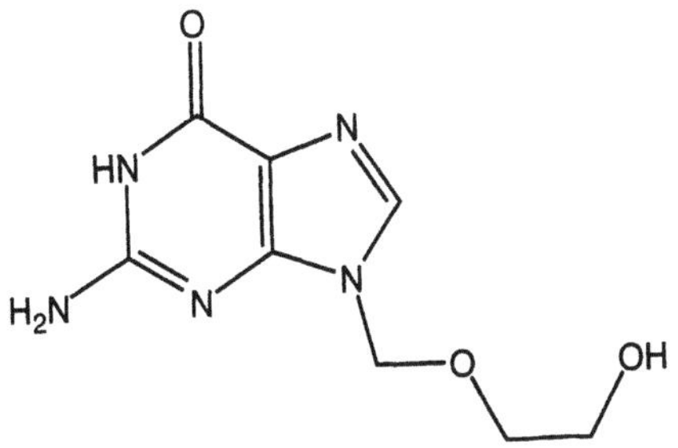

Scheme 3. Acyclovir.

The success of acyclovir demonstrated that useful selectivity for viral enzymes over human host enzymes was a realizable target.

There are now many other DNA synthesis inhibitors in use, e.g., cidofir, idoxuridine, famciclovir, ganciclovir, and trifluorothymidine, and this class of compound makes up the majority of antiviral agents currently available or in clinical trials. However poor selectivity (and the associated toxicity) is still a key problem in this area owing to the similarities of viral and cellular metabolism *(5)*.

By the end of the 1970s, large numbers of compounds had been tested against a variety of viruses, but many had failed to have the required selectivity profile. It became clear that a greater knowledge of virus life cycles would be required to enable the identification of critical functions unique to the virus. More accurate methods of assaying activity and of testing for subtle differences between host and viral processes were also needed. The timely coincidence of the development of molecular biological techniques (allowing a more detailed understanding of the life cycle of viruses and the preparation of useful quantities of viral proteins) and the appearance of a "high-profile" viral disease in AIDS provided the basis for one of the most intensive (and public) scientific endeavors of this century. A worldwide effort to understand the life cycle of HIV immediately followed the discovery of the virus. These studies suggested several processes in which intervention could be expected to lead to therapeutic benefit. Two will be focused on here: HIV reverse transcriptase (RT) and proteinase.

4. HIV RT Inhibitors

An unusual feature of the retrovirus family, of which HIV is a member, is the RT enzyme. This enzyme is essential for replication and has the capacity to generate DNA from RNA. The RNA-dependent DNA polymerase function of the RT provides at least one target for drug discovery. Nucleoside analogs once again proved to be effective inhibitors. Wellcome's experience in the nucleo-

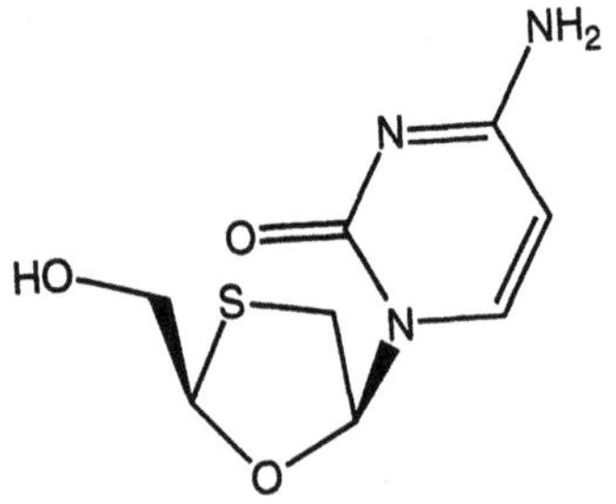

Scheme 4. 3TC.

side field enabled it to rapidly respond to the opportunity provided by HIV and led to the launch of AZT—the first licensed therapy for AIDS *(6)*. However, as with many nucleoside analogs, toxicity was a problem. Several other related compounds followed (e.g., DDC and DDI) but their use was still restricted by dose limiting toxicity. This led to using the compounds in combination, which has proved effective in keeping the virus in check while providing an acceptable side effect profile. A novel approach to the selectivity issue was taken with the nucleoside inhibitor 3TC (*see* **Scheme 4**). In this case, the unnatural enantiomer of the sugar is a more potent inhibitor of RT and is less cytotoxic than the natural enantiomer. This property has been exploited with the development of this compound. The understanding of the mechanistic basis of the action of RT inhibitors and the recognition of a similar function in hepatitis B virus (HBV) (genetically distinct from HIV) has led to active compounds vs HIV RT being tested against HBV to good effect.

Advances in the screening of chemical libraries has led to the discovery of nonnucleoside inhibitors of RT (NNRTIs). Two approaches can be followed. When an appropriate antiviral assay is available compounds can be screened in whole cells. These assays are frequently labor intensive and therefore generally have a lower throughput than isolated enzyme assays. These assays have the advantage that chemical leads generated by this approach have already overcome the barriers of cell penetration and stability.

The discovery of the TIBO class of NNRTIs represents a fine example of this first approach. The problems of lower throughput were reduced by screening smaller focused libraries of compounds. The lead structure for the TIBO class of compound was identified and subsequently optimized (*see* **Scheme 5**) *(7)*.

The discovery of another NNRTI, nevirapine, illustrates the second approach (*see* **Scheme 6**). Here it is no longer necessary to have access to an antiviral assay to discover active entities. Compounds are screened against an isolated enzyme. High throughput of compounds in the screen is a key advantage of this method enabling the testing of thousands of compounds; however, com-

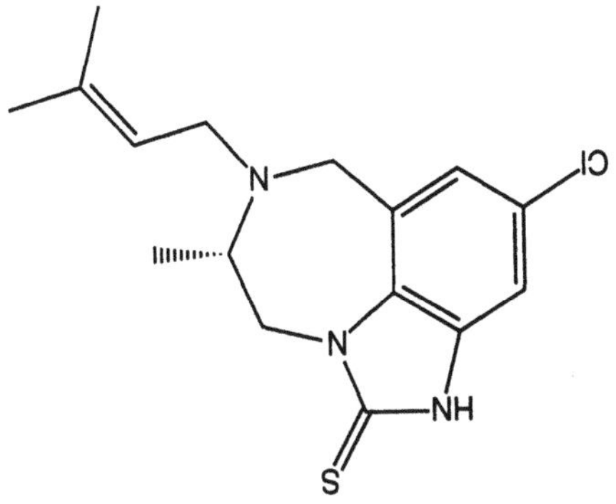

Scheme 5. TIBO R82913.

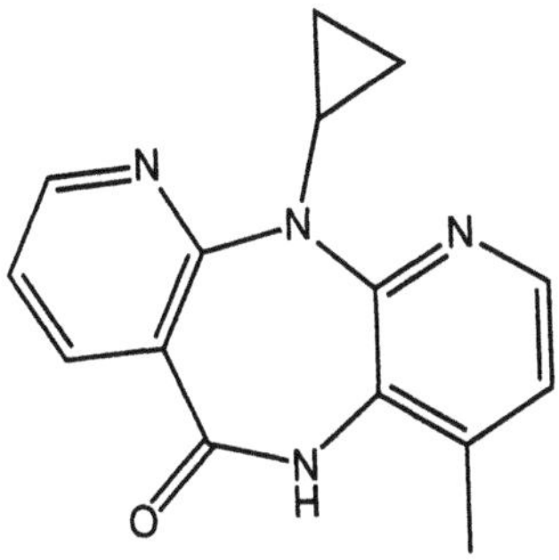

Scheme 6. Nevirapine.

pounds active against the enzyme may lose all their activity in an infected cell or animal. A variety of reasons may be responsible for these failings, e.g., uptake, metabolism, or cellular penetration. In the case of nevirapine, a large library of thousands of compounds was screened against recombinant RT. Having identified an initial hit, medicinal chemists tackled the problem of optimizing the properties and demonstrated that high activity vs the isolated enzyme could lead to good antiviral activity. Screening of a series of related compounds also led to an excellent correlation of anti-HIV activity with inhibition of isolated RT, leading to the conclusion that these compounds were indeed exerting their antiviral effect through RT inhibition *(8)*.

Further NNRTIs have now been discovered *(9)*. None of these compounds require metabolic activation, but they are only active vs HIV-1 RT. Biochemical studies showed that these NNRTIs were noncompetitive inhibitors of RT. That is, in contrast to the nucleoside derivatives, which act as competitive substrates or inhibitors, these compounds do not bind at the active site, but exert their influence on the enzyme via an allosteric mechanism. The techniques of biostructure-based drug design enabled rationalization of much of the work on

RT inhibitors. RT is a heterodimeric enzyme made up of 51 and 61 kDa polypeptides. An X-ray crystallographic structure of the enzyme complexed with nevirapine confirmed the biochemical analyses by indicating that the binding site was close, but distinct from, the polymerase active site. However, conformational changes at the polymerase active site did occur on binding of these inhibitors *(10)*.

Clinical evaluation of nevirapine indicated that resistance emerges rapidly. The nature of the resistance was characterized and specific mutations in the RT were identified. It can be rationalized that as these compounds bind away from the active site, there is less mechanistic pressure for these residues to remain unmutated. Some amino acid residues in the vicinity of the binding site of the NNRTIs are conserved in other retrovirus RTs perhaps implying that they are required for functional protein. This has led to the strategy of using the X-ray structure of the enzyme and inhibitors to design compounds that interact with these residues and, hence, avoid resistance issues *(11)*.

Other NNRTIs complexed with enzyme have now been crystallized and the binding modes compared. Although these molecules are structurally very different, they bind in a similar region to nevirapine *(12)*.

5. HIV Proteinase Inhibitors

The discovery in the mid-1980s that HIV encoded a unique aspartyl proteinase responsible for posttranslational cleavage of the viral polyprotein led to a number of drug research programs in search of inhibitors. These programs represent a paradigm for modern drug discovery—with substrate-based, biostructure-based, and high-throughput screening approaches all successfully employed. In the substrate based approach, knowledge of the cleavage sequence of the natural substrate and the mechanism of enzyme function suggests transition state-based compounds, which traditionally have proven effective for enzyme inhibition. The work in the HIV field has built on studies used to design inhibitors of renin, another aspartyl proteinase. The use of this approach rapidly led to efficacious drugs, e.g., saquinavir (*see* **Scheme 7**) *(13)*. Several proteinase inhibitors designed using this approach have recently received regulatory approval.

While this approach rapidly led to a new treatment for HIV infection, the availability of an X-ray structure of the enzyme complexed to inhibitors allowed theories for improving interactions between inhibitor and enzyme to be developed and tested. Improved interactions allowed other moieties in the inhibitors to be modified, generating compounds with improved pharmacokinetic profiles. This work has culminated in second generation inhibitors exemplified by VX478, in which a structure-based approach using X-ray data has resulted in a compound that retains high affinity for the enzyme but with

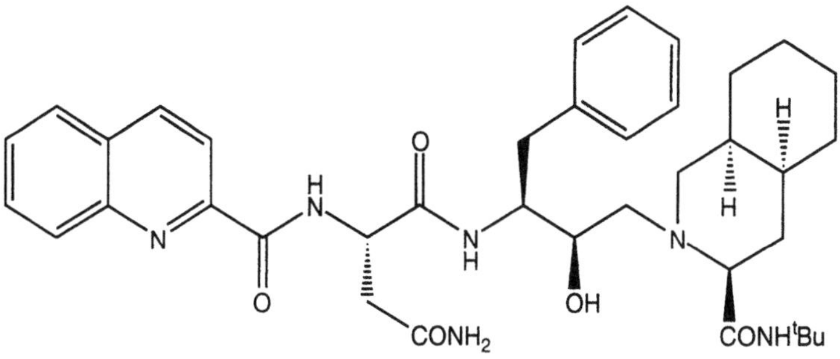

Scheme 7. Saquinavir.

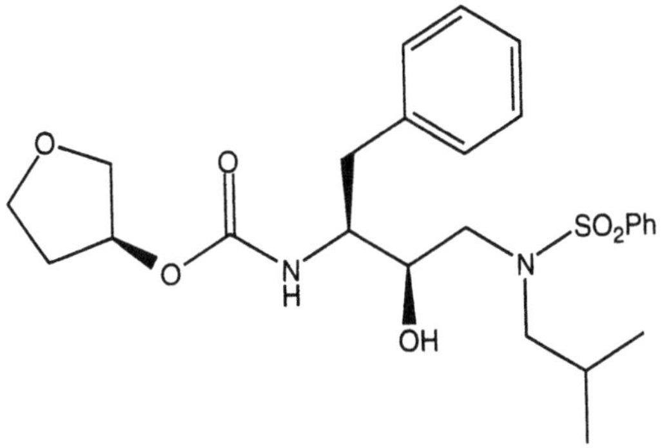

Scheme 8. VX478.

reduced molecular weight (an important feature in hepatic clearance) (*see* **Scheme 8**) ***(14)***. Some of the amide bonds, typically present in first-generation compounds and representing another pharmacokinetic liability, have also been removed.

As had been predicted prior to the determination of the X-ray structure, the proteinase assembles its catalytic machinery using a C2 symmetric homodimer (as opposed to a monomer in renin). The symmetrical nature of the enzyme suggested that C2 symmetric inhibitors might be effective. The X-ray structure also revealed the presence of an "ordered" water molecule bound to two of the carbonyl groups of the inhibitor. Displacement of such a water molecule with an inhibitor should, theoretically, lead to greatly enhanced activity. This theory was exploited with a class of cyclic inhibitors that mimicked the interactions of the water molecule with functionality within the inhibitor leading to highly potent and "compact inhibitors," e.g., XM-323 (*see* **Scheme 9**) ***(15)***.

Finally, the ability to screen large numbers of compounds has also been used in this area leading to the discovery of structurally novel leads. A notable example was the discovery of the pyran shown in **Scheme 10**. The X-ray crys-

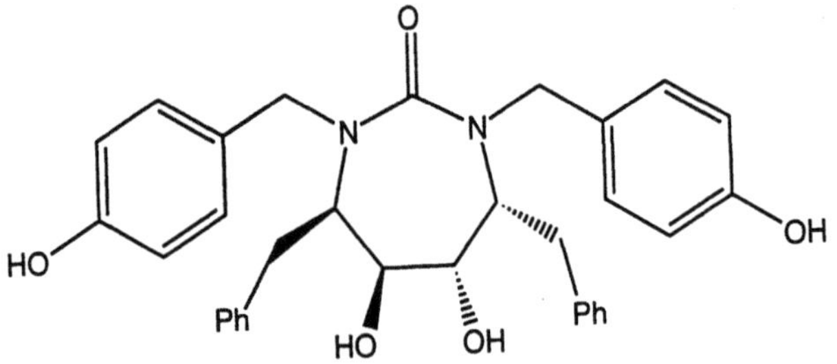

Scheme 9. XM-323.

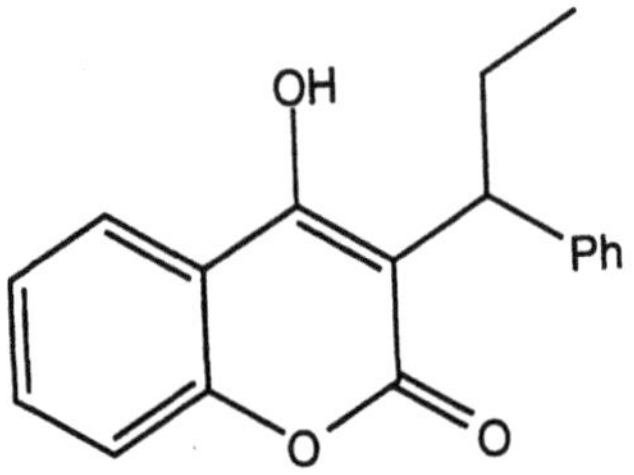

Scheme 10. Pyran.

tal structure of this compound complexed with the enzyme assisted further optimization *(15)*.

Another intriguing application of structural information in the development of better therapies has been in the characterization of resistance in both the HIV proteinase and HIV RT areas. The generation of resistance in HIV is thought to be owing to the poor fidelity of the RTleading to point mutations. Research on the use of different HIV proteinase inhibitors led to the identification of mutations in characteristic but differing positions *(16)*. These mutant proteins have, in some cases, been crystallized, leading to a better understanding of resistance at the molecular level. Frequently the mutation results in loss or gain of only a single methylene in the side chain of one of the amino acids in the proteinase, yet this can have a significant effect on the affinity of the inhibitor for the modified enzyme. These studies have suggested possibilities for the design of subsequent generations of inhibitors that might circumvent the effects of mutation.

6. Influenza Neuraminidase Inhibitors

A fine example of structure-based drug design has been reported for the design of an influenza virus neuraminidase inhibitor (*see* **Scheme 11**). Neuraminidase is an enzyme expressed on the surface of influenza virions and it is thought to be important for the successful release of progeny. Inhibition of

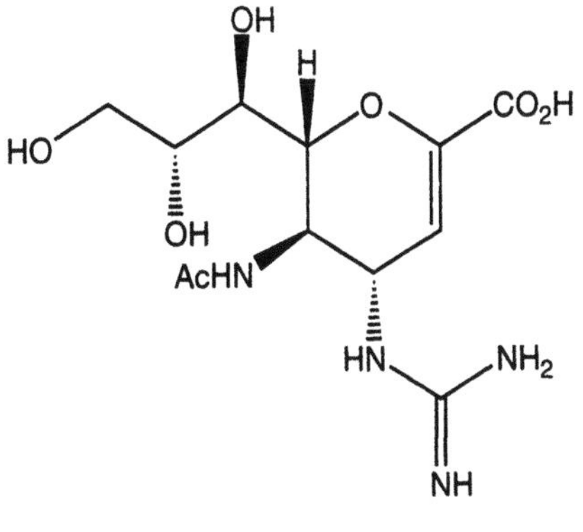

Scheme 11. Neuraminidase inhibitor.

this enzyme should lead to effective therapy against both A and B strains, but selectivity for the viral neuraminidase over human enzymes was an issue. High-resolution X-ray data on the enzyme bound to a weak inhibitor were used to predict areas where extra binding interactions could be added. Synthesis of inhibitors based on this analysis revealed compounds with activity improved by four orders of magnitude and also with very high selectivity ***(17)***. One compound, GG167, is now used in clinical trials.

7. Rhinovirus Canyon Blockers

An early step in any viral life cycle is the attachment of the virus particle to the target cell. Inhibition of this process potentially offers an attractive target for therapeutic intervention. To date, despite several programs based on this approach, none has been successful in producing effective therapies. Attempts at intervening in the rhinovirus life cycle did, however, lead to promising early results ***(18)***. Here, screening provided a lead compound with activity in a virus infectivity assay. Assay data indicated that the likely target was the capsid. Published results using X-ray crystallographic data of whole virions indicated that a second class of compound bound to a "canyon" beneath the surface of the capsid. Combining features from both molecules led to pirodavir—an antiviral with activity against many rhinovirus strains that is also believed to bind in this "canyon" (*see* **Scheme 12**).

8. HSV Ribonucleotide Reductase Inhibitors

As described above, acyclovir is an effective therapy for the treatment of herpes infections. Working on the principle that emerging resistance may be countered by combination therapy, targeting a second enzyme may well provide a useful additional treatment. HSV encodes its own ribonucleotide reductase. A novel approach might be to inhibit this enzyme, which is responsible

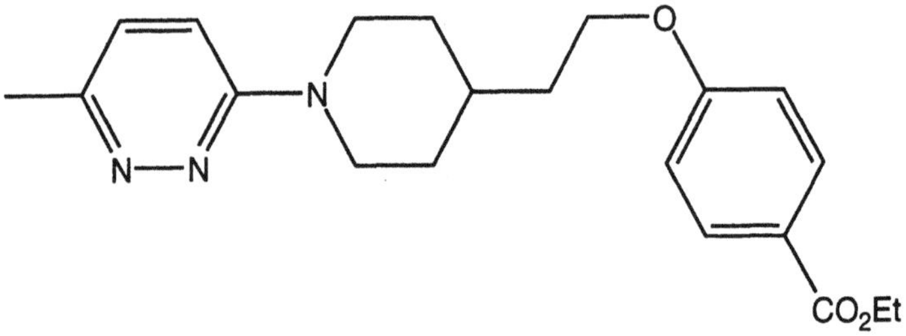

Scheme 12. Pirodavir.

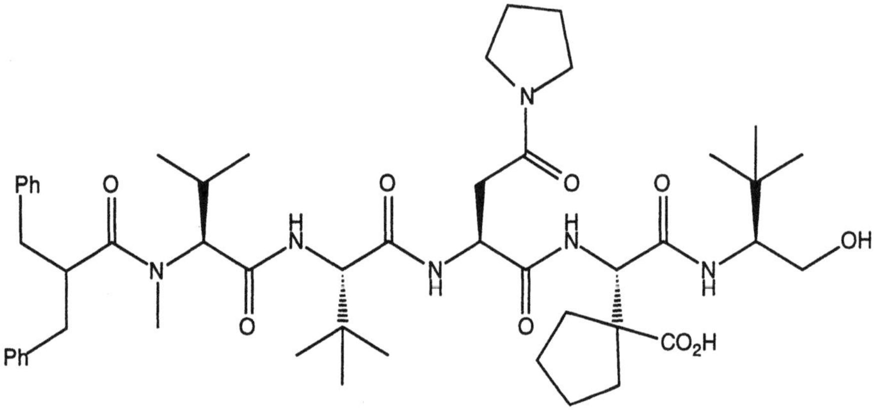

Scheme 13. HSV RR inhibitor.

for the conversion of ribonucleotides to deoxyribonucleotides, the essential building blocks of DNA (*see* **Scheme 13**). HSV ribonucleotide reductase is a tetramer made up of two of each of two types of subunit. It was discovered that a nonapeptide inhibited the function of the enzyme in a reversible but noncompetitive manner, and it was postulated that this molecule competed with the small subunit for the binding site on the large subunit and hence prevented association of the functional complex. A nonapeptide would often be regarded as too large to represent a useful lead for the discovery of compounds active in vivo. However, exceptional increases of activity vs the enzyme have been observed by modification of the side chains of the amino acids in the lead compound demonstrating that large improvements can be attained even without exploiting the benefits of transition state analogs ***(19)***.

9. Antisense

A totally different approach to the design of antiviral therapeutics is the use of antisense oligonucleotides. Here, the mechanistic target for intervention is the messenger RNA, rather than the protein itself. The rules for preparing highly specific agents are those described by Watson and Crick, i.e., the base pairing propensities of the nucleoside bases. In theory the design of highly specific agents relies only on knowing the target gene sequence. Chemical modifications to the sequences are required to resist the destructive actions of host nucleases. Delivery and cellular uptake of compounds, which are frequently highly charged, are also significant issues. Animal studies have, however, demonstrated clear effects and a range of clinical trials are ongoing, which, if successful, will demonstrate a new type of approach to antiviral therapy ***(20)***.

10. Conclusions

Antiviral therapy has made considerable advances over the past four decades. Programs targeting HSV and HIV, in particular, have made excellent contributions and have begun to meet the challenges posed by these viruses. The methods used to produce antiviral drugs have been innovative and varied. A knowledge of the substrate provided an entry for the early polymerase inhibitors. Substrate-based approaches also provided early success in the preparation of the first generation of HIV proteinase inhibitors, but biostructural information, as it became available, has played a key role in the discovery of later classes of compounds. It is interesting to note that for human cytomegalovirus proteinase the X-ray structure had been reported prior to the clinical development of any compound, and for the hepatitis C virus NS3 proteinase, the X-ray structure had been reported prior to the patenting of any inhibitors. Here, it is likely that this information will play a significant role in the first generation of inhibitors. High-throughput screening has been particularly successful for HIV RT inhibitors, generating a range of structurally diverse leads. The methods used to discover drugs, however, are continually evolving, and it will be interesting to see what role high-throughput chemistry using parallel synthesis and robots to make, as well as test, compounds will have.

Viruses have been shown to be particularly adept at developing resistance to drugs, and the effective management of viral diseases may well rely on combination therapy. This may take the form of either targeting a single virus function with multiple agents or using several agents to attack several targets in the life cycle. Many viral diseases still require new treatments. These facts ensure that there will be many new challenges for antiviral drug therapy in the future. The evidence from the past suggests that the challenges will be met.

Acknowledgments

The author wishes to thank Dr. J. S. Mills and Dr. F. X. Wilson for critical reading of the manuscript.

References

1. Sneader, W. (1985) The human herpesviruses, in *Drug Discovery: The Evolution of Modern Medicines,* Wiley, New York, p. 292.
2. Pinto, H., Holsinger, L. J., and Lamb, R. A. (1992) Influenza virus M2 protein has ion channel activity. *Cell* **69,** 517–528.
3. Sneader, W. (1985) *Drug Discovery: The Evolution of Modern Medicines,* Wiley, New York, p. 351.
4. Levine, A. J. (1992) *Viruses,* Scientific American Library, p. 74.
5. Harper, D. R. (1994) Medical applications—antiviral drugs, in *Molecular Virology,* Bios Scientific Publishers, pp. 93–110.
6. Pattishall, K. A. (1993) Discovery and development of zidovidine as the cornerstone of therapy to control human immunodeficiency virus infection, in *The Search for Antiviral Drugs,* Birkhauser, pp. 23–44.
7. Pauwels, R. (1993) Discovery of TIBO, a new family of HIV-1-specific reverse transcriptase inhibitors, in *The Search for Antiviral Drugs,* Birkhauser, Germany. pp. 71–104.
8. Adams, J. and Merluzzi, V. J. (1993) Discovery of Nevinipine, a non-nucleoside inhibitor of HIV-1 reverse transcriptase, in *The Search for Antiviral Drugs,* Birkhauser, pp. 45–70.
9. Romero, D. L. (1994) *Ann. Rep. Med. Chem.* **26,** 123–132.
10. Kohlstaedt, L. A., Wang, J., Friedman, J. M., Rice, P. A., and Steitz, T. A. (1992) Crystal structure at 3.5 angstroms resolution of HIV-1 reverse transcriptase complexed with an inhibitor. *Science* **256,** 1783–1790.
11. Tong, L., Cardozo, M., Jones, P.-J., and Adams, J. (1993) Preliminary structural analysis of the mutations selected by non-nucleoside inhibitors of HIV-1 reverse transcriptase. *Biorg. Med. Chem. Lett.* **3,** 721–726.
12. Jingshan, R., et al. (1995) High resolution structures of HIV-1 RT from four RT-inhibitor complexes. *Nature Struct. Biol.* **2,** 293–302.
13. Roberts, N. A., et al. (1990) Rational design of peptide based HIV proteinase inhibitors. *Science* **248,** 358–361.
14. Navia, M. A., Sato, V. L., and Tung, R. D. (1995) Design of VX-478, a potent inhibitor of HIV protease. *Int. Antiviral News* **3,** 143–145.
15. Boehme, R. E., and Borthwick, A. D., and Wyatt, P. G. (1995) Antiviral agents. *Ann. Rep. Med. Chem.* **30,** 144.
16. Ridky, T. and Leis, J. (1995) Development of drug resistance to HIV-1 protease inhibitors. *J. Biol. Chem.* **270,** 29,621–29,623.
17. von Itzstein, M., et al. (1993) Rational design of potent sialidase-based inhibitors of influenza virus replication. *Nature* **363,** 418–423.
18. Andries, K. (1993) Discovery of piroclavir, a broad spectrum inhibitor of ethnoviruses, in *The Search for Antiviral Drugs,* Birkhauser, Germany, pp. 179–210.
19. Liuzzi, M., et al. (1994) A potent inhibitor of HSV ribonucleotide reductase with antiviral activity in vivo. *Nature* **372,** 695–698.
20. Szymkowski, D. E. (1996) Developing antisense oligonucleotides from the laboratory to clinical trials. *Drug Discovery Today* **1,** 415–428.

2

Laboratory Safety Considerations

Paul M. Feorino, John D. Williamson, and Raymond F. Schinazi

1. Introduction

In the laboratory it is important that potentially pathogenic agents be controlled to protect the laboratory worker from infection and the experiment from contamination. The operation of a safe laboratory depends on many factors: the training and judgement of laboratory personnel; the implementation of protocols, the selection and use of equipment and reagents; and the location and design of the laboratory. These should be integrated in order to provide maximum safety for the personnel without impeding operation of the laboratory.

2. Laboratory-Associated Virus Infections

A survey conducted 20 years ago and based on a total of 3921 cases showed 59% of laboratory-acquired infections had occurred in research laboratories *(1)*. The majority of infections were of laboratory personnel but, in some cases, staff working outside the laboratory were also affected. Other events have emphasized the need for effective biosafety measures. These include: two "escapes" of smallpox virus from laboratories that resulted in members of the public becoming fatally infected; the emergence of new viral diseases with high case-fatality rates; and the recognition that laboratory-based investigations would need to be made on viruses for which no prophylactic or therapeutic measures were available. **Table 1** lists some viruses that have been identified as causal agents of laboratory-acquired infections *(2–4)*.

3. Microbiological Risk Assessment

Factors that can influence the risk of laboratory-acquired infection include: the virus under investigation, laboratory practices being used and the host. The consequences of release of the virus into the environment must also be considered.

From: *Methods in Molecular Medicine, vol. 24: Antiviral Methods and Protocols*
Edited by: D. Kinchington and R. F. Schinazi © Humana Press Inc., Totowa, NJ

Table 1
Laboratory-Acquired Viral Infections

Virus
Ebola virus
Hantaviruses
Hepatitis B virus
Hepatitis C virus
Human herpesviruses
Herpesvirus simiae (B virus)
Human immunodeficiency virus
Lassa virus
Lymphocytic choriomeningitis virus
Marburg virus
Parvovirus B19
Rabies virus
Rift Valley fever virus
Simian immunodeficiency virus
Venezuelan equine encephalitis virus
Vesicular stomatitis virus

Table 2
Infectious Doses for Some Virus Infections (25–50% of Human Volunteers)

Disease or agent	Inoculation route	Dose[a]
Measles	Intranasal spray	0.2
Rhinovirus	Nasal drops	1
Venezuelan equine encephalitis	Subcutaneous	1
West Nile fever	Intramuscular	1
Poliovirus 1	Ingestion	2
Rubella	Pharyngeal spray	10
Influenza A2	Nasopharyngeal	790

[a]Numbers of cell culture infectious doses or animal infectious units.

3.1. Virus

1. Virulence may be defined as the ability of a virus to invade host tissues and cause disease. **Table 2** shows the infectious doses of some viruses are very low (data taken from **ref.** ***3***).
2. Transmissibility: The risk of spread of infection will be determined by the probability of secondary and tertiary cases. This can be assessed by the case-morbidity or case-mortality rates found by epidemiological studies of naturally acquired infection.
3. Latency: Delayed onset of disease with few or no clinical signs during the latent phase may delay recognition that infection has already occurred.

Table 3
Routes of Infection Associated with Laboratory Activities

Route	Laboratory activity
Ingestion (through the mouth)	Mouth pipeting Contaminated articles or fingers placed in mouth Eating, drinking, or smoking
Inoculation (through the skin)	Needle-stick accidents or cuts from sharp objects, such as syringes and glass slides ("sharps accidents")
Contamination (of skin and mucous membranes)	Splashes into mouth, eyes, or nose Splashes on damaged skin Transfer from contaminated fingers to eyes or mouth
Inhalation (through the lungs)	Exposure to aerosols generated by various laboratory procedures

4. Persistence: Continued excretion after infection increases the risk of transmission and may even result in "carriers" of the infection.

3.2. Laboratory Practices

1. Experience of laboratory workers: Training in good microbiological practice is the foundation of safe laboratory procedures; its importance cannot be overemphasized.
2. Type of laboratory: Industrial and research laboratories are more likely to work with large quantities of concentrated viral preparations, which increases the risk of infection following a spillage. Exposure to high virus concentrations may also result in infection by other routes than the natural route of infection.
3. Procedures: The most commonly reported types of activities associated with laboratory-acquired infections are listed in **Table 3**.

3.3. Host

1. Exposure route: Outcome may be affected by route of infection; for example, blood-borne viruses do not readily cause infection by the respiratory route.
2. Individual host characteristics: Compromising factors that can influence the particular consequences of exposure to infection include immune status and pregnancy.
3. Presence in body fluids: An awareness should be maintained of both viral and other, nonviral pathogens that may be present in body fluids (blood, saliva, sputum, semen, and breast milk).
4. Broken biological barriers: Skin is a particularly good barrier against infection, but it is breached by cuts or abrasions.

5. Prophylaxis and chemotherapy: Vaccines and/or drugs, if available, should be used to protect against infection or for treatment if infection is suspected or known to have occurred.

3.4. Environment

1. Vectors: Insects or other animals may become infected following the release of viruses from the laboratory and spread the infection to other animals and/or humans.
2. Environmental factors: The survival of virus particles in a potentially pathogenic state is influenced by ambient temperature and humidity.
3. Population characteristics: Herd immunity resulting from vaccination programs or from infections endemic in the local community, together with other factors, such as social behavior, can affect the spread of infection in the community.

4. Hazard, Risk, and Containment

"Hazard" is the potential danger associated with a particular virus, and "risk" is the probability that the hazard will be expressed as an exposure with the possibility of infection. "Containment" refers to the control measures used to reduce the possibility of exposure. Some authorities categorize viruses according to hazard *(4,5)*, whereas others have drawn up a classification based on risk, which includes such factors as pathogenicity, transmissibility, prophylaxis, and therapeutic measures *(6)*.

4.1. Classification of Viruses by Hazard/Risk Group (see Table 4)

- Hazard/Risk Group 1: A virus that is unlikely to cause human disease and offers no or minimal hazard to laboratory workers.
- Hazard/Risk Group 2: A virus that can cause human disease but is unlikely to be a serious hazard to laboratory workers. Accidental laboratory infection may cause serious infection but effective treatment and preventive measures are available. The risk of spread of infection is limited.
- Hazard/Risk Group 3: A virus that may cause serious human disease and offers a special hazard to laboratory workers. It may present a risk of spread in the community but effective treatment and preventive measures are usually available.
- Hazard/Risk Group 4: A virus that usually causes serious human disease and is extremely hazardous to laboratory workers. It may be readily transmitted from one individual to another causing serious epidemic disease. Effective treatment and preventive measures are not usually available.

5. Biosafety/Laboratory Containment Level Criteria

The hazard of a virus and/or the risks associated with its use in particular laboratory procedures determine the appropriate level of containment. Most classifications are designated in ascending order and include four kinds of laboratories: US Department of Health and Human Services (USDHHS) and the

Table 4
Classification of Viruses on the Basis of Hazard or Risk as Adopted in the European Community (EC), the United Kingdom (UK) and the United States (US)

Virus	EC	UK	US
Dengue viruses types 1–4	3	3	2
Ebola virus	4	4	4
Hantaan (Korean hemorrhagic fever) virus	3	3	3
Hepatitis A virus	2	2	2
Hepatitis B virus	3	3	2
Hepatitis C virus	3	3	2
Hepatitis D virus	3	3	2
Hepatitis E virus	3	3	2
Herpesvirus simiae	3	3	3
Human herpes viruses 1–8	2	2	2
Human immunodeficiency viruses	3	3	2
Human papilloma viruses	2	2	2
Human T-cell lymphotropic viruses I and II	3	3	2
Influenza types A, B, and C	2	2	2
Japanese encephalitis virus	3	3	3
Lassa virus	4	4	4
Marburg virus	4	4	4
Measles virus	2	2	2
Mumps virus	2	2	2
Monkeypox virus	3	3	2
Rabies virus	3	3	2
Vaccinia virus	2	2	2
Variola (smallpox) virus	4	4	4
Venezuelan equine encephalitis virus	3	3	3

World Health Organization (WHO) identify Biosafety Levels 1, 2, 3, and 4 and in the United Kingdom the Advisory Committee on Dangerous Pathogens (ACDP) categorizes Laboratory Containment Levels 1, 2, 3, and 4 *(4–6)*. All share the same objective: to identify biosafety or laboratory containment levels that minimize the risk to the laboratory worker, to the outside community, and to the environment. At Biosafety/Laboratory Containment Level 2, exposure risks to the laboratory worker arise mainly from contact through a contaminated work environment. As the risk of airborne infection increases, Biosafety/ Laboratory Containment Level 3 provides facilities to prevent aerosol transmission. Additional safeguards to protect the outside community and the environment are found at Biosafety/Laboratory Containment Level 4, which is designed to provide both a safe and a secure laboratory for work with the most dangerous human viruses.

Although the Biosafety/Laboratory Containment Level can be determined directly by the Hazard/Risk Group, a strict relationship may not always be required. Some discretion applies to assessment of the infection risks associated with airborne transmission of particular viruses. For example, the USDHHS recommends that a Biosafety Level 2 facility but with Biosafety Level 3 practices and equipment be used for activities with human retroviruses and hepatitis viruses if these viruses are produced in research quantities or are manipulated as concentrated preparations, or if procedures are used that generate droplets or aerosols. In the United Kingdom, the Control of Substances Hazardous to Health Regulations (COSHH) 1994 requires that the minimum Laboratory Containment Level match the Hazard Group. However, work with specified viruses in the ACDP Hazard Group 3 (human hepatitis viruses and human retroviruses), which does not involve their propagation or concentration, can be carried out at a reduced level of containment if the risk of airborne transmission is low. The most important safety precautions applicable to these blood-borne viruses are to minimize contamination of surfaces and avoid the use of instruments or equipment that may accidentally cause cuts, for example, syringes or glass slides. *See* **Table 5** for a summary of biosafety containment requirements.

6. Laboratory Biosafety

The principal element of containment is strict adherence to standard microbiological practices and procedures. They are fundamental to laboratory biosafety at all levels of containment and are designed primarily to protect the laboratory worker by avoiding any activities that are potential sources of infection (*see* **Table 3**). Attention must also be paid to the additional protection provided by safety equipment (primary barriers) and facility design (secondary barriers), particularly with regard to work at Biosafety/Laboratory Containment Levels 3 and 4.

6.1. Standard Microbiological Practices

The following summary is based on the USDHHS publication "Biosafety in microbiological and biomedical laboratories" *(4)*, the UK guidelines "Categorization of biological agents according to hazard and categories of containment" prepared by the ACDP *(5)* and the WHO "Laboratory Biosafety Manual" *(6)*.

1. A biosafety manual is prepared or adopted. Laboratory personnel receive training on potential hazards associated with the work involved, precautions to prevent exposures, and exposure evaluation procedures. Appropriate immunizations

Table 5
Biosafety/Laboratory Containment Level Facility Requirements

Facility requirement	Biosafety/laboratory containment level			
	1	2	3	4
Separated from other activities in the same building	No	No	Yes	Yes
Access restricted to authorized persons	No	Yes	Yes	Yes
Double door entry	No	No	Yes	Yes
Airlock and shower	No	No	No	Yes
Ventilation				
Inward air flow (negative pressure)	No	Yes[a]	Yes	Yes
Filtered air exhaust	No	No	Yes	Yes
Biological safety cabinets				
Classes I and II	No	Yes	Yes	Yes[a]
Class III	No	No	No	Yes
Contains its own equipment	No	No	Yes[a]	Yes
Specified disinfection procedures	Yes	Yes	Yes	Yes
Autoclave				
On site	Yes	Yes	Yes	Yes
In the laboratory	No	No	Yes	Yes
Double-ended	No	No	Yes[a]	Yes
Dunk tank	No	No	No	Yes
Sealable for decontamination	No	No	Yes[a]	Yes

[a]May be required/permitted by particular regulatory authorities

or tests are carried out for infectious agents handled or potentially present in the laboratory. Annual updates or additional training are provided as necessary.

2. Access to the laboratory is restricted to authorized persons. Hazard warning signs on access doors identify the names of personnel authorized to enter and the name(s) and telephone number(s) of person(s) responsible for the laboratory.
3. Laboratory coats or gowns and gloves are worn to prevent contamination or soiling of street clothing and hands. Protective clothing must be removed and left in the laboratory before leaving; if contaminated, it must be decontaminated and cleaned or, if necessary, destroyed.
4. Eating, drinking, smoking, handling contact lenses, and applying cosmetics are not permitted in the laboratory work area. Persons who wear contact lenses in the laboratory also wear goggles or a face shield. Food is stored outside the work area in cabinets or refrigerators designated and used for this purpose only.
5. Mouth pipeting is prohibited; mechanical pipeting devices are used.
6. All procedures are performed carefully to minimize the creation of splashes or aerosols. Biological (microbiological) safety cabinets are used for procedures that may generate aerosols.

7. Special precautions are taken with any contaminated sharp items: needles are restricted in the laboratory for use only when there is no alternative. Plasticware is substituted for glassware whenever possible. Needle-locking syringes or disposable syringe-needle units (i.e., needle is integral to the syringe) are used for injection or aspiration of infectious materials. Used disposable needles must not be bent, sheared, recapped, removed from disposable syringes, or otherwise manipulated by hand before disposal. Nondisposable sharps must be placed in a hard-walled container for transport to a processing area for decontamination, preferably by autoclaving. Syringes that resheath the needle, needleless systems, and other safe devices are used when appropriate. Broken glass must not be handled directly but must be removed by mechanical means, such as a brush, tongs, or forceps.
8. Effective disinfectants are available for immediate use in the event of a spillage and there must be specified disinfection procedures.
9. Laboratory equipment and work surfaces are cleaned with an appropriate disinfectant after work is finished and decontaminated immediately after spills or other contamination by infectious materials. All accidents or incidents must be immediately reported to the laboratory director, medical evaluation provided, and written records maintained.
10. All cultures, stocks, and contaminated wastes must be decontaminated before disposal by an approved method, such as autoclaving. Materials to be decontaminated outside of the laboratory must be placed in a durable, leakproof container and closed for transport from the laboratory. Materials to be decontaminated offsite must be packaged in accordance with any regulations applicable to transport of infectious materials before removal from the facility.
11. Persons wash their hands after removing gloves and before leaving the laboratory. The sink is near the laboratory door and the taps can be operated without being touched by hand. An eyewash facility is readily available.
12. An insect and rodent control program is in effect.

6.2. Safety Equipment (Primary Barriers)

Safety equipment is designed to protect the laboratory worker against accidental exposures to hazardous biological materials. It includes:

1. Personal protective equipment: Safety spectacles and face masks, in addition to laboratory coats or gowns and disposable gloves, offer protection against splashes and spillages. Positive-pressure personnel suits may be worn when working with Hazard/Risk Group 4 agents.
2. Safety pipetting aids: Mouth pipeting is prohibited; it is a potential source of infection either by ingestion or by inhalation. All safety pipetting aids control contamination of the suction end of the pipet and leakage from the pipet tips. Vacuum lines used to aspirate liquids are protected with liquid disinfectant traps and cartridge-type filters (0.45 μm pore size).
3. Biological (microbiological) safety cabinets: In addition to accidental spillages, numerous laboratory procedures—pipeting, mixing, homogenizing, ultrasonic

treatment and centrifugation—can generate aerosols containing virus particles. If aerosol droplets larger than 5 µm in diameter are released during such procedures, they settle rapidly, causing contamination of the hands of the laboratory worker and the immediate working surfaces. Smaller droplets (<5 µm) may remain in suspension in the air for several hours and, if inhaled, they are able to reach the alveoli and initiate infection.

Biological (microbiological) safety cabinets provide additional containment for any procedure likely to generate an aerosol of Risk/Hazard Group 2 viruses and they are obligatory for all work with viruses in Risk/Hazard Groups 3 and 4. There are three types of biological (microbiological) safety cabinets, Classes I, II, and III; all give protection both to the worker and to the environment but only Class II and Class III cabinets also provide a clean work area.

a. Class I cabinet: Open-fronted with operator protection provided by the inward flow of air past the worker and across the work area. This can cause contamination of work materials. Exhaust air is ducted to the outside through High Efficiency Particulate Adsorption (HEPA) filters. Class I cabinets may be used with viruses in Hazard/Risk Groups 2 and 3.
b. Class II cabinets: Also open-fronted with an inward airflow past the worker but the work area is supplied with a vertical laminar downflow of sterile, HEPA-filtered air. Any aerosols generated by the work procedures are entrapped in HEPA filters before the air is exhausted. Class II type A and Class B type 1 cabinets recirculate 70 and 30% of the air, respectively, but no air is recirculated in Class II type B2 cabinets. Class II type B3 cabinets are essentially similar to Class IIA but all plena (internal spaces) are under negative pressure relative to the laboratory. All Class II type B cabinets may be used for work with viruses in Hazard/Risk Groups 2 and 3. In addition, Class IIB cabinets may be used with volatile or toxic chemicals and radioactive substances, although at low levels only with Class IIB type B1 cabinets; Class IIA cabinets are not suitable for such work.

   Horizontal laminar flow cabinets used for product protection, for example, in the pharmaceutical industry, exhaust directly into the face of the operator. This equipment must never be used as a biological (microbiological) safety cabinet.
c. Class III cabinet: Totally enclosed and leak-proof; operated under negative pressure; and the supply air, in addition to the exhaust air, is HEPA-filtered, providing protection of work materials and environment, respectively. The operator works with gloves sealed into the front of the cabinet. Class III cabinets are used with Hazard/Risk Group 4 viruses.

Regular maintenance of biological (microbiological) safety cabinets is essential. National standards, for example, British Standard BS 5726:1992, have been set for their construction, installation and operation. The inward face air velocities of Class I and II cabinets must provide an "operator protection factor" of at least 1×10^5 (for every 100,000 particles released at the working aperture, no more than one should escape into the laboratory). Also, HEPA filters must have a minimal filtration efficiency of 99.997% (for every 100,000 challenge particles generated in a test of a filter and its seal, no more than three should penetrate).

4. Centrifugation. Infectious airborne particles can be released from centrifuges if a centrifuge tube breaks or a centrifuge bucket fails. Their velocity may be so high that these particles are not retained if the centrifuge is placed in a Class I or Class II biological (microbiological) safety cabinet. Centrifuge buckets should be paired by weight and, with tubes in place, properly balanced. Centrifuge tubes should have screw caps and sealed centrifuge (safety) buckets should be used. If a breakage occurs during centrifugation of Risk/Hazard Group 2 viruses, the sealed bucket should be opened in a Class I biological (microbiological) safety cabinet. For centrifugation of viruses in Risk/Hazard Groups 3 and 4, the sealed buckets should be both loaded and opened in a Class I microbiological safety cabinet.

6.3. Facility Design (Secondary Barriers)

The design of a virology laboratory will depend on the risk of transmission of specific viruses. At Biosafety/Laboratory Containment Level 2, exposure risks result mainly from contact through a contaminated work environment; this should be avoidable by strict adherence to standard microbiological practices. As the risk of aerosol transmission increases, other features must be incorporated, such as specialized ventilation systems to assure directional airflow at Biosafety/Laboratory Containment Level 3. A dedicated, non-recirculating ventilation system is required at Biosafety/Laboratory Containment Level 4 and special provisions are made for personnel or materials to enter and leave the laboratory. Laboratories at Biosafety/Laboratory Containment Levels 3 and 4 are separated from other activities in the same building, they are sealable to allow fumigation in the event of a spillage of infectious material outside a biological (microbiological) safety cabinet, and an autoclave is located in the laboratory. At these highest levels of containment, the laboratory must contain its own equipment.

6.3.1. Ventilation Systems

At Biosafety/Laboratory Containment Levels 3 and 4, the laboratory is maintained at a negative air pressure in relation to the external atmosphere. This ensures a continuous airflow into the laboratory. Exhaust air is not recirculated to any other area in the building but is discharged to the outside through a HEPA filter (or equivalent) and dispersed away from occupied areas and air intakes. Any equipment that may produce aerosols is contained in devices that exhaust air through HEPA filters. At Biosafety/Laboratory Containment Level 4 the differential pressure/directional air flow is monitored and alarmed to warn of any malfunction of the system.

A specially designed suit area maintained under negative pressure may be provided in a Biosafety/Laboratory Containment Level 4 facility. Personnel who enter this area wear a positive-pressure suit ventilated by a life-support system that includes alarms and backup breathing air tanks. Entry is through an airlock fitted with airtight doors. A chemical shower is provided to decontaminate the surface of the suit before the worker leaves the area.

6.3.2. Access

Entrance to a laboratory at Biosafety/Laboratory Containment Level 3 is separated from other areas by two sets of self-closing doors. At Biosafety/Laboratory Containment Level 4, access is limited by means of secure, locked doors that lead to outer and inner clothing change rooms separated by a shower. Authorized personnel enter through the outer room, where personal clothing is removed and kept there. Complete personal protective clothing is provided and used by all personnel entering the facility. When leaving the laboratory area, all laboratory clothing is removed in the inner change room and personnel must shower before going to the outer change room, dressing, and leaving the facility.

Supplies and materials needed in the Biosafety/Laboratory Containment Level 4 facility are brought in by way of a double-doored autoclave, fumigation chamber, or airlock, which is appropriately decontaminated between each use. After securing the outer door, personnel within the facility retrieve the materials by opening the inner door. which is secured after materials are brought into the facility.

No materials, except for biological materials that are to remain in a viable or intact state, are removed from the Biosafety/Laboratory Containment Level 4 laboratory unless they have been autoclaved or decontaminated before they leave the facility. Equipment or material that might be damaged by high temperature or steam may be decontaminated by gaseous vapor methods in an airlock or chamber designed for this purpose. Any drains in the floors contain traps filled with chemical disinfectant; sewer vents and other ventilation lines contain HEPA filters.

Biological materials to be removed from the Class III cabinet or from the Biosafety/Laboratory Containment Level 4 laboratory in a viable or intact state are transferred to a nonbreakable primary container and then enclosed in a nonbreakable, sealed secondary container. This is removed from the facility through a disinfectant dunk tank, fumigation chamber or an airlock designed for this purpose.

7. Decontamination

7.1. Disinfectants

In addition to their antiviral properties, it is important to understand the physical and chemical properties of disinfectants so they may be used effectively and safely. Consideration must also be given to the possible harmful effects they may have on the skin, eyes, and lungs.

The most commonly used disinfectants are hypochlorites and phenolics. Hypochlorites are effective against both enveloped and nonenveloped viruses, but their oxidizing action is also directed against other organic matter; for example, serum. Consequently, a solution of sodium hypochlorite for disinfecting pipets should contain 2500 parts per million (ppm) available chlorine, whereas a solution containing 10,000 ppm is needed to decontaminate tissue culture media from virus-infected cell cultures. Hypochlorite solutions corrode some metals, including aluminum, and should not be used on the metal parts of centrifuges or other laboratory equipment. Dilute solutions decay rapidly and need to be freshly prepared from stock solutions on a daily basis. Chlorine-releasing compounds, such as sodium dichloroisocyanurate, are preferable as dry powders for decontamination of spillages.

Phenolic compounds are active against enveloped viruses but their activity against nonenveloped viruses is variable. Most are active in the presence of extraneous protein and are generally used at 2–5% dilutions.

Ethyl alcohol and isopropyl alcohol have similar disinfectant properties. They are active against enveloped viruses but their action against nonenveloped viruses is variable. They are used at concentrations of about 70% in water; it is necessary to have a wetting agent to assist penetration of the alcohols. Such alcohol solutions may be used to disinfect surfaces and to decontaminate centrifuge buckets.

Formaldehyde and glutaraldehyde are good disinfectants that are active against both enveloped and nonenveloped viruses. Because it is noncorrosive, glutaraldehyde is useful for disinfecting metal surfaces. However, both aldehydes are toxic: In the United Kingdom the maximum exposure limit for formaldehyde is 2 ppm and the short-term exposure limit for glutaraldehyde is 0.2 ppm. Formaldehyde affects the eyes and causes respiratory distress and glutaraldehyde can cause sensitization of skin and mucous membranes. Consequently, they are used mainly to disinfect enclosed places: glutaraldehyde to disinfect safety cabinets, and formaldehyde to decontaminate safety cabinets and laboratories.

Many proprietary disinfectants are marketed, and the supplier should always be asked to provide evidence of the product's efficacy. Care should also be taken to ensure a particular disinfectant does not come in contact with other disinfectants or chemicals with which they may react, giving rise to other hazards. For example, carcinogenic compounds can result from interactions between formaldehyde and sodium hypochlorite.

7.2. Autoclaving

Autoclaving is the procedure of choice for decontamination of solid and liquid wastes. Many viruses are relatively heat-labile—HIV is inactivated at

80°C for 1 min—but autoclaves are usually set to decontaminate other heat-resistant microorganisms such as spore-bearing bacilli. Consequently, autoclaving is usually carried out at 121°C for 15 min although higher temperatures and shorter times are also used, for example, 126°C for 10 min or 134°C for 3 min.

References

1. Pike, R. M. (1976) Laboratory-acquired infections. Summary and analysis of 3921 cases. *Health Lab. Sci.* **13**, 105–114.
2. Collins, C. H. (1993) *Laboratory-Acquired Infections.* Butterworth-Heinemann Ltd., Oxford, UK.
3. Sewell, D. L. (1995) Laboratory-acquired infections and biosafety. *Clin. Microbiol. Rev.* **8,** 389–405.
4. Biosafety in microbiological and biomedical laboratories (1993) US Department of Health and Human Services. US Government Printing Office, Washington, DC.
5. Categorisation of pathogens according to hazard and categories of containment (1995) HSE Books, Sudbury, Suffolk, UK.
6. Laboratory biosafety manual (1993) World Health Organization, Geneva, Switzerland.

3

Routine Quality Control Testing of Cell Cultures

Detection of Mycoplasma

Alison Stacey and Glyn Stacey

1. Introduction

The quality of cell cultures and their products is important in scientific research and is also critical where they are used for diagnosis and therapies. Fundamental aspects of quality of cell cultures are purity, correct identity, and freedom from adventitious agents as well as appropriate biological characterization *(1,2)*. Addressing these issues will ensure that experimental data and cell products meet the minimum requirements for scientific accuracy and regulatory approval.

Testing of cell cultures for the presence of key adventitious agents should be routine in any tissue culture facility. Altough bacterial and fungal contaminations can be detected by microscopic and sometimes by macroscopic examination, the detection of mycoplasma and virus contaminants require the use of specific test procedures, including isolation by culture, PCR methods, electron microscopy, and analysis of cytopathic effects.

Microbial contamination can exert numerous effects, and bacterial and yeast contamination will cause nutrient depletion resulting in the death of the cell culture. Although mycoplasma are very fastidious in their growth requirements, contamination with these organisms is known to exert more insidious effects, such as alteration of the growth rate of cells *(3)*, induction of chromosomal aberrations *(4)*, changes in amino acid and nucleic acid metabolism *(5,6)*, and membrane aberrations *(7)*.

The laboratory environment can provide a rich source of bacterial and fungal contamination often focused in damp areas, such as sinks, waterbaths, air

From: *Methods in Molecular Medicine, vol. 24: Antiviral Methods and Protocols*
Edited by: D. Kinchington and R. F. Schinazi © Humana Press Inc., Totowa, NJ

conditioning systems, or materials brought into the laboratory, such as cardboard boxes. However, for mycoplasma the most commonly reported sources of contamination are from human operators (notably with *M. orale* and *M. fermentans*) or cell lines brought in from other laboratories. Historically, animal serum and trypsin were known to be likely sources of mycoplasma; however, most manufacturers of tissue culture reagents now screen to exclude the presence of mycoplasma. The frequency of mycoplasma infection in some tissue culture laboratories may be as high as 100%. Mycoplasma within individual cultures may reach titers of between 10^6 and 10^7 CFU/mL, which is approx 100–1000 times the maximum cell density. It is therefore important to remember that the validity of experimental data, including biochemical and molecular analyses, are at risk because of the overwhelming numbers of mycoplasma relative to the numbers of animal cells in each experiment.

Staff training in aseptic technique and the establishment of a quarantine procedure for cell lines arriving in the laboratory will help to avoid the hazards described above. A prerequisite for mycoplasma-free tissue culture is to use only fully characterized material. This can most readily be achieved by obtaining material from a fully tested source, such as a culture collection. Prior to releasing material to customers, culture collections will have carried out intensive screening of the cells in order to confirm their identity and species of origin. In addition, all cultures will be exhaustively tested for mycoplasma, bacteria, and fungi. Moreover, material supplied by culture collections will ensure that researchers in different laboratories are working with standardized material, enabling direct comparison of results from different laboratories. This is also promoted in culture collections, such as ECACC, where accepted quality management systems, such as BS EN ISO 9000 or Good Laboratory Practice, have been adopted.

The first response to the detection of contamination of any sort should be to discard the material and return to stocks of an earlier passage. However, steps can be taken to reduce the potential for contamination of cell lines. In the first instance care should be taken to avoid handling more than one cell line at any one time. This will significantly reduce the risk of switching or crosscontamination among different cell lines. An important activity to reduce the incidence of microbial contamination is to routinely screen all lines in the facility for the presence of contaminants, such as mycoplasma, bacteria, and fungi. In addition, operating procedures should be adopted that ensure that contaminant-free material is handled in areas remote from contaminated material. Alternatively, if isolated laboratories for infectious work are not available, then a sequence of work progressing from "clean" to "dirty" operations (i.e., "known uncontaminated material" to "untested/unknown" to "known contaminated") with interprocedure disinfection should be adopted. This will ensure that the contaminated material is handled at the end of each day, thereby reducing the potential for contamination.

Mycoplasma is rarely detected in standard bacterial stains (e.g., Gram stain). However, a range of assays are available for their detection. These include DNA staining, isolation by selective culture, specific DNA probes, and, more recently, PCR and ELISA. Protocols for these tests are given in detail below. Each of the tests currently employed has bias toward sensitivity or specificity. Thus, it is recommended that, where possible, two test systems be used in parallel that combine sensitivity and the ability to detect a wide range of species. For bacteria and fungi contaminations, broad-based tests obviously include Gram stain and isolation by culture in broth and on agar plates.

As indicated above, not only is it important to demonstrate that cultures are free of contaminants, but also that they are of the correct origin. Such techniques as isoenzyme analysis and karyotyping can be used routinely to establish the species of origin ***(8)***. Moreover, such techniques as DNA fingerprinting ***(9)*** not only allow the identification of a cell line ***(10)***, but also enable the genetic stability of the material to be monitored during routine and extended culture periods to be studied ***(11,12)***. New applications of the wide range of molecular techniques are being investigated all the time and are leading to the development of useful methods ***(13)***.

Isoenzyme and cytogenetic analysis, like the detection of mycoplasma by DNA staining and culture and the detection of bacteria by broth culture, are recognized by the regulatory authorities, such as the Federal Drug Administration (FDA), and are a prerequisite when applying for product licence. The additional tests required to achieve recognition will obviously incur some additional costs, but the need for quality-controlled cell cultures in both research and commercial situations cannot be underestimated. In addition, in the longer term the increased confidence in the authenticity and quality of the material will ensure that valuable resources, human and financial, are not wasted.

2. Materials

2.1. Reagents and Solutions

1. Carnoy's fixative: 75 mL methanol and 25 mL acetic acid (glacial). Prepare 4 mL of fixative for each sample to be tested. **NB:** Care must be taken when disposing of used fixative.
2. Hoechst stain stock solution (100 mL): Add 10 mg Bisbenzimide Hoechst 33258 to 100 mL of distilled water and allow to dissolve. Filter sterilize using a 0.2 μm filter unit. Wrap the container in aluminum foil and store in the dark at 4°C. **NB:** The toxic properties of Hoechst 33258 are unknown; therefore, gloves should be worn at all times when handling the powder or solutions.
3. Hoechst stain working solution (50 mL): Add 50 μL of stock solution to 50 mL of distilled water. Prepare immediately before use.

4. Mountant: 22.2 mL 0. 1 *M* citric acid and 27.8 mL 0.2 *M* disodium phosphate. Autoclave and then mix with 50 mL glycerol. Adjust to pH 5.5. Filter sterilize and store at 4°C.

2.1.1. Agar Preparation

1. Agar media (prepare fresh as necessary): Dissolve 2.8 g of mycoplasma agar base in 80 mL distilled water, and autoclave at 15 lb/in.^{2} for 15 min.
2. Yeast extract: Dissolve 7 g of yeast extract in 100 mL distilled water, and autoclave as above. Using aseptic technique dispense into 10-mL aliquots and store at 4°C.
3. Pig serum: Using aseptic technique, dispense into 10-mL aliquots and heat-inactivate by incubation of serum at 56°C for 45 min. Store at 4°C.

Prepare the agar as follows:

1. Allow the autoclaved agar media to cool to 50°C and mix with 10 mL of heat-inactivated pig serum and 10 mL yeast extract (both prewarmed to 50°C).
2. Dispense 8 mL/5 cm diameter Petri dish. Seal in plastic bags and store at 4°C for up to 10 d before use.

2.1.2. Broth Preparation

1. Broth media: Dissolve 2 g of mycoplasma broth base in 70 mL distilled water, and autoclave at 15 lb/in.^{2} for 15 min.
2. Yeast extract: Dissolve 7 g of yeast extract in 100 mL distilled water, and autoclave as above. Dispense into 10 mL aliquots and store at 4°C.
3. Horse serum: Dispense into 20 mL aliquots. Store at –20°C. **NB:** Do **not** heat inactivate.

Prepare the broth as follows:

1. Allow the autoclaved agar media to cool to 50°C and mix with 20 mL of horse serum and 10 mL yeast extract (both prewarmed to 50°C).
2. Dispense 1.8 mL per glass vial and store at 4°C. **NB:** Prepared broth may be stored without deterioration for several weeks.

2.1.3. Cell Culture Medium

1. Appropriate cell culture medium. In most cases this will be RPMI-1640.

2.1.4. Antibiotics

The antibiotic of choice:

Agent	Source	Effective concentration
Ciprofloxacin	Bayer	20 mg/L
Mycoplasma removal agent (MRA)	ICN-Flow	0.5 mg/L
Novobiocin	Sigma	44 mg/L
BM Cyclin (two antibiotics)	Boehringer-Mannheim	a. 10 mg/L b. 5 mg/L

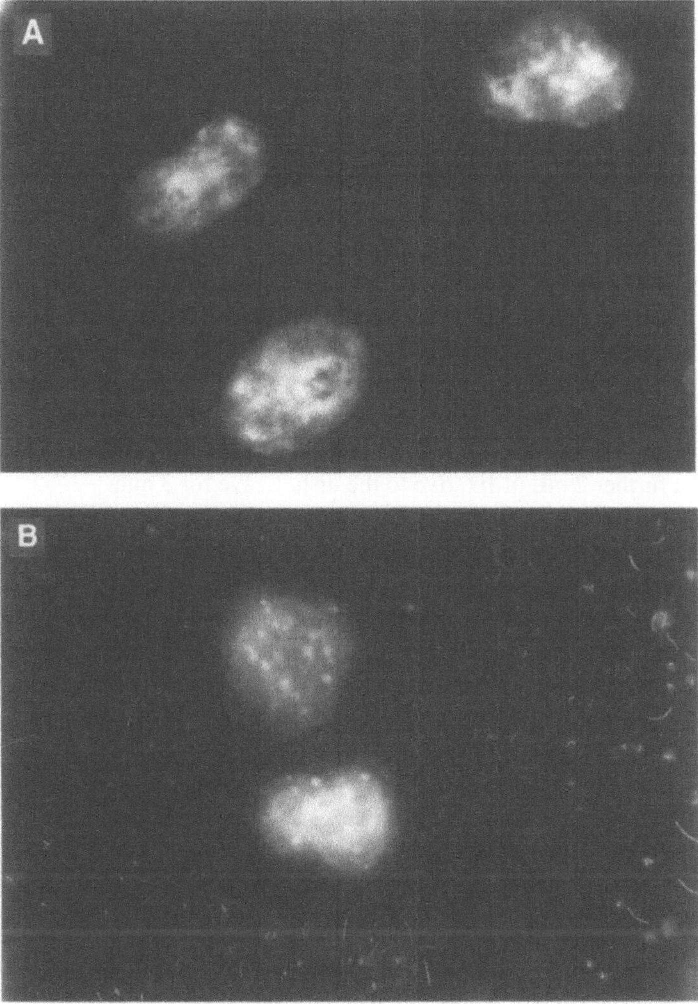

Fig. 1. (**A**) Noninfected cell culture. (**B**) Mycoplasma-infected cell cultures.

3. Methods

3.1. Detection of Mycoplasma by DNA Staining

Prior to testing, cell cultures should undergo at least two passages in antibiotic-free medium, since infection may be masked by the presence of antibiotics. Equally cryopreserved stocks should also undergo two passages in antibiotic-free medium because of the inhibitory effects of cryoprotectants. Suspension cell lines may be used direct. However, cell lines that grow as attached monolayers should be brought into suspension using a standard method of subculture with trypsin and/or EDTA. Cells should be resuspended in the original cell culture medium at a cell concentration of approx 5×10^5 cells/mL.

1. Add 2–3 mL of cell suspension to each of two tissue culture dishes containing glass coverslips. Coverslips should be sterilized by autoclaving prior to placing in the petri dishes. Control dishes: One pair of dishes inoculated with 100 CFU of each of two species of mycoplasma should be included as positive controls (*see* section below on preparation of control organisms). Additionally one pair of dishes should be left uninoculated as a negative control.
2. Incubate at 36 ± 1°C in a humidified 5% CO_2/95% air atmosphere for 12–24 h.
3. Remove one dish and incubate the remaining dish for a further 48 h.
4. Before fixing, examine the cells for the presence of bacterial or fungal contamination.
5. Fix the cells by adding 2 mL of Carnoy's fixative dropwise at the edge of the dish to avoid disturbing the cells. Leave at room temperature for 3 min.
6. Carefully remove the fixative and tissue culture medium to a waste bottle and add a further 2 mL of fixative to the dish. Leave for 3 min.
7. Pipet the fixative to waste.
8. Invert the lid of the dish, and using forceps, rest the coverslip against the lid for 10 min to air-dry.
9. Wearing gloves, return the coverslip to the dish and add 2 mL Hoechst stain (working solution). Shield the coverslip from direct light and leave at room temperature for 5 min.
10. Pipet the stain to a waste bottle.
11. Add one drop of mountant to a labeled slide and place the coverslip cell side down onto the appropriate slide.
12. Examine the slide at ×100 magnification with oil immersion under UV epifluorescence. Cell nuclei will fluoresce. In mycoplasma-negative cultures, the nuclei will be seen against a dark background. In mycoplasma-positive cultures, the cell nuclei will be seen among fluorescing thread-like or coccal structures (**Fig. 1**).

In an alternative system, cells of the test culture can be inoculated onto coverslips preinoculated with an indicator cell line, such as the Vero African Green Monkey cell line. In this case the Vero cell should be inoculated at a cell concentration of 1×10^4 cells/mL and left for 4–24 h prior to addition of the test sample. The major advantage of this system, which overcomes the additional time required to set up, is the increased sensitivity achieved by the increased surface area of cytoplasm in Vero cells, which aids in revealing the mycoplasma. This system also enables the mycoplasma screening of serum and other reagents that can be inoculated directly onto the indicator cell line.

3.2. Detection of Mycoplasma by Culture

1. Using a routine method of subculture, harvest adherent cells with trypsin or EDTA and resuspend in the original cell culture medium at a concentration of approx 5×10^5 cells/mL.

2. Test suspension cell lines directly from a culture at approx 5×10^5 cells/mL.
3. Inoculate an agar plate with 0.1 mL of the test cell suspension and incubate anaerobically at 36 ± 1°C for 21 d.
4. Inoculate a broth with 0.2 mL of the test cell suspension and incubate aerobically at 36 ± 1°C. At approx 7 and 14 d postinoculation, subculture 0.1 mL of the inoculated broth cultures onto fresh agar plates and incubate as above. **NB:** Plates inoculated with 100 CFU of two species of mycoplasma should be included as positive controls (*see below* for the preparation of control organisms). Additionally, one plate should be left uninoculated as a negative control.
5. After 7, 14, and 21 d incubation, the agar plates should be examined under ×40 or ×100 magnification using an inverted microscope for the presence/absence of mycoplasma colonies.

Typically mycoplasma colonies will have a "fried egg" appearance, but this may not be the cases for all strains. However, it is of course necessary to distinguish mycoplasma colonies from "pseudocolonies" and cell aggregates. The use of Dienes stain, which stains true mycoplasma colonies blue but leaves pseudocolonies and fungal and bacterial colonies unstained, can be used. Additionally, by using a sterile bacteriological loop cell aggregates can be disrupted, but mycoplasma colonies will leave a central core embedded in the agar.

4. Positive Control Organisms

Both of the tests described above should be run in parallel with positive controls. In general, three species are used: *M. orale* and *M. hyorhinis* for DNA staining and *M. orale* and *M. pneumoniae* for the culture method. In all cases, the positive control organisms are inoculated at 100 CFU/mL. *See* **Subheading 3.** for preparation of mycoplasma broth and agar.

4.1. Preparation of Stocks of Positive Control Stocks Organisms

1. Thaw existing stocks or reconstitute lyophilised stocks and inoculate 100 µL in to 10 broths. Place at 36 ± 1°C for 5–7 d. Observe daily for changes in broth color.
2. Once a distinct color change has been observed, transfer the entire contents of the broths into 1 mL cryotubes, assign a batch number, and snap-freeze in the vapor phase of liquid nitrogen.

4.2. Enumeration of Control Stocks

1. Thaw an ampule of the batch to be enumerated, serially diluted in tenfold dilutions.
2. Inoculate 3 × 10 µL aliquots of each dilution onto agar plates that have been air-dried for 30 min prior to use. Plates should be labeled with the organism name, the batch number, and the dilution.
3. Plates should then be incubated anaerobically for 2–7 d prior to counting. The time required for colonies to appear depends on the species. As a rough guide 2–3 d are required for *M. hyorhinis,* 4–5 d for *M. orale*, and 5–7 d for *M. pneumoniae.*

4. Using an inverted microscope, count the colonies of the dilution, which should be between 10 and 100.
5. Calculate the number of CFU in the cyropreserved stock using **Eq. 1**:

$$\text{No. of CFU/mL} = (\text{mean no. of colonies counted} \times 100)/(\text{dilution factor}) \quad (1)$$

5. Elimination of Contamination

In the event of cultures becoming infected with mycoplasma, the best course of action is to discard the cultures and following extensive decontamination of the tissue culture cabinets and work surfaces, thereby resuscitating "clean" cell stocks. However, in the case of irreplaceable stocks this may not be practical.

5.1. Elimination of Contamination

1. Culture cells in the presence of the chosen antibiotic(s) for a period of 10–14 d, during which time most cultures will be passaged approx 4 times. Each passage should be performed at the highest dilution of antibiotic that the cell will tolerate following the manufacturer's guidelines.
2. Test the culture for the presence of mycoplasma by a Hoechst stain. If mycoplasma is still detectable, it is unlikely that this antibiotic will be successful and an alternative should be tried on a fresh batch of cells.
3. If the Hoechst stain gives a negative result, then the cells should be cultured in antibiotic-free medium for a period required to conduct 10 passages. Testing should be conducted at every passage to monitor treatment success since mycoplasma may persist at low levels immediately after antibiotic treatment.
4. If the culture is mycoplasma-negative after 10 passages in antibiotic-free medium, the mycoplasma may be considered to have been eradicated and a bank of mycoplasma-free cells should be prepared immediately.

6. Gen-Probe Mycoplasma TC Rapid Detection System

6.1. Introduction

The Gen-Probe Mycoplasma TC Rapid Detection System (Eurogenetics) employs the principle of nucleic acid hybridization to detect mycoplasma in tissue culture. Using in-solution hybridization of ribosomal RNA it is possible to detect positive samples in 3 h or less. The test kit contains a 3H-labeled DNA probe homologs to mycoplasma or acholeplasma ribosomal RNA.

6.2. Method

All operations must be carried out in a designated radioactive area. All reagents used are supplied in each Gen-Probe kit.

1. Pipet 1.5 mL of the cell culture to be tested into an Eppendorf tube and centrifuge at 14,000*g* for 10 min in an Eppendorf centrifuge.
2. Carefully remove the supernatant with a Pasteur pipet, to prevent disturbing the pellet.

3. Add 200 µL of Gen-Probe solution to each tube, and resuspend the pellet by vortexing.
4. Set up controls by pipetting 50 µL of control solutions plus 50 µL of phosphate buffered saline (PBS) into separate microcentrifuge tubes. Add 200 µL of Gen-Probe probe solution to each tube and mix by vortexing as above.
5. Place all tubes (samples and controls) in a waterbath and incubate 72°C for at least 2 h.
6. For each sample and control pipet 5.0 mL of thoroughly mixed separation suspension (bottle is inverted five times before removing each 5 mL unit) into a 7-mL plastic screw cap scintillation vial. **NB:** Any labeling of the vial is only done on the vial's cap.
7. At the end of the incubation transfer the entire contents of each tube into the corresponding scintillation vial containing separation suspension.
8. Briefly vortex each vial and return to the 72°C waterbath for 5 min.
9. Vortex each vial again and then centrifuge at 500*g* for 1 min.
10. Decant all supernatant, ensuring that the pellet is not lost.
11. Wash the pellet by pipeting 5 mL of Gen-Probe wash solution into each vial and briefly vortex to resuspend the pellet.
12. Place vials in the 72°C waterbath for 5 min, remove, and briefly vortex.
13. Centrifuge at 500*g* for 1 min. Remove supernatant without losing the pellet.
14. Repeat the wash process once more.
15. After washing twice, add 5 mL of scintillation solution to each vial and vortex.
16. For the background count, 5 mL of scintillation solution is pipetted into an empty vial.

17a. For the total count, 5 mL of thoroughly mixed (inverted five times) separation suspension is pipetted into a 7-mL plastic screw-cap scintillation vial, centrifuged for 1 min at 500*g*, and the supernatant tipped off without losing the pellet. Then 50 µL of probe solution is added.

b. Add 5 mL of scintillation solution to the vial and resuspend the pellet by vortexing.

18. All the vials are placed in the dark for at least 5 min, removed, and wiped with a clean, damp, paper towel and placed into a scintillation counter. Counts:

$$\text{Total count} = (\text{total count vial} - \text{background vial count}) \times 4\% \text{ hybridization}$$
$$= (\text{sample CPM} - \text{background CPM})/(\text{total count CPM}) \times 100 \quad (2)$$

Positive control should be ≥30% hybridization. Negative and PBS control should be ≤0.2% hybridization. Positive result for mycoplasma is ≥0.4% hybridization.

Note: Occasionally the negative control using the negative control solution produces a hybridization slightly higher than 0.2%, but if the PBS control is still below 0.2% hybridization the results are still valid.

7. Boehringer Mannheim Mycoplasma Detection Kit

7.1. Introduction

The kit is based on the ELISA technique and contains polyclonal antibodies for the detection of four species of mycoplasma found in contaminated cell cultures (*M. orale*, *M. hyorhinis*, *M. arginini*, *A. laidlawii*).

All reagents are supplied with the kit and are stored at 4°C; however, all reagents should have reached room temperature (18–25°C) before use.

1. Pipet 0.25 mL of each capture antibody (one for each mycoplasma species) into two wells for each sample and into one well for each control, according to the information in **Table 1**. Repeat for three other species. Cover microtiter plate with aluminum foil and incubate for 2 h at 37°C.
2. Remove solutions by inverting microtiter plate and then tapping on a clean dry paper towel. Pipet 0.25 mL of blocking solution into all antibody coated wells and incubate at 37°C for 30 min.
3. Remove solutions as above. Wash wells three times with 0.25 mL washing solution buffer and finally remove washing buffer thoroughly.
4. To 2 mL of each sample add 0.5 mL sample buffer. For the negative control, add 0.25 mL of sample buffer to either 1 mL of either sterile media analogs to the sample or 1 mL of washing buffer.
5. Pipet 0.2 mL of prepared sample into the eight designated sample wells. Pipet 0.2 mL of negative and positive control (as supplied) into each of the designated wells. Cover the microtiter plate with aluminum foil and incubate overnight at 4°C.
6. Wash plate as above.
7. Pipet 0.2 mL each detection antibody solution in turn into the appropriate wells. Cover the microtiter plate with aluminum foil and incubate at 37°C for 2 h.
8. Wash plate as above.
9. Pipet 0.2 mL of streptavidin–AP solution into all antibody-coated wells. Cover the microtiter plate with aluminum foil and incubate for 1 h at 37°C.
10. Wash plate as above.
11. Pipet 0.2 mL substrate solution into all antibody-coated wells and incubate for 1 h at 18–25°C.
12. Read the results using an ELISA reader set at 405 nm.

7.2. Comparison of Mycoplasma Detection Methods

The tests which are available commercially are generally straightforward to use and provide results within 1–2 d. In addition the results are generally easy to interpret. However, as with all diagnostic tests a small proportion of tests will yield false positive results, false negative results, and equivocal results, which should be borne in mind.

Most of the tests discussed above will detect all species of mycoplasma and closely related organisms, such as *A. laidlawii*. The table below shows a comparison of the methods described above. Isolation by culture will detect all species except for *M. hyorhinis,* which is noncultivable ***(14)***. The range of species which may be detected with the commercially available ELISA method described is much restricted since the ELISA assay, while allowing a positive identification of the contaminating mycoplasma species, detects only four species (*M. orale*, *M. hyorhinis*, *M. arginini*, and *A. laidlawii*).

Table 1
Placement of Controls and Samples for Mycoplasma Detection

	M. orale	*M. hyorhinis*	*M. arginini*	*A. laidlawii*	5	6	7	8	9	10	11	12
A	Positive control	Positive control	Positive control	Positive control								
B	Negative control	Negative control	Negative control	Negative control								
C	Sample 1	Sample 1	Sample 1	Sample 1								
D	Sample 1	Sample 1	Sample 1	Sample 1								
E	Sample 2	Sample 2	Sample 2	Sample 2								
F	Sample 2	Sample 2	Sample 2	Sample 2								
G												
H												

Table 2
Comparison of Different Techniques Used for the Detection of Mycoplasma Infection

Test	Sensitivity	Detection range	Speed	Cost/test, excluding staff time	Regulatory authority approval	Special equipment requirements
DNA stain	10^3–10^4 CFU	All species	1 d	<£2	FDA[a] only	Microscope
Culture	1 CFU	All cultivable species (excludes *M. hyorhinis*)	2–4 wk	£2	EP[b] and FDA[a]	None
Gen-probe	10^3–10^4 CFU	All species	1 d	£15–20	None	Scintillation counter
ELISA	10^3–10^4 CFU	Four species only	2 d	£2–5	None	ELISA reader

[a]EP: European pharmacopoeia.
[b]FDA: Federal Drug Administration (USA).

Poor sensitivity of a detection method may result in a low-level contamination being missed. The tests described generally show a threshold of detection of at least 10^4 CFU/mL of sample. Greater sensitivity can be obtained with the culture method, which has a theoretical detection threshold of 1 CFU/mL of sample for cultivable species. However, in order to achieve this level of sensitivity, a culture period of 4 wk is necessary; this should be combined with the use of a second, more sensitive test, such as PCR or culture. In addition, cultures should be tested every time they are recovered from nitrogen storage since mycoplasma may proliferate more quickly than animal cells.

Economic factors are clearly important when selecting a test method. The price per test can vary significantly depending on the system used (*see* **Table 2,** *opposite page*). The Gen-probe assay currently costs £300 for 20 tests and the ELISA system is £200 for 96 tests (including positive and negative controls). In addition, the shelf life of a "kit" once opened should be borne in mind, since this can be quite restrictive. The DNA staining and culture methods have a relatively low cost per test as compared with the commercial kits; however, the interpretation of results requires a significant level of training and experience. A further consideration is the need for specialist equipment. As can be seen from **Table 2**, all the tests described except for the culture method require specialist equipment, thus adding an additional setup cost.

On final analysis the choice of technique used will be largely based on the availability of skilled staff and the frequency of testing required. For a larger number of tests DNA staining techniques will probably represent the most cost-effective way of providing a comprehensive screening system provided adequate training of staff. Training for all of the tests described is also available through culture collections, which can also provide mycoplasma testing services to regulatory approved standards (ECACC Newsletter, 1997).

References

1. Doyle, A., Morris, C. B., and Melling, J. M. (1989) Animal cell culture collections and the supply of authenticated cultures and services for industry and research, in *Biotechnology and Engineering Reviews,* vol. 7, Intercept, Andover, UK.
2. Stacey G. N., Hoelzl, H., Stephenson, J. R., and Doyle, A. (1997) Authentication of animal cell cultures by direct visualisation of DNA, Aldolase gene PCR and isoenzyme analysis. *Biologicals* **25,** 75–83.
3. McGarrity, G. J., Phillips, D., and Vaidya, A. (1980) Mycoplasma infection of lymphocyte cultures: infection with *M. salivarium. In Vitro Cell. Dev. Biol.* **16,** 346–356.
4. Aula, P. and Nichols, W. W. (1967) The cytogenetic effects of mycoplasma in human leucocyte cultures. *J. Cell. Physiol.* ***70,*** 281–290.
5. Stanbridge, E. J., Hayflick, L., and Perkins, F. T. (1971) Modification of amino acid concentrations induced by mycoplasmas in cell culture medium. *Nature* **232,** 242–244.

6. Levine, E. M., Thomas, L., McGregor, D., Hayflick, L. V., and Eagle, H. (1968) Altered nucleic acid metabolism in human cell cultures infected with mycoplasma. *Proc. Natl. Acad. Sci. USA* **60,** 583–589.
7. Wise, K. S., Cassell, G. H., and Action, R. T. (1978). Selective association of murine T lymphoblastoid cell surface alloantigens with *M. hyorhinis. Proc. Natl. Acad. Sci. USA* **75,** 4479–4483.
8. O'Brien, S. J., Kleiner, G., Olsou, R., and Shannon, J. E. (1977) Enzyme polymorphisms as genetic signatures in human cell cultures. *Science* **195,** 1345–1348.
9. Jeffreys, A. J., Wilson, V., and Thein, S. L. (1985) Individual-specific 'fingerprints' of human DNA. *Nature* **316,** 76–79.
10. Stacey, G. N., Bolton, B. J., and Doyle A. (1992) DNA fingerprinting transforms the art of cell authentication. *Nature* **357,** 261,262.
11. Stacey, G. N., Bolton, B. J., Morgan, D., Clark, S. A., and Doyle, A. (1992) Multilocus DNA fingerprint analysis of cell banks: Stability and culture identification in human B lymphoblastoid and mammalian cell stocks. *Cytotechnology* **8,** 13–20.
12. Racher, A. J., Stacey, G. N., Bolton, B. J., Doyle, A., and Griffiths, J. B. (1994) Genetic and biochemical analysis of a murine hybridoma in long-term continuous culture, in *Animal Cell Technology: Products of Today, Prospects for Tomorrow* (Spier, R. W., Griffiths, J. B., and Berthold, W., eds.), Butterworth-Heinemann, Oxford, UK, pp. 69–75.
13. Stacey, G. N. (1997) Standardisation in animal cell technology. *Folia Microbiol.* **42,** 113–116.
14. Razin, S. (1994) DNA probes and PCR in diagnosis of mycoplasma infection. *Mol. Cell. Probes.* **8,** 497–511.

I

Hepatitis Virus

4

Hep AD38 Assay

A High-Throughput, Cell-Based Screen for the Evaluation of Compounds Against Hepatitis B Virus

Robert W. King and Stephanie K. Ladner

1. Introduction

Approximately 5% of the world's population has been infected with hepatitis B virus (HBV). Ten percent of these adults will become chronic carriers, as will 95% of the infants infected perinatally. Those that do become chronically infected with HBV are at increased risk of developing liver dysfunction, cirrhosis, and liver failure *(1)*. In addition, they also have a greater incidence of heptocellular carcinoma *(2)*. Approximately two million chronic carriers die annually from liver disease attributed to infection by HBV *(3)*.

Human HBV, which is a member of the *hepadnavirus* family, has a circular partially double-stranded DNA genome of approx 3000 bp in length. In the nucleus of the infected cell, the HBV genome is converted into a completely double-stranded, covalently closed circular DNA species *(4)*. This DNA serves as the template for the transcription of the pregenomic and messenger RNAs. The viral messenger RNAs are translated into the viral surface antigen, core antigen, polymerase, and X protein. The surface antigen is found in the envelope of the mature virion, whereas the core antigen forms the virion nucleocapsid. The HBV polymerase has several functions. It transcribes the genomic DNA from the pregenomic RNA, digests the pregenomic RNA template, produces the partially double-stranded DNA molecule found within the mature virion, and plays a role in the assembly of the core particle *(5,6)*. Additionally, the HBV polymerase acts as a primer for DNA synthesis during reverse transcription and is covalently attached through a tyrosine residue to the 5' end of

From: *Methods in Molecular Medicine, vol. 24: Antiviral Methods and Protocols*
Edited by: D. Kinchington and R. F. Schinazi © Humana Press Inc., Totowa, NJ

the minus strand of the viral DNA *(7)*. The function of the X protein has not been elucidated. However, it has homology to eukaryotic transactivating factors and may act to regulate the expression of the viral genes *(8)*.

Currently, duck HBV polymerase has been the only HBV target successfully formatted into a high throughput, in vitro assay to detect inhibitors of HBV replication (*see* Chapter 6). To screen large chemical libraries for compounds that inhibit any one of the many steps that make up the HBV replication cycle, including those that are not catalyzed by the HBV polymerase (i.e., viral RNA transport, translation and turnover, capsid assembly, and virus egress), a high-throughput, cell-based screen was created using the Hep AD38 cell line *(9)*. The Hep AD38 assay is run in a 96-well microtiter plate format and can be completed in approx 1 wk. The assay, if run as described below, allows one person to screen approx 100 compounds for anti-HBV and anticellular activities per week.

The mode of action of a compound that tests positive in the Hep AD38 assay could be either the inhibition of a specific step in the HBV replication cycle or the repression of the inducible promoter responsible for the transcription of pregenomic RNA in the Hep AD38 cell line. To differentiate between these two possiblities, positive hits from the Hep AD38 assay are screened in the Hep AD43 cell line, a stably transfected Hep G2 cell line that contains the *Eschericha coli lac z* gene under the control of the same tetracycline-responsive promoter used to create the Hep AD38 cell line. If a compound inhibits HBV replication in the Hep AD38 cell line but does not inhibit β-galactosidase activity in the Hep AD43 cell line, one can assume that it acts to specifically inhibit one or more steps of the HBV replication cycle.

2. Materials

1. Hep AD38 cells.
2. Hep AD43 cells.
3. Hep AD38 seeding medium: DMEM/F12 supplemented with 10% fetal bovine serum (FBS), 50 μg/mL penicillin, 50 μg/mL streptomycin, 100 μg/mL kanamycin (P/S/K), 400 μg/mL G418, and 0.3 μg/mL tetracycline.
4. Hep AD38 assay medium: Dulbecco's modified Eagle's medium (DMEM)/F12 supplemented with 10% FBS and P/S/K.
5. Hep AD43 seeding medium: DMEM/F-12 supplemented with 10% FBS, P/S/K, 100 μg/mL zeocin (Invitrogen, San Diego, CA), 800 μg/mL G418, and 0.3 μg/mL tetracycline.
6. Hep AD43 assay medium: DMEM/F12 supplemented with 10% FBS, P/S/K, 100 μg/mL zeocin, and 800 μg/mL G418.
7. Dulbecco's phosphate-buffered saline (DPBS).
8. Trypsin:ethylenediaminetetra-acetic acid (EDTA) (Gibco-BRL Life Technologies, Gaithersburg, MD).
9. MTS (Owen's reagent) solution: Dissolve 42 mg of MTS [3-(4,5-dimethylthiazol-2-yl)-5-(3-carboxymethophenyl)-2-(4-sulfophenyl)-2H-tetrazolium] into 21 mL of

DPBS in a light protected container. Adjust pH to 6.0–6.5 and sterile filter through 0.2-µm membrane.
10. Phenazine methosulfate (PMS) at 0.92 mg/mL in DPBS.
11. MTS/PMS Solution: Mix 100 µL of PMS solution with 2 µL of MTS solution just prior to use.
12. Molecular Devices VMax Kinetic Microplate Reader equipped with 405- and 490-nm wavelength filters.
13. 96-well tissue-culture plates (Costar, Cambridge, MA).
14. T162 tissue-culture flasks (Costar).
15. 2X Denaturing solution: 2 *M* NaOH, 20X saline sodium citrate (SSC), 1% NP40 (added fresh just before use).
16. Neutralization solution: 1 *M* Tris-HCl (pH 7.2–7.4), 2 *M* NaCl.
17. 20X SSC; 2X SSC *(**10**)*.
18. Nytran Plus nylon membrane (Schleicher and Schuell, Keene, NH), product no. 77419.
19. 96-well dot-blotting apparatus.
20. Ultraviolet crosslinker.
21. Hybridization solution: 5X SSC, 5X Denhardt's Reagent, 20 m*M* $NaPO_4$, pH 6.5, 50% Formamide, 1% sodium dodecylt sulfate (SDS), 250 µg/mL salmon sperm DNA.
22. Megaprime DNA Labeling System (Amersham Corp., Arlington Heights, IL), product no. RPN1607.
23. Chroma Spin + TE-30 Columns (Clontech Laboratories, Inc., Palo Alto, CA), product no. K1321-1.
24. GS-363 Molecular Imaging System (Bio-Rad, Hercules, CA).
25. β-Galactosidase Enzyme Assay System (Promega, Madison, WI), product no. E2000.

3. Methods

3.1. Cell Line Maintenance

Hep AD38 cells are maintained in Hep AD38 seeding medium in T162 flasks. They are passaged weekly at a 1:10 ratio with medium being replaced once between passages.

1. Wash the cell monolayer with 3–5 mL of trypsin:EDTA.
2. Add 3 mL of fresh trypsin:EDTA and incubate at room temperature for 4 min.
3. Dislodge the cells by tapping the flask several times against your hand.
4. Add 17 mL of seeding medium to the cell suspension and pipet up and down with a 10-mL pipet to break up clumps.
5. Transfer 2 mL of cell suspension to each T162 flask and add 40–50 mL of seeding medium.

3.2. Hep AD38 Assay

3.2.1. Assay for Anti-HBV Activity

1. Place 100 µL of Hep AD38 cell suspension (6×10^5 viable cells/mL of Hep AD38 seeding medium) into each well of a 96-well microtiter plate, and incubate at 37°C for 3 d.

2. Remove the medium from the wells and wash the cell monolayers three times with 100 µL of warmed (37°C) DPBS.
3. To the proper wells, add 100 µL of HepAD38 assay medium that contains either test or control compounds at the desired concentrations (*see* **Fig. 1** for example of templates for testing compounds at two, three, and six concentrations). Include several wells with Hep AD38 assay medium alone to serve as "virus only" controls. Incubate the plates at 37°C for 3 d.
4. On d 3, wash the cells once with warmed DPBS and add fresh medium containing the appropriate compound to the wells.
5. After 24 h, transfer the supernatants to v-bottomed 96-well plates and remove cellular debris by centrifugation (15 min, 2500 rpm at 4°C, Sorvall RT-6000D). Transfer 90 µL of the clarified supernatants to new v-bottomed plates and store at –70°C for quantification of HBV DNA.

3.2.2. Cytotoxicity Assay

1. Add 100 µL of DPBS and 20 µL of MTS/PMS solution to the cell monolayers from **step 5** of **Subheading 3.2.1.**
2. Incubate at 37°C for at least 1 h or until color develops.
3. Read the absorbance at 490 nm on a microplate reader to assess cell viability.

3.3. Detection of Human HBV DNA

3.3.1. Dot-Blotting Procedure

1. Thaw the supernatants that were collected in **step 5** of **Subheading 3.2.1.** and add 90 µL of 2X denaturation solution to each well, pipeting up and down several times to mix.
2. Incubate at room temperature for 20 min.
3. Cut the nylon membrane to size and prepare it for blotting by wetting it first with distilled water and then 20X SSC.
4. Dot-blot the denatured supernatants on to the nylon membrane as directed by the manufacturer of the blotting apparatus.
5. Wash the blot with 200 µL of neutralization solution per well followed by 200 µL of 20X SSC.
6. Remove the blot from the blotting apparatus, rinse it briefly in 2X SSC, and then crosslink the DNA to the nylon filter by UV irradiation.

3.3.2. Probe Preparation and Hybridization Procedure

1. Prehybridize the blot at 42°C for ≥1 h in 20 µL of hybridization solution.
2. Prepare a ^{32}P-labeled probe by random priming (Amersham Megaprime DNA Labeling System) using a portion of the HBV genome as a template (*see* **Note 4**). Purify the probe through a Clontech Chroma Spin column as directed by the manufacturer.
3. Denature the probe by boiling for 5 min and add it immediately to the hybridization solution. Hybridize the nylon filter overnight at 42°C.
4. Wash the nylon filters twice with 50 mL of 2X SSC, 0.1% SDS at room temperature for 20 min and twice with 50 mL of 0.2X SSC, 0.1% SDS at 65°C for 20 min.

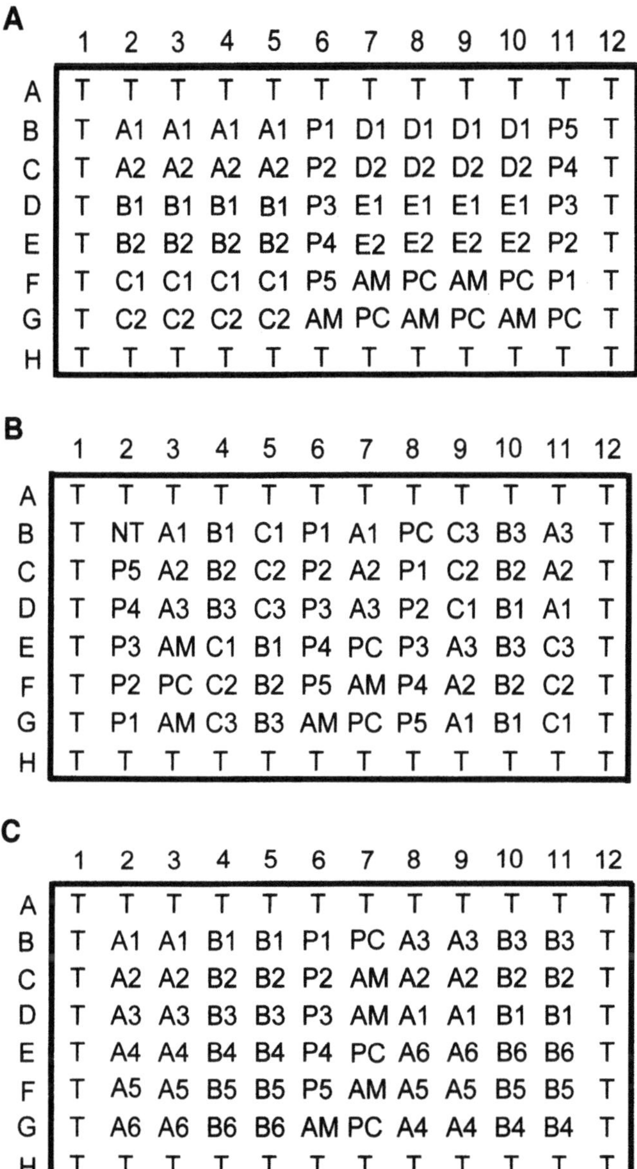

A

	1	2	3	4	5	6	7	8	9	10	11	12
A	T	T	T	T	T	T	T	T	T	T	T	T
B	T	A1	A1	A1	A1	P1	D1	D1	D1	D1	P5	T
C	T	A2	A2	A2	A2	P2	D2	D2	D2	D2	P4	T
D	T	B1	B1	B1	B1	P3	E1	E1	E1	E1	P3	T
E	T	B2	B2	B2	B2	P4	E2	E2	E2	E2	P2	T
F	T	C1	C1	C1	C1	P5	AM	PC	AM	PC	P1	T
G	T	C2	C2	C2	C2	AM	PC	AM	PC	AM	PC	T
H	T	T	T	T	T	T	T	T	T	T	T	T

B

	1	2	3	4	5	6	7	8	9	10	11	12
A	T	T	T	T	T	T	T	T	T	T	T	T
B	T	NT	A1	B1	C1	P1	A1	PC	C3	B3	A3	T
C	T	P5	A2	B2	C2	P2	A2	P1	C2	B2	A2	T
D	T	P4	A3	B3	C3	P3	A3	P2	C1	B1	A1	T
E	T	P3	AM	C1	B1	P4	PC	P3	A3	B3	C3	T
F	T	P2	PC	C2	B2	P5	AM	P4	A2	B2	C2	T
G	T	P1	AM	C3	B3	AM	PC	P5	A1	B1	C1	T
H	T	T	T	T	T	T	T	T	T	T	T	T

C

	1	2	3	4	5	6	7	8	9	10	11	12
A	T	T	T	T	T	T	T	T	T	T	T	T
B	T	A1	A1	B1	B1	P1	PC	A3	A3	B3	B3	T
C	T	A2	A2	B2	B2	P2	AM	A2	A2	B2	B2	T
D	T	A3	A3	B3	B3	P3	AM	A1	A1	B1	B1	T
E	T	A4	A4	B4	B4	P4	PC	A6	A6	B6	B6	T
F	T	A5	A5	B5	B5	P5	AM	A5	A5	B5	B5	T
G	T	A6	A6	B6	B6	AM	PC	A4	A4	B4	B4	T
H	T	T	T	T	T	T	T	T	T	T	T	T

Fig. 1. 96-well microtiter plate templates for screening compounds in quadruplicate at two, three, and six concentrations. **(A)** The two-concentration template. **(B)** The three-concentration template. **(C)** The six-concentration template. T: Hep AD38 seeding medium containing tetracycline; AM: Hep AD38 assay medium; PC: positive control for virus inhibition (a known inhibitor of HBV replication at its established EC_{90}); P1–P5: PC for dose response (a known inhibitor of HBV replication that is serially diluted using threefold dilutions); A–E: letter designation for the compounds being screened (the number following the letter represents different concentrations of the compound).

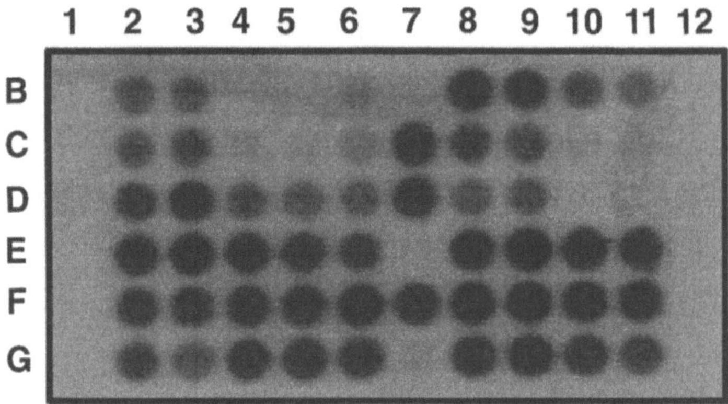

Fig. 2. Autographic results of the assay of two compounds for anti-HBV activity in the Hep AD38 assay. The compounds were tested in quadruplicate at six concentration, as shown in **Fig. 1C**. The two compounds were tested at 30, 10, 3, 1, 0.3, and 0.1 μg/mL. The dose response PC was CDG at 0.1, 0.03, 0.01, 0.003, and 0.001 μg/mL, and the PC for virus inhibition was 3TC at 0.3 μ*M*.

5. Expose the nylon filters to a molecular imager screen for four hours and scan on a phosphorimager to obtain the data (*see* **Fig. 2** for an example of a typical result).
6. To determine the percent inhibition of HBV replication, subtract the background value (i.e., counts of radiation detected from the nylon filter itself) from all control and experimental values. Divide the average values of the experimental wells (i.e., cells treated with test compounds) by the average value for the "virus only" control (i.e., cells not treated with compound or tetracycline during the experiment) and multiply this number by 100.

3.4. Assay for Inhibition of the Tetracycline-Responsive Promoter

3.4.1. Hep AD43 Assay

1. Place 100 μL Hep AD43 cell solution (1 × 10^5 cells/mL of Hep AD43 seeding medium) into each well of a 96-well microtiter plate. Incubate for 3 d at 37°C.
2. Wash cells three times with warmed (37°C) DPBS. Add 100 μL of Hep AD43 assay medium containing either test or control compound to the proper wells.
3. After 3 d incubation at 37°C, wash the cells one time with warmed DPBS and add fresh medium and compound.
4. Incubate the cells an additional 24 h at 37°C, wash two times with cold DPBS and add 50 μL of Reporter Lysis Buffer (RLB) (β-Galactosidase Enzyme Assay System) to each well.
5. Place the plates on a rocking platform for 20 min at room temperature. Complete cell lysis by pipetting the contents of each well several times with a multichannel pipeter.
6. Transfer cell lysates to the wells of a v-bottomed microtiter plate and clarify them of cellular debris by centrifugation (15 min, 2500 rpm at 4°C; Sorvall RT-6000D).

Transfer the supernatant fluid to a new microtiter plate and store at –70°C or place on ice if they are to be assayed immediately for β-galactosidase activity.

3.4.2. β-Galactosidase Assay

β-galactosidase activity is assayed using the β-Galactosidase Enzyme Assay System (Promega). A standard curve is generated using the β-galactosidase control that is provided with the kit. This standard curve allows one to calculate the level of β-galactosidase activity in Hep AD43 cells treated with the test compounds.

1. Thaw components of the kit and the cell lysates (if frozen) and place on ice.
2. Dilute each cell lysate 30-, 100-, and 300-fold in 1X RLB. Keep samples on ice until **step 4**.
3. Place 50 µL of 2X assay buffer into each well of a flat-bottom microtiter plate.
4. Add 50 µL of the diluted cell lysates to the proper wells
5. Add 50 µL of the β-galactosidase standard curve dilution series to the proper wells. Prepare the standard curve dilution series as follows:
   a. Dilute β-galactosidase standard 1:10,000 in 1X RLB.
   b. Dilutions for the standard curve:

      i. 1 mU β-galactosidase: 10 µL diluted β-galactosidase + 40 µL RLB.
      ii. 2 mU β-galactosidase: 20 µL diluted β-galactosidase + 30 µL RLB.
      iii. 3 mU β-galactosidase: 30 µL diluted β-galactosidase + 20 µL RLB.
      iv. 4 mU β-galactosidase: 40 µL diluted β-galactosidase + 10 µL RLB.
      v. 5 mU β-galactosidase: 50 µL diluted β-galactosidase + 0 µL RLB.

6. Mix samples by pipeting the contents of each well several times with a multichannel pipeter.
7. Incubate the plate at 37°C for 30 min. (If a yellow color has not developed in the positive controls (PCs), continue incubation until the color appears.)
8. Stop the reaction by adding 150 µL 1 *M* calcium carbonate to each well. Mix the contents of the wells with a multichannel pipeter.
9. Read the absorbance of the samples at 405 nm in a plate reader.
10. Plot A_{405} vs the level of β-galactosidase activity in the standards to determine the level of β-galactosidase activity in compound-treated cells.

4. Notes

1. As with all cell lines, it is important to maintain consistent culture conditions for the Hep AD38 cell line. In particular, it is important to validate one's lots of FBS and medium prior to use in the assay to ensure good and consistent virus production. In addition, the authors find that different lots of trypsin:EDTA have variable effects on cell viability. Thus, before using a new lot of trypsin:EDTA, its effect on cell viability should be determined.
2. The assay format of 3 d of compound treatment/medium change/1 additional day of treatment increases the sensitivity of the assay over a format that consists of a 4-d treatment period without media change. The inclusion of an additional 3-d treatment

period followed by a medium change (7 d of compound treatment total) increases the amount of virus produced, but does not affect the sensitivity of the assay.

3. The authors have had varied success with nylon membranes from different vendors, and recommend the membrane listed in **Subheading 2.** for optimal results.
4. The authors' radioactively labeled probe is produced from a 2.8-kbp DNA fragment of the nonrepetitive region of the HBV genome. This is generated by polymerase chain reaction amplification of a cDNA copy of the genome of HBV, strain ayw using sense (5'-ACTCAGTTACGTCAACACTAATACGGGCCTAAA-3') and antisense (5'-TGGGTCGACACGGTGGTCTCCATGCGACGT-3') primers.
5. The peak absorbance of the products of the β-galactosidase/ONPG reaction is approx 420 nm. However, wavelengths ranging from 405 to 430 nm can be used satisfactorily to monitor β-galactosidase activity.

References

1. Dudley, F. J., Sheuer, P. J., and Shelock, S. (1972) Natural history of hepatitis associated antigen positive chronic liver disease. *Lancet* **ii,** 1388–1393.
2. Beasley, R. P. and Hwang, L.-Y. (1994) Epidemiology of heptocellular carcinoma, in *Viral Hepatitis and Liver Disease* (Vyas, G. N., Dienstag, J. L., and Hoofnagle, J. H., eds.), Grune & Stratton, New York, pp. 209–224.
3. World Health Organization (1990) WHO reports decry of neglect of world health problems. *ASM News* **56,** 358,359.
4. Seeger, C., Summers, J., and Mason, W. S. (1991) Viral DNA synthesis, in *Current Topics in Microbiology and Immunology,* vol. 168. Springer-Verlag, Berlin, pp. 41–66.
5. Wang, G. H. and Seeger, C. (1993) Novel mechanism for reverse transcription in hepatitis B viruses. *J. Virol.* **67,** 6507–6512.
6. Hirsch, R. C., Lavine, J. E., Chang, L.-J., Varmus, H. E., and Ganem, D. (1990) Polymerase gene products of hepatitis B viruses are required for genomic RNA packaging as well as for reverse transcription. *Nature (London)* **344,** 552–555.
7. Wang, G. H. and Seeger, C. (1992) The reverse transcriptase of hepatitis B virus acts as a protein primer for viral DNA synthesis. *Cell* **71,** 633–670.
8. Rossner, M. T. (1992) Hepatitis B virus X-gene product: a promising transcriptional activator. *J. Med. Virol.* **36,** 101–117.
9. Ladner, S. K., Otto, M. J., Barker, C. S., Zaifert, K., Wang, G.-H., Guo, J.-T., Seeger, C., and King, R. W. (1997) Inducible expression of human hepatitis B virus in stably transfected hepatoblastoma cell: a novel system for screening potential inhibitors of HBV replication, submitted for publication.
10. *Current Protocols in Molecular Biology,* vol. 3 (1995) (Janssen, K., series ed.), Wiley, New York, pp. A.2.5.

5

Hepatitis B Virus Cell Culture Assays for Antiviral Activity

Karen Schmidt and Brent Korba

1. Introduction

Hepatitis B Virus (HBV) is a causative agent of both acute and chronic hepatitis, a major etiologic factor of primary hepatocellular carcinoma, and a serious global health problem, with over 240 million estimated chronically infected individuals. Although there are several promising antiviral agents currently in clinical trials, alpha interferon remains the only licensed drug for the treatment of chronic HBV infection. Several cell lines and cell culture assays have been developed to identify potential therapeutics against chronic HBV infection. One of these cell lines, 2.2.15 *(1)*, has been developed into a standardized assay, by the authors' laboratory, that has been repeatedly shown to be an accurate model of chronic cellular HBV replication and a predictive model of antiviral response for chronic hepadnaviral infection in vivo *(2–5)*. This assay system, described here, is currently that used by the National Institutes of Health-National Institute of Allergy and Infectious Diseases (NIH-NIAID) (contract NO1-AI-45195) as an in vitro screen for antiviral agents against HBV replication.

The 2.2.15 cell line was derived through transfection of cloned HBV DNA (subtype AYW) into the well-characterized human hepatoblastoma cell line HepG2 which exhibits many of the properties of normal liver cells *(1)*. When optimally cared for, this cell line, at confluence, secretes relatively consistent high levels (1–3 × 10^7/mL/24 h period) of HBV virion particles, which have been shown to cause both acute and chronic infection and disease in chimpanzees *(6)*, and reliably responds to various antiviral agents, as evidenced by a decrease both in the level of virus secreted and reductions in various intracellular forms of replicating viral DNA.

From: *Methods in Molecular Medicine, vol. 24: Antiviral Methods and Protocols*
Edited by: D. Kinchington and R. F. Schinazi © Humana Press Inc., Totowa, NJ

However, the careful maintenance of this cell line is crucial for its effectiveness in revealing potential antiviral activities. This chapter discusses, in detail, important aspects of the culture system used in the authors' laboratory since 1989 that are essential for the application of 2.2.15 cells for use as a reliable and reproducible tool to study the activities of compounds that directly disrupt cellular production of HBV.

2. Materials

Whenever possible, all materials should be prepared sterile and solutions passed through 0.22-μ filters. All chemical and radioactive materials and waste are to be handled and discarded in accordance with each individual's current institutional safety procedures.

1. RPMI-1640 (without L-glutamine).
2. L-Glutamine.
3. Fetal bovine serum (FBS).
4. Trypsin-versine solution.
5. HEPES-buffered saline (HBS).
6. G418 (Genticin™, Gibco-BRL, Gaithersburg, MD).
7. 3TC (lamivudine, (–)β-L-2',3'-dideoxy-3'-thiacytidine).
8. Dimethyl sulfoxide (DMSO) (tissue culture grade).
9. Formaldehyde (37%, Sigma-Aldrich, Milwaukee, WI).
10. Neutral red dye.
11. Acetic acid/EtOH (1% glacial acetic acid [GAA]/50% EtOH in H_2O).
12. Dulbecco's phosphate-buffered saline (DPBS) with calcium and magnesium.
13. Filtered, sterile distilled water.
14. NaOH.
15. 20X SSC.
16. NaCl.
17. HCl.
18. 0.5 *M* phosphate buffer, pH 6.5.
19. 2.0 *M* Tris-HCl, pH 7.4.
20. 20% SDS.
21. 20% Sarkosyl.
22. Glycine.
23. Dextran sulfate.
24. Denhardt's solution (2% polyvinylpyrolidone, 2% bovine serum albumin [Pentax™, fraction V]).
25. 4.0 *M* Guanidine thiocyanate.
26. βME (2-mercaptoethanol, gel electrophoresis grade).
27. TE:10 m*M* Tris-HCl, pH 8.0/25 m*M* ethylenediaminetetra-acetic acid (EDTA).
28. Buffered phenol, pH 7.4 (molecular biology grade).
29. Chloroform.

30. Isopropanol.
31. Ammonium acetate.
32. 6X Bromophenol blue tracking dye: 0.25% bromophenol blue, 30% glycerol in TE.
33. TAE (Tris-acetate-EDTA running buffer).
34. Agarose (standard low–m_r).
35. Plastic pipets (1 mL to 50 mL, sterile, individually wrapped).
36. 5 in. Glass Pasteur pipets.
37. 96-Well tissue culture plates.
38. 24-Well tissue culture plates.
39. Tissue culture flasks (75, 150 cm^2).
40. 10-, 250-, 500-µL pipet tips.
41. Eppendorf centrifuge tubes (1.5, 2.0 mL).
42. 1.1-mL strip tubes in strips of 8 and 12 tubes (sterile) (Continental Laboratories, San Diego, CA).
43. Dialysis membranes (12,000-mol-wt cutoff) for microdialysis apparatus (Gibco-BRL).
44. Nitrocellulose (two sizes: 96-well plate and 12 × 15 cm).
45. Blotting and wicking paper.
46. 1.0-kb Ladder (size markers, Gibco-BRL).
47. Proteinase K (10 mg/mL TE).
48. *Hin*dIII (50 U/µL) and 10X buffer.
49. Kit for radioactive labeling (^{32}P) of DNA hybridization probe.
50. Deionized formamide: Molecular biology grade formamide (Fluka) is mixed with 150 g/L of AG-X-100 mixed bed resin (Bio-Rad, Hercules, CA) for 1 h at room temperature (covered, in a chemical hood). The deionized formamide is filtered (with gentle vacuum) over Whatman filter paper twice (one filtering will not remove all the resin). Deionized formamide is stored in 50-mL aliquots in screw-capped tubes at –70°C and can be kept for up to 1 yr.
51. HBV hybridization probe: A 3.2-kb full genome length HBV fragment is retrieved from a restriction digest of a plasmid clone (e.g., pAM6 *[7]*) electrophoresed in a 1% agarose gel and isolated by the procedure of choice. Store at –20°C.
52. HBV gel standard: 1.0 µL of HBV standards (100 ng/mL) plus 5 µL of tracking dye and 14 µL of TE (per lane). HBV standards are made by performing separate *Bam*HI and *Eco*RI digests of cloned HBV DNA. The digests are combined in equimolar amounts and stored at –20°C. This produces several HBV fragments (positive hybridization controls) as well as a non-HBV plasmid DNA fragment (negative hybridization control). For example, the authors use pAM6 ***(8)***, which produces HBV DNA fragments of 3.2, 1.85, and 1.35 kb, as well as a plasmid fragment of 4.3 kb. This mixture serves as a positive and a negative hybridization control, a size standard, and a quantitation standard that occupies only one lane of a gel.
53. HBV media standards. Collect culture medium (RP2, *see* **Subheading 3.1.** for formulation) from confluent non-G418-treated 2.2.15 cells and store frozen at –70°C. Pool aliquots as necessary (typically 1–2 L) and centrifuge at 7000*g*, 10 min to remove cellular debris. Add the supernatant to an Amicon "stirred cell" (8400 series) fitted with a YM100 membrane (cat. no. 13642) 400 mL at a time.

Filter at approx 20 psi nitrogen with constant stirring, at 4°C (approx 3–5 h), ensuring that the membrane is not allowed to dry. This will result in approx a 40-fold concentration by volume. HBV DNA content in the concentrated sample is quantitated by blot hybridization against a known standard quantity of HBV DNA standard (*see* **Note 1**).

54. 12-Channel 50–300-μL pipeter.
55. 6-Channel 200–100 μL pipeter.
56. Various pipeters for 0.1–1000 μL vol.
57. Mechanical or electric pipet-aids.
58. Hemacytometer.
59. Lab jacks or similar supports.
60. Dot blot apparatus (96-well format with 30-mm openings).
61. 28-Place microdialysis apparatus (Gibco-BRL).
62. 6-L Flasks.
63. Microtube racks.
64. Savant Rotoevaporator.
65. Vacuum source.
66. Microcentrifuge (18 place, 16,000*g* max. force, 30-min timer).
67. Tube rocker/mixer.
68. Rotary platform.
69. 4°C refrigerator.
70. –20 and –70°C freezers.
71. –135°C freezer or liquid nitrogen freezer.
72. Gel electrophoresis apparatuses.
73. Gel electrophoresis power supplies.
74. Blot transfer apparatus/plastic ware.
75. Ultraviolet (UV) transilluminator with camera.
76. OSHA approved chemical fume hood.
77. OSHA approved biosafety (BS) cabinet (tissue culture hood).

3. Methods

3.1. Guidelines for the Culture of 2.2.15 Cells

Cell cultures should be handled aseptically, *without antibiotics*, and in contained facilities (BS level II). The basal culture medium used for the culture of 2.2.15 cells is RPMI-1640. FBS is added at either 2 or 4% final concentration, may be obtained from any reliable source, and need not be heat inactivated or lot tested. L-Glutamine is added to a final concentration of 4 m*M*. Complete culture medium can be stored at 4°C for up to 4 wk. Cells are grown and maintained at 37°C in a 5% CO_2 humidified atmosphere.

Flasks and plates are routinely seeded at a density of 3–5 × 10^4 cells/cm^2. This seeding density will produce confluent cultures in 3–5 d. Seeding densities of approx 1 × 10^4 cells/cm^2 are permissible and will prolong time to confluence. Seeding densities lower than this will usually lead to colonies with a heavily "piled up" appearance. Cells in this condition rarely produce sufficient virus for screening and do not always respond appropriately to antiviral agents. At confluence, cells should be at a density of 3–5 × 10^5 cells/cm^2 and produce their maximal and relatively stable levels of HBV *(1,2)*. A confluent, "healthy" T-75 flask, grown in medium with 4% FBS can be subcultured in up to six, 96- or 24-well flat-bottomed plates. Cells should not be continually maintained in G418. However, they should be "reselected" for G418-resistance after every 3–4 passages.

Care must be taken not to overtrypsinize the cells when removing them from the tissue culture surface. The 2.2.15 cells are "sticky" and have a natural tendency to clump. Aggregated cells do not grow well and are difficult to count. The 2.2.15 cells also perform better in reseeding and cryopreservation procedures if they receive fresh medium 24 h before trypsinization.

The passaging of cells should be held to a minimum. The authors routinely do not use cells that have been passaged more than six times after recovery from cryopreservation. This limits the potential for genetic drift, produces highly reproducible results in different experiments performed years apart, and minimizes the potential for bacterial or fungal contamination. This laboratory philosophy requires that fairly large stocks (30–50 vials) of a limited number of cell passages be made and used as parental passages.

Active cultures should be checked approximately every 6 mo for mycoplasma contamination using any of several standard commercial kits. Cultures that are intended for cryopreserved stocks should be selected for G418-resistance and checked for mycoplasma contamination immediately prior to freezing.

1. To make culture medium:
   a. Thaw stock bottles of FBS at room temperature or at 4°C.
   b. Filter FBS through a 0.45-µm Nalgene cellulose acetate filter, and store in 25-mL aliquots in screw-capped tubes at –70°C. FBS may be kept for up to 2 yr. Do not freeze-thaw aliquots more than twice.
   c. For growth medium (4% FBS) (RP4): Add 20 mL of FBS and 10 mL of L-glutamine to 500 mL of RPMI-1640 (without glutamine), and filter through an 0.22 µm cellulose acetate (or nylon) filter. Store at 4°C.
   d. For the maintenance of confluent cultures and for drug treatment (2% FBS) (RP2): add 10 mL of FBS and 10 mL of L-glutamine to 500 mL of RPMI-1640 (without glutamine) and filter through an 0.22 µm cellulose acetate (or nylon) filter. Store at 4°C.
2. To maintain stock cultures: Feed cells with RP4 two to three times a week. A 75-cm^2 (T-75) flask receives 12–15 mL of culture medium per feeding, a 150-cm^2 flask receives 25–30 mL. Cells can generally be maintained at confluence with this feeding schedule for 2–3 wk without loss of viability (*see* **Note 3**).
3. To reselect cells for G418 resistance: The 2.2.15 cell line was transfected with a vector that confers resistance to the neomiycin analog, G418. Although the HBV

DNA in 2.2.15 cells is very stable, it is recommended that resistance to G418 be confirmed occasionally (every three to four passages, and any cell passage that is to be cryopreserved). To do this:

a. Seed cells at a low density (1×10^4 cells/cm^2) in RP4.
b. Add fresh RP4 containing 330 µg/mL G418 after 2, 3, and 7 d of culture.
c. Change back to RP4 (without G418) after 10 d of culture and continue to culture as normal. Cells will reach confluence after another 3–5 d of culture. Do not cryopreserve cells until the culture has been maintained in G418-free medium for at least 48 h (viability will be reduced significantly if this is not done).

4. To plate cells for an assay or to passage cells (T-75 flask):
   a. Remove the culture medium.
   b. Wash with 10 mL HBS.
   c. Add 2.0 mL Trypsin-Versine solution and gently roll solution over tissue culture surface three to four times.
   d. Immediately remove all but 100–200 µL of the trypsin, and incubate at room temperature, rapping the side of the flask, until the monolayer just begins to lift off (1–3 min).
   e. Add 10–12 mL of RP4, pipet vigorously, using the force of the medium to remove the cells if necessary. Pipet up and down several times with the pipet tip near, but not touching the inside surface of the flask. Do not centrifuge cells for routine passaging or reseeding.
   f. For routine passaging, transfer 1–2 mL to a fresh flask and add additional (prewarmed) RP4.
   g. For 96-well or 24-well plates, transfer resuspended cells to a sterile 50-mL centrifuge tube. Immediately count 10 µL of the cell suspension in a hemacytometer to determine the concentration. Adjust concentration of cells to 2×10^5/mL. Plate cells immediately at 100 µL/well for 96-well plates or 600 µL/well for 24-well plates (approx 3–4×10^4/cm^2).
5. To cryopreserve cells:
   a. Label cryovials (self-standing style with inside threads on cap are preferred); 5–6 vials per T-75 flask are usually required.
   b. Trypsinize cells as described **step 4a–e**.
   c. Centrifuge cells at 500*g* at room temperature in a sterile conical tube (15 or 50 mL) for 3 min (no brake), and remove the supernatant.
   d. Gently resuspend the cells at 2–3×10^6 cells/mL of cell freezing medium A (Biofluids). Add an equal volume of cell freezing medium B (Biofluids). Gently mix cells and immediately aliquot at 1.0 mL per cryovial.
   e. Place cryovials immediately into an appropriate freezing canister (e.g., Nalgene "Cryo 1" freezing container containing isopropanol) and incubate at –70°C overnight. The next day, transfer vials into liquid nitrogen or a –135°C freezer. Cells should remain viable for at least 8–10 yr.
6. To recover cells from cryopreservation:
   a. Thaw cryopreserved cells for 1–2 min at 37°C.

b. Immediately upon full thawing, cells are transferred to a flask with prewarmed RP4 culture medium. One cryovial should be sufficient for two T-75 tissue culture flasks, which should grow to confluence in 5–7 d.

3.2. Drug Setup and Treatment

3.2.1. "Primary" or "Screening" Assay (96-Well Plate Format)

This assay format is well suited to the screening of test compounds for potential antiviral activity. The assay provides a minimal assessment of antiviral activity by measuring the levels of HBV virion release from the cells, as well as providing a measurement of cytotoxicity (*see* **Subheading 3.2.2.**). Two rows of cells will be required for each compound, plus four rows for the assay controls (two for untreated, and two for positive antiviral control (e.g., 3TC). After treating for 9 d, the media are harvested from the antiviral plates and transferred to 96-well U-bottomed plates. They are then centrifuged, and supernatant is transferred to tubes for dot-blot hybridization analysis of HBV virion DNA. The medium is aspirated off of the toxicity plates and discarded. Toxicity plates are then incubated with neutral red dye (methylthiouracil [MTT] can also be used if preferred), washed with DPBS, developed with an acetic acid/ethanol solution, and assayed in a plate reader.

There are many opinions regarding what concentration ranges to use for these assays. The authors have found that nucleoside analogs (about which no other information is known) should be tested for antiviral activity at an initial concentration of 10 μ*M*, with a 10-fold dilution series (10–0.1 μ*M*). Drugs should be tested for toxicity at as high a concentration as the compound's solubility and the toxicity of the diluent (frequently DMSO) allows. The 2.2.15 cells will tolerate 2–3% DMSO for up to 10 d with little loss of viability *(2)*. For nucleoside analogs, the authors routinely use an initial concentration of 1000 μ*M* with a threefold dilution series (1000–30 μ*M*).

1. Seed 2.2.15 cells into 96-well, flat-bottomed tissue culture plates as described in **Subheading 3.1., step 4.** Duplicate plates will be used for the antiviral treatments for each test compound (up to eight compounds per pair of plates). After 3–4 d, cells should be confluent and medium should be yellow in color. Remove the medium and replace it with 100 μL of RP2 24 h before the beginning of drug treatment.
2. To set up compounds for antiviral treatment:
   a. For each compound, a total of four concentrations will be examined. This will require nine sets of four sterile, 1.1-mL minitubes (36 tubes/compound). Into the first tube of each set, aliquot sufficient compound to make up 700 μL (for 10-fold dilution series) or 980 μL (for 3.3-fold dilution series) of the highest test concentration. Leave the other tubes empty.

b. The sample aliquots for the last day of treatment are to be set up at a 3X concentration of the other aliquots. This is done to provide sufficient material for DNA analysis (*see* **Subheading 3.3.1.**).
c. Cover the tubes with the rack lids, label appropriately, and store the racks at –20°C or the appropriate temperature for the test compounds. If compounds are stored at 4°C, cover the tops of the tubes with a sheet of parafilm to prevent evaporation. This procedure prevents multiple freeze-thaw cycles of stock solutions of the test compound, and ensures that all nine daily test aliquots are treated in an identical manner with respect to temperature variations.

3. To set up compounds for toxicity treatment: For each compound, a total of four concentrations will be examined. This will require nine sets of four sterile, 1.1-mL minitubes (36 tubes/compound). Into the first tube of each set, aliquot sufficient compound to make up 465 µL of the highest test concentration. Leave the other tubes empty. Cover the tubes with the rack lids, and store the racks at –20°C or at an appropriate temperature. Tubes for the last day of treatment for toxicity testing contain the same amount of compound as used the previous days (not 3X as for the antiviral assays).
4. To make the compound dilution series for antiviral treatment.
   a. For a 10-fold dilution series: To the first (compound containing) tube, add 700 µL of RP2 (175 µL × 4). Add 630 µL (210 µL × 3) RP2 culture medium to the remaining three tubes. Mix the first tube by pipeting up and down with a pipetman (a multichannel pipetman permits the simultaneous processing of multiple compounds). Serially transfer 70 µL of test compound-containing medium from the first tube to the other three tubes, taking care to thoroughly mix each tube before transferring medium.
   b. To make a 3.3-fold dilution series: Add 960 µL (160 µL × 6) of RP2 to the first tube (containing the aliquot of compound) and 640 µL (160 µL × 4) of RP2 to each of the empty tubes. Serially transfer 280 µL of test compound-containing medium from the first tube to the other three tubes.
5. The cytotoxicity of test compounds is analyzed in a 3.3-fold dilution series as follows. Add 485 µL (155 µL × 3) of RP2 to the first tube (containing the aliquot of compound) and 310 µL (155 µL × 2) of RP2 to each of the three remaining tubes. Serially transfer 150 µL of test compound–containing medium from the first tube to the other three tubes.
6. To initiate the treatments,
   a. Remove the culture medium. Minimize the time that the cell monolayers are without medium.
   b. Add 100 µL of each dilution of every compound to each of six wells (three wells/plate) using the configuration listed in **Table 1** as an example. Start with the lowest concentration and use the same tips to add the higher concentrations. The untreated cells receive 100 µL of RP2 per well (untreated cells need to be carried on only one pair of the antiviral assay plates).
   c. Repeat treatments daily for 9 d. For the last day of treatment, add an additional 200 µL of RP2 to each well of the antiviral assay plates after the wells are treated with the test compounds (a total of 300 µL medium per well).

Table 1
Design of Drug-Treatment Plate

	Columns 1–3	Columns 4–6	Columns 7–9	Columns 10–12
Row A		Untreated cells		
Row B	Drug 1 @ 1X	Drug 1 @ 1/10X	Drug 1 @ 1/100X	Drug 1 @ 1/1000X
Row C	Drug 2 @ 1X	–	–	–
Row D	–	–	–	–
Row E	–	–	–	–
Row F	–	–	–	–
Row G	–	–	–	–
Row H	–	–	–	Drug 7 @1/1000X

7. A single plate will be used for the toxicity treatments for each test compound (up to seven compounds per plate since the top row will be reserved for untreated cells on every toxicity plate). To initiate the treatments, remove the culture medium, and add 100 µL of each dilution of every compound to each of three wells, using a configuration similar to that used for the antiviral treatments. The untreated cells receive 100 µL of RP2 per well. Repeat daily for 9 d.
8. To terminate the assay and harvest samples for quantitative analysis of HBV virion DNA, remove the culture medium 24 h following d 9 of treatment, and store the culture medium in 96-well U-bottomed culture plates. Cover the U-bottomed plates tightly with parafilm to prevent evaporation. Store these samples at 4°C until blotting is performed. Samples can eventually be transferred to –20°C for long-term storage.

3.2.2. Assay for Effects on Intracellular HBV Replication (24-Well Plate Format)

This assay format serves to further define the action of potential antiviral agents by permitting an assessment of the levels of intracellular HBV DNA replicative forms. This type of assay is usually performed on compounds that are initially screened in the 96-well plate format because the effective antiviral concentrations observed in those experiments can be used as a guide for this type of assay (which is considerably more labor intensive and costly). In general, a three- to fivefold higher concentration of compound will be needed than that observed in the antivirion assay to produce similar levels of effects on intracellular HBV DNA replication. The 2.2.15 cells are seeded in 24-well plates for this assay and treated for 9 d. The medium is collected at the end of the treatment period for analysis of HBV virion DNA. For analysis of intracellular HBV DNA, the monolayers are lysed with guanidine thiocyanate/sarkosyl/βME, dialyzed, digested with SDS/proteinase K, extracted with phenol and chloroform, and precipitated with sodium acetate/isopropanol. The intracellular DNAs are then resuspended, digested with *Hin*dIII, subjected to gel electrophoresis, and transferred to nitrocellulose for hybridization analysis. A detailed description of the intracellular HBV DNA forms present in 2.2.15 cells and their application to this assay can be found in **ref.** ***8***.

1. Seed 24-well culture plates as described in **Subheading 3.1., step 4**. The day before the addition of compounds, change the medium to RP2 (0.5 mL per well). As in the 96-well plate assay, duplicate plates are used. A total of two wells on each plate are treated with each dilution of compound (four wells per dilution).
2. To set up compounds for antiviral treatment:For each compound, a total of four concentrations will be examined. This will require nine sets of four sterile, 1.1-mL minitubes (36 tubes per compound). Into the first tube of each set, aliquot sufficient compound to make up 2.2 mL of drug-containing medium (additional medium to make up the proper total volume will be added at the time of cell treatment (*see* **step 4**). Tubes for the last day of treatment for toxicity testing contain the same amount of compound as used the previous days (not 3X as for the 96-well plate assay). Cover the tubes with the rack lids, and store the racks at –20°C or at an appropriate temperature.
3. Usually, compounds in this assay are tested in a 3.3-fold dilution series. To make this dilution series, add 720 µL (240 µL × 3) of medium to the first tube. Add 460 µL (230 µL × 2) of medium to the remaining three tubes. Serially transfer 200 µL from the first tube to the remaining three tubes.
4. Treat wells from the lowest concentration of drug to the highest, adding 100 µL of RP2 to each of the four wells. Add an additional 400 µL of RP2 (without drugs) to each well. (A 200–1000 µL multichannel pipetman can be used to add the additional culture medium.) Continue changing culture medium and adding test compounds each day for a total of 9 d.
5. Twenty-four hours following the final addition of compound, collect the culture medium and store in new 24-well plates. Transfer a 250-µL aliquot of each stored culture medium sample to 96-well U-bottomed culture plates (one plate can hold samples from up to four 24-well plates), and store at 4°C until dot-blotting is performed.
6. The cell monolayers are then lysed for analysis of intracellular HBV DNA as described in **Subheading 3.3.2.**

3.2.3. Neutral Red Dye Determination of Drug Toxicity

The antiviral effect of any compound must be measured against its toxicity. Once cells are seeded and treated following the guidelines above, a neutral red dye uptake assay *(2)* is performed to assess toxicity. Other assays of cytotoxicity (e.g., MTT) can be substituted for the procedure described below. Note that this procedure assesses toxicity under culture and treatment conditions that are identical to those used for the antiviral analyses, thereby permitting a determination whether the reductions in virus observed are caused by a specific antiviral effect, or most likely, by a cytotoxic effect on the host cell under the conditions of the antiviral treatment. Because the cultures, by necessity, are at confluence, the cytotoxic effects of the test compounds will probably be reduced relative to the cytotoxic effects that would be expected for actively dividing cells.

1. Treat cultures on the designated toxicity plates as described in **Subheading 3.2.**
2. Carefully remove the culture medium 24 h following d 9 of treatment. Fully remove the monolayer in the top left three wells (row A, columns 1–3). These wells will be used as "blanks" for the plate reader.
3. Add 100 µL of DPBS (containing 0.01% neutral red dye) to each well, including the empty wells. Incubate the 96-well plate in the tissue culture incubator for 30 min.
4. Remove the dye carefully and gently. The authors frequently use a multichannel pipetman since the monolayers can become fragile after incubation with neutral red dye. Add 200 µL of DPBS to all the wells, taking care not to displace the monolayers. Remove the DPBS and add 100 µL of 50% EtOH/1% glacial acetic acid (in H_2O) to each well. Mix the plates for 15 min on an orbital platform shaker (120–150 rpm) to allow for full extraction of the dye from the cells.
5. Read optical absorbance at 510 nm in an enzyme-linked immunosorbent assay type plate reader. Use the three empty wells to set the background. Calculate an average absorbance value for the nine untreated cultures on a plate. Express the absorbance of dye for the treated cultures on the same plate as a percentage of that value. Repeat for each individual plate.

3.3. Analysis of HBV DNA

3.3.1. Extraction and Preparation of Culture Medium Samples for Dot-Blot Hybridization

To affix HBV DNA to nitrocellulose membranes for quantitation, the culture media samples from the end of the treatment period are centrifuged and transferred to 1.1-mL tubes. These samples are then denatured with NaOH/20X SSC, transferred onto nitrocellulose membranes using a dot-blot manifold, neutralized with Tris-HCl/NaCl, and then rinsed with 20X SSC. The membranes are then air-dried and vacuum desiccated at high temperature to fix the DNA onto the membranes for hybridization analysis.

1. Centrifuge the culture medium samples from the 96-well assay in the U-bottomed plates at 1500*g* for 10 min at 4°C. Remove a 100-µL aliquot from the top of each well and transfer to a 1.1-mL plastic strip tubes. Store these samples at 4°C until blotting is performed and transfer remaining media samples to –20°C for long-term storage. For media samples from the 24-well plate assay, transfer 200 µL and discard the media remaining in the U-bottom plates. (Take care not to pipet from the bottom of the wells, which contains cell debris that can produce false positives.)

2. Prepare a fresh solution of 2.0 *M* NaOH/20X SSC (200 μL per sample) by dissolving NaOH directly in sterile 20X SSC and filtering through a 0.220-μm nylon filter (NaOH will dissolve acetate or nitrocellulose filters). This solution must be made fresh the day of use.
3. To each medium sample, add 100 μL of 2.0 *M* NaOH/20X SSC. If the media aliquots have been stored at 4°C, allow them to come to room temperature before adding the NaOH solution (approx 20 min).
4. Incubate at room temperature for 30 min (longer periods, e.g., 60–90 min will not affect the results).
5. Hydrate nitrocellulose membranes by soaking in sterile filtered water for 1–2 min and then in sterile 20X SSC for 3–5 min at room temperature. (Membranes may soak in SSC for several hours). Handle nitrocellulose with unpowdered gloves to prevent contamination of the membranes.
6. Assemble a dot-blot manifold (the authors use the Convertible Manifold [Gibco-BRL] with a 96-well format and 30-mm openings) according to the instructions, using one sheet of hydrated nitrocellulose. Load all samples into the manifold wells and then apply moderate vacuum until the samples just enter the membrane. Too much vacuum will produce poor transfer of DNA; samples should take a minimum of 30 s to enter the membrane.
7. Immediately after the samples have entered the membrane, add approx 0.4 mL of 1.0 *M* Tris-HCl (pH 7.4)/2 *M* NaCl (sterile and filtered through an 0.22-μm nylon filter) to each sample well and allow it to enter the membrane. Then add approx 0.4 mL of sterile, filtered 20X SSC to each well and allow it to enter the membrane.
8. Remove the nitrocellulose membrane from the apparatus and rinse in 2X SSC for 3–5 min, and then air-dry for 5–10 min.
9. Bake the membranes in a vacuum oven (20–30 PSI) at 80°C for 30 min. Store membranes at room temperature in a plastic bag or container until they are used in the hybridization procedure (membranes can be stored for several weeks without loss of signal). Hybridize for HBV DNA as described in **Subheading 3.3.4.**

3.3.2. Extraction of DNA Samples from Cell Monolayers

Cellular DNA is extracted, resuspended, restriction enzyme digested, and electrophoresed in a 1% agarose gel, and transferred via Southern blot technique to nitrocellulose membranes. The nitrocellulose is baked, prehybridized, hybridized, washed, quantitatively analyzed for radioactivity, and exposed to film.

1. At the end of the treatment period, remove the culture medium as described in **Subheading 3.2.2., step 5.** Add 0.5 mL of 4.0 *M* guanidine thiocyanate (Sigma-Aldrich [cat. no. 50980F])/7% βME (gel electrophoresis grade) to each well and swirl the plate. Add 50 μL of 20% sarcosyl (in H_2O), swirl to mix, and incubate the plate at 60°C for 5 min. Add βME to the guanidine thiocyanate stock just before using (freeze and thaw the stock solution only once after addition of 2-βME).

2. Transfer each culture lysate to a well of a microdialysis apparatus (Gibco-BRL, 28-place apparatus set up with a 12,000 mol wt cutoff membrane). Dialyze samples against 6 L of 50 m*M* Tris, pH 7.2, 5.0 m*M* Na_2EDTA, over 60–75 min at room temperature (buffer elevation approx 30 cm above the apparatus). samples will become slightly cloudy and volume will increase to approx 600 µL.
3. While the samples are dialyzing, add 10 µL of 20% SDS to one 2.0-mL Eppendorf centrifuge tube for each well lysate, and preheat the tubes to 50°C for at least 5 min. After dialysis, transfer the cell lysates to these tubes. Add 50 µL of proteinase K (10 mg/mL in TE), mix well, and incubate the tubes for 60 min at 50°C. A white precipitate may form in the tubes on transfer of the lysates; this will disappear after approx 10 min incubation at 50°C. Mix tubes again after the first 10 min of incubation to help resolubilize this SDS precipitate.
4. Following digestion with proteinase K, extract samples for 5 min (with gentle mixing) with 1.0 mL buffered phenol (pH 7.4 with 50 m*M* Tris-HCl/5 m*M* Na_2EDTA). Centrifuge for 1 min (maximum speed) in a microcentrifuge.
5. Remove phenol (lower) layer with a sterile Pasteur pipet. Genomic DNA is frequently trapped in the interface at this stage of preparation. Therefore, it is imperative that the interface remains in the tube. This may require that approx 50 µL of the phenol remains in the tube. If the separation of the organic and aqueous layer is difficult to see, incubate the tubes for approx 30 s in a 50°C water bath.
6. Extract DNA samples for 5 min with 1.0 mL of chloroform/tube. Centrifuge for 1 min and remove chloroform (lower) layer. Remove the interface with the chloroform.
7. To each tube, add 75 µL of 4.0 *M* sodium acetate, pH 5.5, and then add 1.0 mL of isopropanol. Mix very well and incubate overnight at –20°C. Alternatively, samples can be incubated in a dry ice/ethanol bath for 1 h (thaw samples for 5 min at room temperature before centrifugation).
8. Centrifuge samples for 20 min in a microcentrifuge at maximum speed. Pour off and discard the supernatant, and invert the tubes on a paper towel for 1–2 min. Dry the pellets in a Savant Rotoevaporator for 3–5 min, or air-dry (inverted) for 60 min.
9. Resuspend the DNA pellet in 85 µL of sterile, filtered distilled H_2O. Place on an orbital platform shaker (120–150 rpm) or tube mixer for 30 min at room temperature. Store the DNA samples at either 4°C (up to 10 d) or longer at –20°C.

3.3.3. Preparation of Gels for Southern Blot Analysis

To show diagnostic changes in HBV replicative DNA intermediates, the cellular DNA must be efficiently digested with the restriction enzyme *Hin*dIII (which does not digest HBV DNA). Following the separation of the various forms of DNA by gel electrophoresis, the DNA must be transferred to nitrocellulose to be analyzed. For efficient transfer, the DNA must first be denatured by incubation in acid and alkaline, and the gel neutralized (to preserve the integrity of the nitrocellulose) and permeated with transfer buffer. (Alternatively, DNA can be transferred to nitrocellulose or nylon membranes using electrophoretic techniques.) Following transfer, the nitrocellulose membranes are vacuum desiccated at high temperature to fix the DNA to the membrane, and incubated with an HBV-specific probe to discriminate HBV DNA forms.

1. Prepare digests of DNA samples following the general format below: 85 µL DNA solution, 10 µL 10X reaction buffer, 5 µL restriction enzyme (*Hin*dIII) (10–20 U/µg DNA), for a total 100 µL of reaction volume. Tap tubes to mix and pulse centrifuge (5 s). Incubate digests for 2 h at 37°C.
2. Pour one 1% agarose gel in TAE buffer for every 24 DNA samples. Use 110 mL of agarose mixture for each leveled gel apparatus (12 × 15 cm surface area). Insert two 14-place, 2-mm combs; one at the top and one in the middle of the gel. Allow gel to harden (15–20 min) and carefully remove the combs (*see* **Note 5**). Flood the gel and buffer chamber with enough TAE buffer to cover the gel with approx 0.5–1.0 cm of buffer.
3. Add 10 µL of 6X bromophenol blue tracking dye to each sample, and incubate at 70°C for 5 min. Load 20 µL of 1.0-kb ladder size markers into the two far left-hand wells, and 20 µL of the HBV markers into the two far right-hand wells. Load 50 µL of each cellular DNA sample into the remaining wells. Run the gel at 100 V for approx 1–1.5 h at room temperature. Stop electrophoresis when the bromophenol blue dye front is approx 2 cm from the bottom of each of the running areas. Store the remaining cellular DNA samples at –20°C.
4. Remove the gel from the electrophoresis apparatus, cut off the 1.0-kb ladder lane, and stain with ethidium bromide (0.1 µg/mL 1X TAE buffer) for 5 min. Destain in water for at least 15 min, and photograph the lane with a fluorescent ruler on a UV transilluminator.
5. To prepare for transfer of the DNA to nitrocellulose, incubate each gel in 250 mL of the series of solutions listed next at room temperature on an orbital platform shaker at 40–50 rpm.
   a. 2 min in 0.1 *N* HCl.
   b. 30 s in dH_2O (rinse wells with flowing water).
   c. 15 min in 0.5 *M* NaOH/1.5 *M* NaCl (made fresh).
   d. 15 min in 0.5 *M* NaOH/1.5 *M* NaCl.
   e. 30 s in dH_2O (rinse wells with flowing water).
   f. 20 min in 0.5 *M* Tris-HCl, pH 7.2/1.5 *M* NaCl.
   g. 20 min in 0.5 *M* Tris-HCl, pH 7.2/1.5 *M* NaCl.
   h. 15 min in 20X SSC.

   Transfer each gel to one hydrated (*see* **Subheading 3.3., step 5**) nitrocellulose membranes with 450 mL of 20X SSC over 16–18 h using blotting (approx 20 sheets) and wicking (1 sheet) filter papers (Gibco-BRL). Maintain contact between the gel and the nitrocellulose and filter papers by placing a 500-mL bottle of water on top of the blotting paper.
6. After transfer is completed, label and mark the location of the lanes on the nitrocellulose with a ball-point pen or nitrocellulose marker. Soak the membranes in 2X SSC for 1–2 min and air-dry on a paper towel for 5–10 min. Bake the membranes at 80°C for 30 min, under vacuum (20–30 PSI), and store at room temperature. Hybridize the membranes as described in **Subheading 3.3.4.**

Table 2
Formulas for Prehybridization and Hybridzation Solutions

	Prehybridization buffer (100 mL)	Hybridization buffer (100 mL)
Deionized formamide	30 mL	30 mL
100X Denhardt's solution	5 mL	5 mL
0.5 *M* phosphate buffer, pH 6.5	4 mL	4 mL
20X SSC	15 mL	15 mL
10% Glycine (electrophoresis grade)	10 mL	–
50% Dextran sulfate (in H_2O)	–	0 ml
Sterile, filtered distilled H_2O	36 mL	36 mL

3.3.4. Nick Translation of Probe and Hybridization of Membranes

A gel-purified 3.2-kb full genome length, *Eco*RI fragment HBV DNA is labeled with ^{32}P and used as a blot hybridization probe. The blot membranes are then prehybridized, hybridized, washed to remove excess probe, air-dried, quantitatively analyzed for radioactivity, and exposed to film.

1. Use the formulas given in **Table 2** to make up the prehybridization and hybridization solutions. These solutions can be stored at 4°C for up to 10 d.
2. Label the 3.2-kb HBV DNA fragment with ^{32}P using any appropriate procedure and store at –20°C. Calculate the amount of probe needed: $1–2 \times 10^6$ dpm/mL hybridization buffer, using 5.0 mL of buffer per dot-blot membrane, and 7.5 mL per Southern gel membrane (approx 50–100 μL/cm^2).
3. Incubate nitrocellulose membranes briefly (15 min) at 42°C in prehybridization buffer (incubations overnight will not harm the membranes). The authors normally prehybridize for only the amount of time required for the denaturation of the labeled hybridization probe (*see* **step 4**).
4. Place the labeled probe in a water bath and heat to boiling (make sure the top of the tube is mechanically held in place to prevent opening). Boil probe for 5 min (time starts once boiling begins). Immediately submerge the probe into an ice water bath for 2–3 min. Add the required volume of denatured probe to the hybridization mixture and mix very well.
5. Remove the prehybridization buffer from the membranes, add the hybridization buffer (with labeled fragment), and incubate at 42°C for 36–72 h. (Shorter times, such as 18 h, are acceptable for slots or rehybridization; however, 40–45 h is optimal for initial hybridizations).
6. To remove excess probe, heat hybridization wash buffer (0.1X SSC/ 0.1% SDS, 600–750 mL/filter total) to 60–65°C. Remove the membranes from the hybridization mix, rinse each one with 5–10 mL of wash buffer from a squirt bottle, and place them immediately in a container of wash buffer (200–250 mL/filter). Two or three membranes may be washed together. Do not let membranes dry before washing is complete.

7. Incubate the membranes in wash buffer (250 mL/membrane) for 20 min at 60–65°C. Pour off wash buffer (into an appropriate container). Repeat the incubations, washing membranes a total of three times. Turn membranes over after each wash. Rinse the membranes with distilled H_2O (in a squirt bottle) after the final wash and air-dry (5–10 min).
8. Wrap each membrane, backed with precut support paper, in Saran™ wrap (do not substitute with another brand), and expose to Kodak Biomax™ X-ray film for 24–48 h at –70°C with a Biomax™ MS enhancing screen. Analyze filters on a beta scanner (InstantImager™, Packard Instruments) for approx 1–2 h.

4. Notes

1. Approximately a twofold loss of HBV DNA (as compared to the theoretical starting concentration) frequently occurs during this process. The final product is diluted to a standard concentration of 10 ng HBV DNA/mL with RPMI-1640 (without FBS). The concentration is then rechecked by blot hybridization. The adjusted standard pool is stored at –70°C in 5-mL aliquots in screw-capped tubes and is stable for at least 5 yr.
2. Centers or Disease Control-NIH guidclincs (HHS publication [CDC] 93-8395) specify the use of BS level II containment for work with infectious HBV. Vaccination of all laboratory personnel is also recommended.
3. Use of FBS concentrations above 5% in RPMI-1640 is detrimental to 2.2.15 cells as assayed by growth rates and colony forming assays. Although cells can be maintained for 2–3 wk in 2% FBS at confluence, growing cultures will not survive with <4% FBS. Confluent cultures can be maintained in as little as 1% FBS, but the monolayers become fragile and detach easily after several days.
4. Variations of the 9-d treatment regimen can be performed. However, in our experience, nucleoside analogues require daily additions of compound for maximal effectiveness. Shorter periods of treatment will require substantially more compound to induce antiviral effect (*see* **ref. *8*** for examples of kinetic patterns). Limiting treatment to only 5 d, e.g., will increase the EC_{90} of 3TC and several other nucleosides approx five- to 10-fold over that observed after 9 d of treatment.
5. Spraying the combs with 2% SDS (in H_2O) with a squirt bottle makes it easier to remove the combs from the agarose without producing holes in the bottoms of the wells.
6. Ethidium bromide causes a relatively high background in the gel following hybridization with the HBV probe; therefore, it is strongly recommended that the sample lanes not be stained.
7. Methods of quantitation other than the listed beta scanner and the use of Biomax™ film can be used (e.g., Kodak X-OMAT AR film, AMBIS beta scanner, phosphorimager, densitometric scans on films, and so on). However, the authors have found that these items are, by far, the most sensitive and efficient tools for quantitation of HBV DNA in this assay system.

References

1. Sells, M. A., Zelent, A. Z., Shvartsman, M., and Acs, G. (1988) Replication intermediates of hepatitis B virus in HepG2 cells that produce infectious virions. *J. Virol.* **62,** 2836–2844.
2. Korba, B. E. and Gerin, J. L. (1992) Use of a standardized cell culture assay to assess activities of nucleoside analogs against hepatitis B virus replication. *Antiviral Res.* **19,** 55–70.
3. Korba, B. E. and Gerin, J. L. (1995) Antisense oligonucleotides are effective inhibitors of hepatitis B virus replication *in vitro. Antiviral Res.* **28,** 225–242.
4. Korba, B. E. (1996) *In vitro* evaluation of combination therapies against hepatitis B virus replication. *Antiviral Res.* **29,** 49–52.
5. Korba, B. E. and Boyd, M. R. (1996) Penciclovir is a selective inhibitor of hepatitis B virus replication in cultured human hepatoblastoma cells. *Antimicrob. Agents Chemother.* **40,** 1282–1284.
6. Acs, G., Sells, M. A., Purcell, R. H., Price, P., Engle, R., Shapiro, M., and Popper, H. (1987) Hepatitis B virus produced by transgected Hep G2 cells causes hepatitis in chimpanzees. *Proc. Natl. Acad. Sci. USA* **84,** 4641–4644.
7. Moriarty, A. M., Hoyer, B. H., Shih, J. W.-K., Gerin, J. L., and Hamer, D. H. (1981) Expression of the hepatitis B virus surface antigen gene in cell culture by using a simian virus 40 vector. *Proc. Natl. Acad. Sci. USA* **78,** 2606–2610.
8. Korba, B. E. and Milman, G. (1991) A cell culture assay for compounds which inhibit hepatitis B virus replication. *Antiviral Res.* **15,** 217–228.

6

A Rapid Microtiter Assay for Duck Hepatitis Virus Reverse Transcriptase

Michael J. Otto and Richard A. Whitaker

1. Introduction

The duck hepatitis B virus (DHBV) genome contains a *pol* gene that codes for the viral polymerase protein. This enzyme, which is essential for the replication of the virus, has multiple activities including an RNA directed DNA polymerase or reverse transcriptase (RT) activity, an RNase H activity, and a DNA-directed DNA polymerase activity. The assay described in this chapter is designed to measure the ability of test compounds to inhibit the RNA-directed DNA polymerase activity of the DHBV *pol* gene product. The assay is based on research performed in the laboratory of Dr. Christoph Seeger *(1)* and on the observation that the ε stem loop structure in the pregenomic RNA is required for initiation of DNA synthesis *(2–4)*.

The DHBV *pol* gene product is produced by in vitro transcription of a cDNA copy of the DHBV genome and subsequent translation of the RNA using an in vitro rabbit reticulocyte translation system. Aliquots of the translated polymerase are monitored, without further purification, for RNA-dependent DNA polymerase activity. The activity is monitored by measuring the incorporation of [^{35}S]-labeled deoxynucleotide triphosphate (dNTP) into nascent DNA.

The assay described herein is capable of detecting at least three of the multiple functions of the polymerase. These are the initiation of DNA synthesis, the translocation of the initiation DNA-*pol* complex, and the extension of the genomic negative-strand DNA using a portion of the pregenomic RNA as template. The initiation of DNA synthesis by DHBV *pol* is unusual in that the polymerase protein acts as a primer and the first nucleotide incorporated (dGTP) is covalently linked to a tyrosine residue near the N-terminus of the

From: *Methods in Molecular Medicine, vol. 24: Antiviral Methods and Protocols*
Edited by: D. Kinchington and R. F. Schinazi © Humana Press Inc., Totowa, NJ

protein *(5)*. Compounds that inhibit either initiation or extension can be detected in this assay by using [α-^{35}S]dATP since the third and fourth residues in the nascent DHBV DNA strand are adenosines. Inhibition of either initiation or extension would result in a reduction in the incorporation of the radioactively labeled precursor into product DNA. The extent of DNA synthesis is determined by quantifying the amount of [α-^{35}S]-labeled nucleic acid bound to a diethylaminoethyl (DEAE) membrane using a Bio-Rad Molecular Image System or, alternatively, by X-ray film autoradiography.

2. Materials

1. Qiagen columns.
2. *Eco*RV (Promega).
3. *Sty*I (Promega).
4. *Afl*II (Promega).
5. RNasin (Promega).
6. Ribonucleotide triphosphates: ATP, GTP, CTP, and UTP (USB).
7. SP6 polymerase (Ambion).
8. T7 RNA polymerase (Promega).
9. DH5α transformation competent *Escherichia coli* (Gibco-BRL).
10. LB agar plates.
11. Luria broth.
12. Ampicillin (Sigma).
13. Rabbit reticulocyte lysate (RRL) (Promega).
14. [α-^{35}S]dATP, >1000 Ci/mmol (Amersham).
15. Deoxyribonucleotide triphosphates: dGTP, dCTP, and dTTP (USB).
16. NA 45 DEAE membranes (Schleicher & Schuell).
17. 10X TMN buffer: 100 m*M* Tris-HCl, pH 7.5, 20 m*M* $MgCl_2$, 30 m*M* NaCl.
18. 20X SSC buffer: 0.3 *M* sodium citrate, pH 7.0, 3 *M* NaCl.
19. TE buffer: 10 m*M* Tris-HCl, pH 7.6, 1 m*M* ethylenediaminetetra-acetic acid (EDTA).
20. Diethylpyrocarbonate- (DEPC) treated H_2O.
21. 2X SSC buffer: 30 m*M* sodium citrate, pH 7.0, 0.3 *M* NaCl.
22. EDTA/SSC stop solution: 10 mL 0.5 *M* EDTA plus 40 mL 2X SSC.
23. Phenol (saturated with 10 m*M* Tris-HCl, pH 8.0).
24. Ethanol.
25. Polypropylene microtiter plates, 96-well U-bottomed (Costar).
26. Clear plastic packing tape.
27. Water bath set at 30°C.
28. Pharmacia GeneQuant RNA/DNA Calculator or equivalent.
29. –20°C Freezer.
30. 96-well dot blotter (Bio-Rad).
31. 14 × 14 cm plastic "sandwich" boxes with lids (Rubbermaid).
32. Gel drier (Bio-Rad).
33. Bio-Rad Molecular Image System.

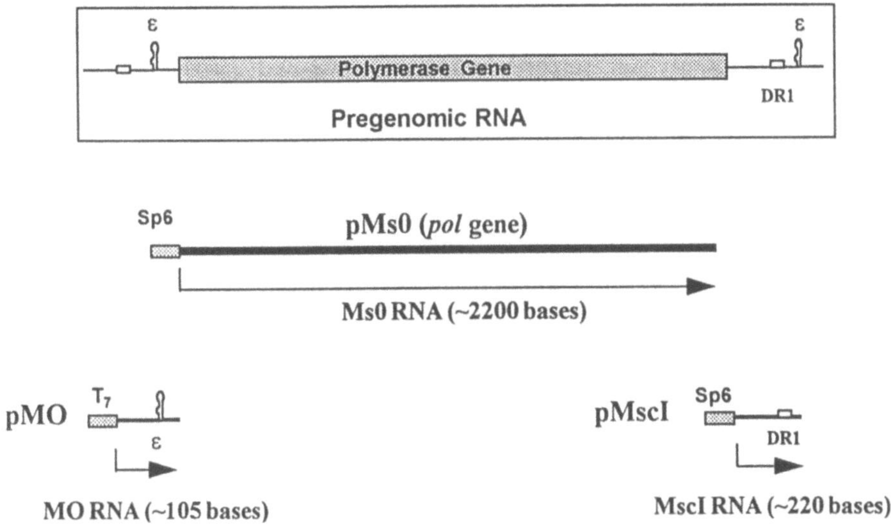

Fig. 1. Plasmids and RNAs used in duck hepatitis virus polymerase assay.

3. Methods

3.1. Plasmid DNA Preparation

Plasmids pMs0, pJP, and p*Msc*I were provided by Christoph Seeger (*see* **Fig. 1**).

Plasmids Ms0 and *Msc*I were utilized without modification. Plasmid JP, which contains a cDNA copy of the entire HBV genome, was used to construct plasmid MO, which contains a cDNA copy of the 5' terminal portion of the DHBV genome. A DNA fragment corresponding to the 5' end of DHBV pregenomic RNA was generated by polymerase chain reaction (PCR) from plasmid JP. The resulting PCR product was blunt end cloned into the *Apa*I site of Pgem7Z, and the correct orientation was determined by sequencing. This pMO construct allows transcription utilizing T7 RNA polymerase.

1. Plasmids are propagated by transforming the DNA into competent DH5α cells according to the supplier's protocol.
2. Plate transformed DH5α cells on LB agar with 100 µg/mL of ampicillin, and grow overnight at 37°C.
3. Inoculate a single colony into 3.0 mL of Luria broth with 100 µg/mL of ampicillin, and grow with shaking for 6–8 h at 37°C.
4. Dilute culture into 250–500 mL of Luria broth with 100 µg/mL of ampicillin, and grow overnight.

5. Collect cells by centrifugation in a Sorvall GSA rotor at 8000 rpm for 5 min.
6. Isolate and purify plasmid DNA from cells using Qiagen columns according to the manufacturer's instructions.
7. Quantitate the plasmid DNA concentration using a Pharmacia GeneQuant RNA/DNA Calculator or equivalent method.
8. Prepare plasmid DNAs for in vitro transcription reactions by digestion with the appropriate restriction enzyme using buffers as provided by the vendor.

Plasmid	Enzyme
pMO	*Eco*RV
pMS0	*Afl*II
p*Msc*I	*Sty*I

9. Digestion of plasmid DNAs (100 µL-reaction): 26 µL of plasmid DNA (~1 µg/µL), 55 µL of DEPC H_2O, 10 µL of 10 X enzyme buffer, and 9 µL of restriction enzyme (~10 U/µL).
10. Incubate for 2 h at 37°C.
11. Analyze one aliquot of each DNA by agarose gel electrophoresis to check for complete digestion.
12. Phenol extract digested plasmid DNAs two times and ethanol precipitate.
13. Resuspend precipitated DNAs in TE buffer, pH 7.6, at a concentration of approx 1 µg/µL.
14. Store DNAs at –20°C.

3.2. Preparation of Duck Hepatitis Virus RNAs by In Vitro Transcription

All reagents are kept on ice until initiation of reaction. The following protocol describes the preparation of the DHBV RNAs required for both the in vitro translation of DHBV *pol* and for the DHBV RT assays.

1. Prepare 5X transcription buffer in DEPC-treated H_2O: 200 m*M* Tris-HCl, pH 7.5, 30 m*M* $MgCl_2$, 10 m*M* spermidine. Autoclave and store at –20°C
2. Prepare reaction mix: 16.0 µL of 5X reaction buffer, 32.0 µL of NTP mix (2.5 m*M* each ATP, GTP, CTP, and UTP), 0.8 µL of bovine serum albumin (BSA) (10 mg/mL), 8.0 µL of dithiothreitol (DTT) (100 m*M*), and 1.0 µL of RNasin (total 57.8 µL).
3. For transcription reactions for MS0, MO, and *Msc*I RNAs, *see* **Table 1** (prepare these reactions at room temperature to prevent spermidine from precipitating the DNA).
4. Add 2 µL of Sp6 polymerase (20 U/µL) to the Ms0 and MO reactions and 4 µL to the *Msc*I reaction.
5. Incubate the reactions in a water bath for 2 h, 40°C for Sp6 and 37°C for T7.
6. Freeze reactions at –70°C.

3.3. In Vitro Translation of Duck Hepatitis Virus Polymerase

All reagents are kept on ice until initiation of reaction. The following protocol describes the preparation of enough DHBV RT for 88 assays in a microtiter

Table 1
Transcription Reactions for MS0, MO, and *MscI*

Component	MS0	MO	*Msc*I (μL)
DNA (1 μg/μL)[a]	2.4	2.0	4.0
DEPC H_2O	1.15	1.55	3.1
Reaction mix	14.45	14.45	28.9
Total	18.0	18.0	36.0

[a]Prepared as described in **Subheading 3.1.**

Table 2
Translation Master Mixes

Component	"Hot" 1	"Cold" 27
RRL	7.0	189 mL
[^{35}S]Methionine (1000 Ci/mmol)	1.0	0 μL
Amino acid mix minus methionine	0.4	0 μL
RNasin (40 U/μL)	0.25	6.75 μL
Complete amino acid mix	0	10.8 μL
DEPC-treated dH_2O	1.0	54 μL
Total	9.65	260.55 μL[a]

[a]This is sufficient to prepare enough enzyme for 88 (i.e., one microtiter plate) DHBV RT reactions.

plate as described below. Two translations are often run in parallel. One small reaction containing [^{35}S]methionine is run to monitor the synthesis of the DHBV polymerase by sodium dodecyl sulfate-polyacrylamide gel electrophoresis (SDS-PAGE). A larger reaction is run to produce the DHBV polymerase required for the RT assay.

1. Two translation master mixes are prepared (*see* **Table 2**).
2. For "hot" reactions transfer 9 μL of [^{35}S] translation master mix to microcentrifuge tubes on ice.
3. Add 0.5 μL of MS0 RNA (from transcription reaction above) and 0.5 μL of MO RNA (from transcription reaction above) to this tube.
4. For "cold" reactions, transfer 252 μL of cold translation master mix to microcentrifuge tubes on ice.
5. Add 14 μL of MS0 RNA and 14 μL of MO RNA to this tube.
6. Incubate both tubes in a water bath at 30°C for 60 min.
7. To the "hot" reaction, add 10 μL 2X SDS sample buffer and process for SDS-PAGE.
8. The cold reaction should be frozen and stored at –70°C until needed for DHBV RT assay.

Table 3
Reverse-Transcriptase Master Mix

Component	Number of reactions 1	112
dNTP stock solution	0.625	70 µL
[α-^{35}S]ATP (>1000 Ci/mmol)	0.625	70 µL
10X TMN buffer	1.250	140 µL
RNasin (40 U/µL)	0.125	14 µL
*Msc*I RNA (prepared as above)	0.250	28 µL
DEPC-treated dH_2O	0.275	30.8 µL
Total	3.15	352.8 µL

3.4. Duck Hepatitis Virus RT Assay

3.4.1. RT Reaction

All reagents are kept on ice until initiation of reaction. The following is the set up for an assay performed in a 96-well microtiter plate. In this format, multiple compounds can be assayed for their ability to inhibit the activity of the DHBV RT. The concentrations of reagents for each individual reaction are also given.

1. Prepare reaction plate by placing 0.6 µL of 10% DMSO in DEPC dH_2O or 0.6 µL of test compounds dissolved in 10% DMSO in DEPC dH_2O per well. Four wells with DEPC dH_2O should serve as controls, two for $t = 0$ and two for $t = 30$ min. Cover the plate with clear plastic packing tape and keep on ice.
2. Prepare dNTP stock solution of dCTP, dTTP, and dGTP containing 0.1 m*M* of each.
3. Prepare RT master mix (*see* **Table 3**).
4. Prepare a master reagent plate on ice for use with an eight-channel micropipet as follows:
   a. Aliquot 44.1 µL of RT master mix in each of eight wells of a 96-well microtiter plate.
   b. Aliquot 31.5 µL of the RRL containing translated DHBV RT (RRL + RT) into each of eight additional wells of the microtiter plate.
   c. Remove tape from reaction plate and keep plate on ice.
   d. Using an eight-channel pipet, deliver 3.15 µL of the RT master mix from the reagent plate to each well of the reaction plate.
   e. To the wells designated as the $t = 0$ samples, add 100 µL of the stop solution (100 m*M* EDTA in 2X SSC).
   f. Using an eight-channel pipet, deliver 2.25 µL of the RRL + RT from the reagent plate to each well of the reaction plate with stirring action.
   g. Cover the plate with tape.
   h. Incubate the reaction plate at 30°C in water bath for 30 min.

i. Remove tape and stop reaction by adding 100 μL of stop solution per well.
j. At this point, plates can be frozen at –20°C if not blotting immediately.

3.4.2. Dot Blotting

1. If reaction plates are frozen, thaw at room temperature.
2. Prewet the NA 45 DEAE filter in 2X SSC.
3. Assemble Bio-Rad dot blotter with NA 45 DEAE filter in place.
4. Transfer 95 μL of each reaction well to the corresponding wells of the dot blotter.
5. In the dot blotter, wash each well two times with 200 μL of 2X SSC.
6. Remove filter from dot blotter, and soak face down in 4X SSC for 20 min at room temperature in plastic sandwich box.
7. Wash filter for 2 min in 95% ethanol in plastic box.
8. Wash filter for 2 min in dH_2O in plastic box.
9. Wash filter for 2 min in 95% ethanol in plastic box.
10. Dry filter face up in gel drier for 15 min at 50°C.
11. Expose dried filter to phosphorimage screen and quantify radioactivity bound to filter.
12. $T = 0$ samples serve as background controls. $T = 30$ samples serve as positive activity controls.
13. Inhibition by test compounds is calculated by the following equation:

$$\% \text{ inhibition} = [1 - (T/C)] \times 100 \quad (1)$$

where: T = (Counts in test sample) – (Counts in $t = 0$ sample); and C = (Counts in $t = 30$ sample) – (Counts in $t = 0$ sample). Counts are as determined by the phosphorimager.
14. Alternatively dried filters can be exposed to X-ray film and the developed film scanned by densitometer or estimated by eye.

References

1. Wang, G. H., Zoulim, F., Leber, E. H., Kitson, J., and Seeger, C. (1994) Role of RNA in enzymatic activity of the reverse transcriptase of hepatitis B viruses. *J. Virol.* **68,** 8437–8442.
2. Wang, G. H. and Seeger, C. (1992) The reverse transcriptase of hepatitis B virus acts as a protein primer for viral DNA synthesis. *Cell* **71,** 663–670.
3. Wang, G. H. and Seeger, C. (1993) Novel mechanism for reverse transcription in hepatitis B viruses. *J. Virol.* **67,** 6507–6512.
4. Tavis, J. E., Perri, S., and Ganem, D. (1994) Hepadnavirus reverse transcriptase initiates within the stem-loop of the RNA packaging signal and employs a novel strand transfer. *J. Virol.* **68,** 3536–3543.
5. Zoulim, F. and Seeger, C. (1994) Reverse transcription in hepatitis B viruses is primed by a tyrosine residue of the polymerase. *J. Virol.* **68,** 6–13.

7

Assays for Measuring Hepadnaviral Supercoiled DNA

Stephen A. Locarnini and Gilda M. Civitico

1. Introduction

A major reason for treatment failure during antiviral therapy of chronic hepatitis B infection is thought to be the persistence of the key replicative intermediate, the viral covalently closed circular (CCC) or supercoiled DNA *(1,2)*. Investigators studying the structure and function of hepadnaviral CCC DNA *(3)* have provided evidence that suggests that this structure exists in the nucleus of infected hepatocytes as a heterogeneous population of viral minichromosomes, which range from half to fully chromatinized, thought to be owing to their association with variable numbers of nucleosomes.

Most of what we know about hepatitis B virus (HBV) replication has been extrapolated from studies with the two major hepadnaviral animal models: the duck and the woodchuck. The unusual replication strategy of HBV was originally elucidated using the duck system, but the woodchuck model has proven to be a more useful disease system. Both animal models have been used for the evaluation of antiviral agents in in vitro and in vivo studies.

In cultured primary duck hepatocytes (PDH) congenitally infected with duck hepatitis B virus (DHBV), all major viral replicative intermediates are generated, and CCC DNA, present initially at a low copy number, is amplified in the PDH after a few days in culture *(4,5)*. The amplification of CCC DNA in vitro provides an alternative to liver analysis for studying the structure of this molecule and its sensitivity to potential antiviral agents.

In this chapter, procedures are described for the enrichment and isolation of CCC DNA and total DNA from both cultured PDH and fresh and frozen liver (or other organ) specimens. The technique for the former is essentially a modified Hirt *(6)* high-salt extraction *(5)*. Detection of the replicative intermediates is by Southern blot hybridization analysis, which can be performed using

From: *Methods in Molecular Medicine, vol. 24: Antiviral Methods and Protocols*
Edited by: D. Kinchington and R. F. Schinazi © Humana Press Inc., Totowa, NJ

labeled single-stranded RNA or double-stranded DNA probes. The replicative intermediates are visualized by autoradiography and quantitation is done by microdensitometry of autoradiographs and/or directly by means of a phosphorimager. Provided that certain experimental conditions are met, drug-induced alterations in the levels of viral DNA replicative intermediates and in the CCC DNA species may be analyzed, allowing comparisons of the antiviral effects of different drugs to be made within a single study and between different studies *(2,7–9)*.

2. Materials

Chemicals should be analytical grade or the purest grade commercially available. All aqueous solutions should be prepared in sterile, distilled, deionized water, and all (except sodium dodecyl sulfate [SDS], glycogen, and enzymes) are autoclavable and are stable at room temperature unless otherwise stated. All equipment should be sterile or sterilized before use. Gloves should be worn for all procedures. Phenol and chloroform are toxic and should be handled in a fume hood and disposed of safely.

1. 1.5-mL microfuge tubes (phenol resistant).
2. 50-mL centrifuge tubes (phenol resistant).
3. Phosphate-buffered saline (PBS).
4. CCC DNA lysis buffer: 10 m*M* Tris-HCl pH 7.4, 10 m*M* ethylenediaminetetra-acetic acid (EDTA), 0.5% SDS.
5. 2.5 *M* KCl.
6. Total DNA lysis buffer: 50 m*M* Tris-HCl, pH 8.0, 10 m*M* EDTA, 150 m*M* NaCl, 0.5% SDS.
7. Chloroform.
8. 50 m*M* Tris-HCl (pH 7.5) buffered phenol. Make up in batches and store frozen at –20°C in 50-mL aliquots. Thaw before use.
9. Tris-buffered phenol: chloroform (1:1). Make up as required; can be stored for several days at 4°C.
10. Absolute ethanol.
11. 70% ethanol in distilled water
12. TE buffers (10:10): 10 m*M* Tris-HCl, pH 7.5, 10 m*M* EDTA, (10:2): 10 m*M* Tris-HCl, pH 7.5, 2 m*M* EDTA.
13. 10% SDS.
14. 1 *M* Tris-HCl, pH 7.5.
15. 0.5 *M* EDTA, pH 8.0.
16. Glycogen stock 20 mg/mL in TE 10:10. Stored frozen at –20°C.
17. Proteinase K (20 mg/mL stock in distilled water). Store frozen in 0.5-mL aliquots at –20°C.
18. RNase A (DNase free) 5 mg/mL stock in distilled water. Store frozen in small aliquots at –20°C.

19. Loose fitting 20-mL vol glass Dounce tissue homogenizers.
20. Forceps.
21. Sterile disposable scalpels.
22. Pronase. Store at 4°C as powder; make up as required.
23. Tissue DNA lysis buffer: 200 m*M* Tris-HCl, pH 7.5, 2 m*M* EDTA, 250 m*M* NaCl, 1% SDS.
24. 20X Nicking solution (50 m*M* Na acetate, pH 4.2). Dilute to 1X immediately before use.
25. Gel soak 1: 0.1 *N* NaOH, 1.5 *M* NaCl. Prepare fresh as required.
26. Gel soak 2: 0.1 *M* Tris-HCl pH 7.5, 1.5 *M* NaCl.
27. 10X saline sodium citrate (SSC): 1.5 *M* NaCl, 1.5 *M* Na citrate, pH 7.0.

3. Methods

PDH can be prepared from the livers of 1–7-d-old ducklings congenitally infected with DHBV. Hepatocytes are isolated by collagenase perfusion and then purified from other hepatobiliary elements by Percoll gradient centrifugation ***(10)***. Purified PDH are seeded onto tissue culture plastic at an appropriate seeding density, allowed to adhere, and are then maintained in Leibovitz 15 medium (Gibco-BRL, Gaithersburg, MD) supplemented with 5% fetal bovine serum (FBS), 15 m*M* HEPES, insulin, glucose, hydrocortisone hemisuccinate, penicillin, and streptomycin as described by Tuttleman et al. ***(4)***, with medium changes every 2 d. Hepatocytes cultured in this manner are viable for at least 2 wk after plating out.

3.1. Extraction and Purification of DHBV DNA from Cultured Cells

After approx 5 d of culturing, congenitally infected hepatocytes begin to show an accumulation in the levels of viral DNA. In a typical experiment, total DHBV DNA levels will show a 10-fold increase whereas CCC DHBV DNA will increase 50-fold over a 2 wk period (*see* **Fig. 1**). PDH prepared from virus-free birds can also be *de novo* infected and are permissive to infection for several days postplating ***(4,5)***. This allows infection parameters to be more carefully regulated and also allows greater flexibility, particularly when planning experiments designed to investigate early events in viral replication.

To distinguish DHBV CCC DNA from other viral replicative intermediates, a modified salt extraction of the extracts must be performed, which enriches for viral DNAs noncovalently bound to protein ***(5)***.

3.1.1. Extraction of DHBV CCC DNA from Cultured PDH

1. Remove the culture medium and wash the primary hepatocyte monolayers free of residual medium with sterile PBS.
2. Lyse cells in CCC DNA lysis buffer (0.5 mL/1 × 10^7 cells) and scrape lysate into 1.5-mL microfuge tubes. If lysates are not going to be analyzed immediately, they can be stored for several months at –80°C.

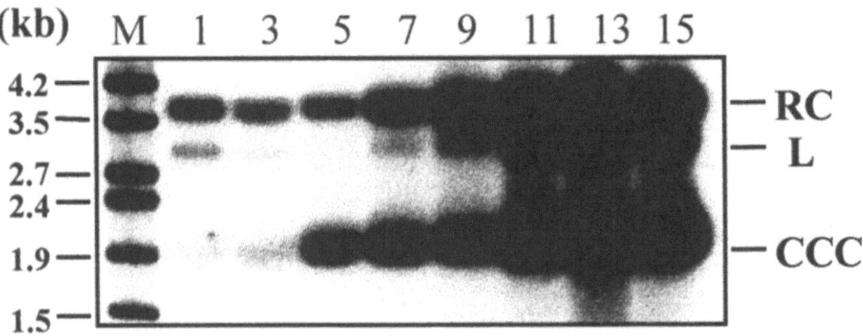

Fig. 1. Time-course study of the accumulation of DHBV CCC DNA in PDH congenitally infected with DHBV. PDH cultures were harvested from d 1 to 15 post-plating and selectively extracted to enrich for viral CCC DNA. The DNA was analyzed by Southern blot hybridization using a full length, double-stranded DHBV probe labeled with ^{32}P.

3. Add 1/4 vol of 2.5 *M* KCl to the lysates, gently mix, and allow to stand at room temperature for 30 min.
4. Centrifuge at 12,500*g* for 15 min and collect supernatant, carefully avoiding the precipitate.
5. Extract the supernatant twice with an equal volume of Tris-buffered phenol, followed by one extraction with chloroform; vortex extracts briefly, centrifuge at 12,500*g* for 10 min, and collect the aqueous phase.
6. Add 1 µL of glycogen carrier to the extracted supernatants, followed by 2 vol of absolute ethanol, invert to mix, and then allow to precipitate at room temperature for 1 h.
7. Collect precipitated DNA by centrifugation at 12,500*g* for 15 min, and then wash once with 70% ethanol.
8. Remove as much of the ethanol as possible from the microfuge tube using a pipet tip and allow the pellet to dry at room temperature (if the pellets are small, this should take only a few minutes) or under vacuum.
9. Redissolve the pellet in 10:2 TE (20 µL/1 × 10^7 cells).
10. DNA isolated using this method is now ready for analysis by Southern blot hybridization (*see* **Subheading 3.3.**).

3.1.2. Extraction of Total DHBV DNA from Cultured PDH

1. Remove medium and wash monolayers as in **step 1** of **Subheading 3.1.1**.
2. Lyse the cells in total DNA lysis buffer (0.5 mL/0.5 × 10^7 cells) and scrape lysate into 1.5-mL microfuge tubes. If lysates are not going to be analyzed immediately, they can be stored for several months at –80°C.

3. Digest the lysates with 0.5 mg/mL (final) of proteinase K at 45°C for 1 h.
4. Deproteinize samples by two extractions with Tris-buffered phenol:chloroform, followed by one extraction with chloroform (as in **step 5** of **Subheading 3.3.1.**).
5. Add 2 vol of absolute ethanol, mix, and allow to stand at room temperature for 1 h. Collect the precipitated DNA by centrifugation at 12,500*g* for 15 min, and then wash once with 70% ethanol.
6. Remove as much of the ethanol as possible from the microfuge tube using a pipet tip, and allow the pellet to dry, as in **step 8** of **Subheading 3.1.1.**
7. Redissolve the pellet in 10:10 TE (20 µL/0.5 × 10^7 cells).
8. DNA isolated using this method is now ready for analysis by Southern blot hybridization (**Subheading 3.3.**).

3.2. Extraction of DHBV DNA from Liver Tissue

When in vivo experiments in infected adult ducks are performed, the methods described for the isolation of DHBV DNAs from cell culture material are modified slightly to accommodate a larger volume of cellular material. Although the protocol here describes the extraction of liver tissue, most tissues could be successfully extracted using this method. The DNA isolated using these methods may then be analyzed by Southern blot hybridization.

Quantitation and standardization of the amounts of total DNA isolated from each tissue sample must also be performed prior to analysis by Southern blot hybridization so that the amounts of total DNA loaded into each lane are equivalent and so that the autoradiographic signals obtained after Southern blot hybridization are directly comparable. This is not required for the analysis of DNA isolated from tissue culture as the number of PDH extracted are standardized at the time of seeding. By recording the exact weight of the tissue extracted, it is possible to calculate the viral load per cell in each sample.

3.2.1. Preparation of Liver Material for DNA Extraction

1. Thaw a piece of liver on a piece of filter paper. Blot off excess moisture and remove any clotted blood and surface fat using a sterile disposable scalpel and sterile forceps before chopping the tissue finely. Weigh out approx 300 mg of chopped tissue (accurately record the exact weight). During handling, the tissue sample(s) to be extracted should be kept cold on ice for as much of the procedure as possible to minimize degradation of the DNA in the samples.
2. Place tissue in a sterilized, prechilled, loose fitting, 20-mL glass Dounce tissue homogenizer and add 5 mL of ice-cold 10:10 TE to the grinding chamber.
3. Gently grind tissue (on ice), slowly rotating the pestle with each downward stroke and taking care to avoid frothing, until there are no more lumps. Between 10 and 15 strokes should be adequate. It is possible to make a count of the nuclei at this stage (*see* **Note 2**).
4. Divide the homogenate into 2 × 2.5 mL aliquots in 50-mL (phenol resistant) centrifuge tubes; one each for DHBV CCC DNA (**Subheading 3.2.2.**) and total DNA extractions (**Subheading 3.2.3.**).

3.2.2. Extraction of DHBV CCC DNA from Liver Homogenate

1. Add a further 1.25 mL of TE to the 2.5-mL aliquot of liver homogenate, followed by 250 µL of 10% SDS and finally 1 mL of 2.5 *M* KCl, gently mixing contents after each addition.
2. Mix well and leave at room temperature for 30 min.
3. Centrifuge at 10,000*g* (*see* **Note 1**) for 20 min at room temperature and collect supernatant, carefully avoiding the precipitate.
4. Extract the supernatant twice with an equal volume of Tris-buffered phenol, followed by one extraction with chloroform; invert extracts 20 times to mix, and then centrifuge at 5000*g* for 10 min and collect the aqueous phase.
5. Add 2 vol of absolute ethanol and precipitate DNA overnight at –20°C.
6. Collect the precipitated DNA by centrifugation at 5000*g* for 30 min, then wash twice with 70% ethanol. Gently pour off ethanol and washes to avoid dislodging the DNA pellet.
7. Invert the tube onto a piece of tissue to drain off residual ethanol.
8. Dry the pellets under vacuum for 15–30 min, and then redissolve the DNA pellets in 150 µL of 10:2 TE.
9. The amount of total DNA in the sample can be quantitated using a fluorometer; using this method, a fixed amount of a DNA intercalating dye is added to a series of known double-stranded DNA samples. The amount of dye that binds is directly proportional to the amount of DNA in the sample, which fluoresces when exposed to a particular wavelength of light produced by the fluorometer. A standard curve is constructed using the fluorometric readings, from which the concentration of unknown DNA samples can be calculated. If a fluorometer is unavailable, the concentration of DNA in a sample can be calculated by spectroscopy; the optical density (OD) of a 10-µL aliquot is read at 260 and 280 nm. An OD of 1 at 260 nm corresponds to 50 µg/mL of double-stranded DNA. After the DNA concentration in a sample has been calculated, the sample volumes should be adjusted so that the final concentration in the sample extracted for CCC DNA is 10 µg/10 µL.

3.2.3. Extraction of Total DHBV DNA from Liver Homogenate

1. To the 2.5-mL aliquot of liver homogenate, add 2.5 mL (1 mg/mL) pronase in tissue DNA lysis buffer.
2. Mix well and then incubate at 37°C for 30 min.
3. Extract the supernatant twice with an equal volume of Tris-buffered phenol:chloroform followed by one extraction with chloroform; invert extracts 20 times to mix, centrifuge at 5000*g* for 10 min, and collect the aqueous phase.
4. Add 1/25 vol of 5 *M* NaCl, followed by 2 vol of absolute ethanol. Precipitate DNA overnight at –20°C.
5. Collect precipitated DNA by centrifugation at 5000*g* for 30 min, and wash twice with 70% ethanol. Avoid dislodging the DNA pellets.
6. Invert the tube onto a piece of tissue to drain off residual ethanol.
7. Dry pellets under vacuum for 15–30 min, and then redissolve DNA pellet in 500 µL of 10:10 TE.

8. In a microfuge tube, digest half the total DNA with RNase A at a final concentration of 0.1 mg/mL for 1 h at 37°C. The remainder of the DNA can be stored at –20°C.
9. Deproteinize digests by extracting twice with Tris-buffered phenol:chloroform, followed by one extraction with chloroform; vortex the extracts briefly, centrifuge at 12,500*g* for 10 min, and collect the aqueous phase.
10. Add 1/25 vol of 5 *M* NaCl, followed by 2 vol of absolute ethanol. Precipitate DNA for 30 min at room temperature.
11. Pellet the precipitated DNA by centrifugation at 12,500*g* for 15 min.
12. Remove as much of the ethanol as possible from the microfuge tube using a pipet tip and allow the pellets to dry under vacuum for 15–30 min.
13. Redissolve the total DNA pellet in 200 µL of 10:10 TE.
14. Calculate the DNA concentration in the sample, as in step 9 of **Subheading 3.2.2.** Adjust the final volumes so that the final concentration of DNA in the sample extracted for total DNA is 1 µg/10 µL

3.3. Analysis of DHBV DNAs

For visualizing viral replicate intermediates, in particular DHBV CCC DNA, isolated using the techniques described in **Subheadings 3.1.1.** and **3.2.2.**, the DNA samples are analyzed by agarose gel electrophoresis and Southern blot hybridization. When DHBV CCC DNA is to be analyzed, at the completion of electrophoresis the gel must first be treated with a mildly acidic reagent (sodium acetate), which depurinates the DNA, produces single-stranded nicks, and converts the DHBV CCC DNA, *in situ*, to the relaxed circular form. The DNA is then denatured with alkali, and the alkali is neutralized. These procedures ensure efficient transfer of the CCC DNA to the hybridization membrane. Details of probe preparation and filter hybridization are not described here because the choice of conditions, hybridization mix, probe, and label will depend on the materials available to individual laboratories; detailed methods are described in such publications as *Current Protocols in Molecular Biology* ***(11)***.

3.3.1. Southern Blot Hybridization

1. Subject 10 or 1 µg of extracted CCC DNA or total DNA, respectively (isolated from whole tissue), or a 10-µL aliquot of CCC or total DNA isolated from tissue culture material, together with suitable DHBV DNA controls and DNA molecular size markers, to electrophoresis through 1.5% agarose slab gels in an appropriate buffer at 60 V for approx 3 h using standard techniques ***(12)***.
2. Soak the gel in 1X nicking solution (use sufficient solution to totally immerse the gel) for 30 min at room temperature, with frequent agitation.
3. Rinse the gel in distilled water, and then soak it for a further 30 min in fresh 1X nicking solution at 52°C.
4. Denature the DNA by incubation in gel soak 1 (sufficient to cover gel) for 30 min at room temperature, with frequent agitation. Rinse the gel in fresh gel soak 1 solution, and then repeat this procedure.

5. Neutralize the gel by soaking it in gel soak 2 for 30 min at room temperature, with frequent agitation. Rinse the gel in fresh gel soak 2 solution, and then repeat this procedure.
6. Set up a capillary transfer pyramid using negatively charged nylon membrane and 10X SSC as the transfer buffer. Allow to transfer overnight. Fix the DNA to the membrane by baking or ultraviolet crosslinking
7. Probe preparation, hybridization, and autoradiography ***(11)***.

3.3.2. Quantitation and Data Analysis

Quantitation of autoradiographic images may be achieved by using a scanning densitometer or computer-assisted image processor. In each case, the relationship between image density and amount of bound probe should be calibrated using internal standards, and should ideally be linear over the range of interest. Alternatively, radioactivity can be quantitated more directly by cutting out and counting specific membrane regions, or by use of a phosphorimager. Signals generated by these latter methods are usually linear over very large ranges.

There are at least two alternatives for assessing activity of potential anti-HBV agents from this type of data: (1) if a range of drug concentrations is used, activity may be assessed by regression analysis of dose-response plots (which may not, however, be linear or even monotonic); (2) if at least three replicate results from untreated control cultures are obtained, the significance of drug-induced alterations in HBV DNA levels can be estimated statistically. Provided that there is no contribution from drug cytotoxicity, the significance of any measured drug-induced alteration in HBV DNA decreases as the intra-assay "noise" increases. As a rough guide, drug-induced changes in HBV DNA begin to become significant (at $p < 0.05$ level) when they exceed 1.25 times the control range.

4. Notes

1. To pellet the protein-DNA complexes generated in this step, a high-speed centrifugation step is required. Most benchtop type centrifuges with rotors/adapters able to accommodate the larger 50-mL tubes are unable to spin at the required *g*-force. It is therefore suggested that a Midrange or Ultracentrifuge (e.g., Beckman TJ-6 series, Beckman Instruments, Palo Alto, CA), together with the appropriate rotor and centrifuge tubes, be used for this step.
2. As an alternative to DNA quantitation, a nuclei count can be performed on the liver homogenate (in 10:10 TE), prior to treatment with detergent, to standardize the amount of DNA present in a liver tissue extraction. To a 100-µL aliquot of tissue homogenate, add 1 µL of a 10 mg/mL stock solution of ethidium bromide. Using a fluorescence microscope, count the number of nuclei using a hematocytometer. From this the number of nuclei in the original sample can be calculated. DNA (either total or CCC DNA enriched) extracted from the equivalent of 3×10^6 nuclei are then loaded into each lane for Southern blot hybridization analysis. Assuming thatthere are 5×10^{-6} µg of total cellular DNA per duck hepatocyte ***(12)***, the amount of total DNA loaded can be calculated.

References

1. Hirota, K., Sherker, A. H., Omata, M., Yokosuka, O., and Okuda, K. (1987) Effects of adenine arabinoside on serum and intrahepatic replicative forms of duck hepatitis B virus in chronic infection. *Hepatology* **7,** 24–28.
2. Mason, W. S., Cullen, J., Saputelli, J., Wu, T.-T., Liu, C., London, W. T., Lustbader, E., Schaffer, P., O'Connell, A. P., Fourel, I., Aldrich, C. E., and Jilbert, A. R. (1994) Characterization of the antiviral effects of 2'carbodeoxyguanosine in ducks chronically infected with duck hepatitis B virus. *Hepatology* **19,** 398–411.
3. Newbold, J. E., Xin, H., Tencza, M., Sherman, G., Dean, J., Bowden, S., and Locarnini, S. (1995) The covalently closed duplex form of hepadnaviral genome exists *in situ* as a heterogeneous population of viral minichromosomes. *J. Virol.* **69,** 3350–3357.
4. Tuttleman, J., Pugh, J., and Summers, J. (1986) *In vitro* experimental infection of primary duck hepatocyte cultures with duck hepatitis B virus. *J. Virol.* **58,** 17–25.
5. Wu, T.-T., Coates, L., Aldrich, C., Summers, J., and Mason, W. S. (1990) In hepatocytes infected with duck hepatitis B virus, the template for viral RNA synthesis is amplified by an intracellular pathway. *Virology* **175,** 255–261.
6. Hirt, B. (1967) Selective extraction of polyoma DNA from infected mouse cell cultures. *J. Mol. Biol.* **119,** 487–506.
7. Luscombe, C., Pederson, J., Bowden, S., and Locarnini, S. (1994) Alterations in intrahepatic expression of duck hepatitis B viral markers with ganciclovir therapy. *Liver* **14,** 182–192.
8. Wang, Y., Luscombe, C., Bowden, S., Shaw, T., and Locarnini, S. (1995) Inhibition of duck hepatitis B virus DNA replication by antiviral chemotherapy with ganciclovir-nalidixic acid. *Antimicrob. Agents Chemother.* **39,** 556–558.
9. Lin, E., Luscombe, C., Wang, Y-Y., Shaw, T., and Locarnini, S. (1996) The guanine nucleoside analogue penciclovir is active against chronic duck hepatitis B virus infection *in vivo. Antimicrob. Agents Chemother.* **40,** 413–418.
10. Bishop, N., Civitico, G., Wang, Y., Guo, K., Gust, I. D., and Locarnini, S. (1990) Antiviral strategies in chronic HBV infection: I. Establishment of a suitable *in vitro* system using the duck hepatitis B virus model. *J. Med. Virol.* **31,** 82–89.
11. Moore, D. (1995) Preparation and analysis of DNA, in *Current Protocols in Molecular Biology,* vol. 1 (Ausubel, F. M., Brent, R., Kingston R. E., Moore, D. D., Siedman, J. G., Smith, J. A., and Struhl, K., eds.), Wiley, New York.
12. Jilbert, A., Freiman, J., Burrell, C., Holmes, M., Gowans, E., Roweand, R., Hall, P., and Cossart, Y. (1988) Virus-liver cell interactions in duck hepatitis B virus infection: A study of virus dissemination within the liver. *Gastroenterology* **95,** 1375–1382.

8

Assays for Hepatitis B Virus DNA- and RNA-Dependent DNA Polymerase Activities

Timothy Shaw and Stephen A. Locarnini

1. Introduction

Genomes of the hepatitis B viruses (HBVs) consist of approx 3.2 kb of partly double-stranded DNA containing three or four overlapping open reading frames, the largest of which encodes the viral polymerase (Pol) protein. After entry into the cell and uncoating, the viral genome is transported to the nucleus where it is converted into a covalently closed circular (CCC) or supercoiled molecule by cellular repair mechanisms. The viral CCC DNA is transcribed, presumably by host cell RNA polymerase II, into unspliced, capped polyadenylated mRNA species from which viral proteins are transcribed. In addition, terminally redundant 3.5-kb RNA transcripts, which function as pregenomes, are produced and exported to the cytoplasm where they are packaged into viral core particles in which reverse transcription, pregenome degradation, and duplication occurs, reproducing the partly double-stranded HBV genome (for recent review, *see* **ref.** ***1***). Besides its essential role in HBV genome replication, HBV Pol is also involved in virus assembly, and because hepadnaviruses do not encode enzymes functionally equivalent to deoxynucleoside kinases *(2)*, functions associated with HBV Pol are probably the only virus-specific targets for antiviral activity of nucleoside analogs. In vitro assays for inhibition of HBV Pol functions by deoxynucleoside triphosphate (dNTP) analogs are useful indicators but, because of restrictions imposed by hepatocyte enzymology, provide no guarantee of potential anti-HBV activity of the parent (deoxy)nucleoside analogs in intact cells *(2)*.

From: *Methods in Molecular Medicine, vol. 24: Antiviral Methods and Protocols*
Edited by: D. Kinchington and R. F. Schinazi © Humana Press Inc., Totowa, NJ

1.1. HBV DNA Pol

Hepadnaviral Pol proteins are multifunctional and contain four domains, namely (in order from amino to carboxy terminus) terminal protein, spacer, polymerase, and RNaseH, respectively. Known functions include (1) acting as a primer for first (–) strand DNA synthesis; (2) synthesizing first-strand DNA from RNA pregenome (reverse transcriptase or RNA-dependent DNA polymerase [RDDP] activity); (3) degrading viral RNA in resulting RNA-DNA hybrids (RNase H activity); and (4) copying second- (+) strand DNA from the (–) strand DNA template (DNA-dependent DNA polymerase [DDDP] activity). In addition, multiple Pol domains appear to be required for proper assembly of the pregenomic RNA molecule and associated Pol into cytoplasmic core particles ***(1)***.

Unfortunately, the enormous difficulties associated with isolating useful quantities of purified protein from HBV virions has hindered biochemical studies of the HBV Pol. However, Oberhaus and Newbold ***(3)*** have described an *in situ* activity gel assay that will detect RDDP, DDDP, and RNaseH activities of DHBV Pol, and several groups have recently cloned Hepadnaviral *Pol* genes and succeeded in expressing full-length recombinant Pol proteins in vitro ***(4–6)***. The recombinant proteins have been shown to be capable of priming and extending first- (–) strand HBV DNA, but not completing it, and RNase H and DDDP activities of recombinant proteins have yet to be convincingly demonstrated at the time of this writing.

1.1.1. Endogenous HBV DNA Polymerase Assays

Endogenous HBV polymerase assays measure the ability of the viral polymerase to incorporate dNTPs into viral replicative intermediates present within viral core particles. If the cores are derived from secreted virions, the assay measures predominantly DDDP activity, whereas if the particles are isolated from cytosol of infected cells, the assay measures predominantly RDDP activity. In these assays, one dNTP is usually radiolabeled, and polymerase activity is detected by scintillation counting of radioactivity incorporated into acid-precipitable material, presumed to be HBV DNA. In most published assay methods, a large excess of unlabeled dNTPs is present (*see* **Note 1**). In addition to dNTP substrates, reaction mixtures used for polymerase assays typically contain a buffer (usually Tris-HCl, pH 7.5–8.0), a monovalent salt (usually KCl), essential divalent metal ions (Mg^{2+} or Mn^{2+}), a reducing agent (dithiothreitol [DTT] or 2-mercaptoethanol), and a nonionic detergent (usually Nonidet-P40 or Triton X-100). Concentrations of individual components of the reaction mixture in different published assay methods vary considerably.

2. Materials

Chemicals should be analytical grade or the purest grade commercially available. All aqueous solutions should be prepared in sterile, distilled, deionized, ultrafiltered water (prepared using a MilliQ water purification unit [Millipore, Bedford, MA] or similar apparatus). Solutions and reagents are stable at room temperature unless specifically stated otherwise. All equipment should be sterile or sterilized before use.

1. DTT stock solution, 100 m*M* (1.55 g DDT in 100 mL water; dispense in small aliquots and store frozen at –20°C).
2. Tris-HCl (tris[hydroxymethyl]aminomethane), 1 *M* stock, pH 7.6. Dissolve 121 g Tris base in 800 mL water, adjust pH to 7.6 with 0.1 *M* HCl, and add water to 1 L.
3. Ethylenediamine tetraacetic acid (EDTA) 500 m*M* stock (pH 8.0). Dissolve 186.1 g Na_2 EDTA·$2H_2O$ in 700 mL water; adjust pH to 8.0 with 10 *M* NaOH (≈ 50 mL), and add water to 1 L.
4. Nonidet-P40.
5. 1 *M* stock potassium chloride (74.6 g KCl, water to 1 L).
6. 100 m*M* magnesium chloride (2.3 g $MgCl_2 \cdot 6H_2O$, water to 100 mL).
7. 100 m*M* manganese chloride (1.98 g $MnCl_2 \cdot 4H_2O$, water to 100 mL).
8. 100 m*M* sodium pyrophosphate (44.6 g $Na_4P_2O_7 \cdot 10H_2O$, water to 1 L).
9. Glass microfiber or paper disks (Whatman [Maidstone, UK] GF/A or DE81, respectively).
10. Non-dNTP inhibitors: aphidicolin (10 mg/mL in water), phosphonoformic acid (10 mg/mL in water), actinomycin D (10 mg/mL in ethanol). Store frozen, protected from light, in small aliquots. Make up 400 μg/mL solutions just before use.
11. Trichloroacetic acid (TCA) stock 50% (w/v). (500 g TCA, water to 1 L).
12. RNase (10 mg/mL; ≈500 U/mL) stock in water. Store frozen in small aliquots at –20°C. (Crude RNase is adequate; no need to boil or autodigest.)
13. 5 mg/mL DNase I (≈10,000 U/mL) stock in water. Store frozen in small aliquots at –20°C.
14. Polyethylene glycol (PEG) 8000 50% (w/v) in 500 m*M* NaCl.
15. Phosphate buffered saline (PBS).
16. Dounce homogenizer (20–50 mL vol).
17. 5 *M* NaCl (292.2 g NaCl, water to 1 L).
18. Absolute ethanol.
19. Sucrose 10, 20, 30, 50, and 60% (w/v) (≈0.3, 0.6, 0.9, 1.5, and 1.8 *M*, respectively) in 50 m*M* Tris-HCl, pH 7.6. Store frozen at –20°C.
20. 4X polymerase buffer (40 m*M* Tris-HCl, 1 *M* KCl).
21. dNTP solutions, ultrapure: can be purchased as >95% purity, 100 m*M* solutions of lithium or sodium salts at pH 7.0. Store frozen in small aliquots at –80°C. Purity of solutions and possible degradation of stored solutions may be checked by high-pressure liquid chromatography.

22. dNTP trio solution, 4X: each of three or four unlabeled dNTPs in 5 m*M* $MnCl_2$ or 50 m*M* $MgCl_2$. (Omit the dNTP corresponding to the dNTP label to be used.) Store frozen in small aliquots at –80°C.
23. dNTP substrate solution, 4X: Prepare immediately before use. Add labeled dNTP to dNTP trio solution. For α-[^{32}P]-dNTPs (specific activity ≈3000 Ci/m*M*; 10 mCi/mL), add 100 μCi/mL (≈0.33 μ*M*); for [^{3}H]-dNTPs (labeled on purine or pyrimidine base; specific activity ≈10 Ci/m*M*), add 10 μCi/mL (≈10 μ*M*) (*see* **Note 1**).
24. dNTP duo solution, 4X: 1 m*M* each of two unlabeled dNTPs in 5 m*M* $MnCl_2$ or 50 m*M* $MgCl_2$. (Omit both the dNTP corresponding to the dNTP label to be used and the natural dNTP corresponding to the dNTP analog to be used as inhibitor.) Store frozen in small aliquots at –80°C (*see* **Note 2**).
25. Kinetic substrate solution: Prepare as for dNTP substrate solution above, but using dNTP duo solution instead of dNTP trio solution.
26. Heating block.
27. Proteinase K (20 mg/mL) in distilled water. Store frozen in small aliquots at –20°C.
28. Chloroform.
29. 1.5-mL microfuge tubes (phenol resistant).
30. 50 m*M* Tris-HCl–buffered phenol, pH 7.6. Make up in batches and store frozen at –20°C in 50-mL aliquots. Thaw immediately before use.
31. Tris-buffered phenol:chloroform (1:1). Make up as required.
32. 10% (w/v) sodium dodecyl sulfate (SDS) in water.

3. Methods

3.1. Isolation of HBV Virions and Core Particles from HBV Producer Cells

3.1.1. Isolation of HBV Virions from Culture Medium

1. Grow 2.2.15 cells *(7)* (or cells of another HBV producer line) to confluence in RPMI medium plus 10% fetal bovine serum (*see* **Note 3**).
2. When cells are confluent, change medium to RPMI + 2% fetal calf serum.
3. Change medium every 3 or 4 d for 12–16 d, and collect and store cell culture supernatant at –80°C.
4. Save cell monolayers at the end of incubation for preparation of cytoplasmic core particles (*see* **Subheading 3.1.2.**).
5. Clarify collected cell culture supernatant by centrifugation for 10 min at 2000*g*.
6. To 4 vol of cell culture supernatant, add 1 vol of 50% PEG 8000 in 500 m*M* of NaCl (final concentrations, 10% and 100 m*M*, respectively); keep at 4°C overnight.
7. Pellet HBV virions by centrifugation for 15 min at 15,000*g*.
8. Resuspend pellets in 20–25 mL of Tris-HCl. Add ≈5 U/mL each of DNase I and RNase; incubate 30–60 min at 37°C.
9. Add 1 mL of 500 m*M* EDTA (final concentration, 25 m*M*) and continue incubation for a further 15–30 min.
10. Clarify by centrifugation for 10 min at 2000*g*.

11. Layer the supernatant onto three-step sucrose gradients (consisting of 6 mL each 10, 20, and 30% (w/v) sucrose in 50 m*M* of Tris-HCl in Beckman SW28 tubes (Beckman Instruments, Palo Alto, CA).
12. Pellet viral particles by centrifugation overnight (16–20 h) at 4°C in an SW28 rotor at 140,000*g*.
13. Resuspend virus pellets by brief sonication in 1 mL water, then dispense in small aliquots, and store frozen at –80°C.
14. Estimate and record the concentration of HBV DNA in a small aliquot of the HBV virion preparation by slot-blot hybridization in parallel with known standards.

3.1.2. Isolation of HBV Core Particles from HBV Producer Cells

1. At the end of incubation (*see* **step 4** of **Subheading 3.1.1.**) rinse cell monolayers once with sterile PBS, then add ≈0.5–1.0 mL 5% sucrose, 50 m*M* Tris-HCl, pH 7.6, 5 m*M* DTT per million cells, and harvest cells by scraping.
2. Homogenize thoroughly using a Dounce homogenizer.
3. Pellet cell debris and nuclei by centrifugation for 10 min at 2000*g*.
4. Layer the supernatant over two-step sucrose gradients (consisting of 6 mL each 50 and 60% (w/v) sucrose in 50 m*M* of Tris-HCl) in Beckman SW28 tubes.
5. Concentrate the HBV particles by centrifugation overnight (16–20 h) at 4°C in an SW28 rotor at 140,000*g*.
6. Recover the 50% sucrose layer, which contains the HBV core particles, add DNase I and RNase, and incubate as described in **step 8** of **Subheading 3.1.1.**
7. Continue as described in **steps 9–14** of **Subheading 3.1.1.**

3.2. Isolation and Purification of HBV Virions from Infected Serum

1. If available, select pretreatment sera having high-titer HBsAg for further screening for HBV DNA by dot-blot hybridization. Pool sera with high HBV DNA levels and clarify by centrifugation for 10 min at 400*g* (*see* **Note 4**).
2. Pellet virions by centrifugation overnight through a discontinuous sucrose gradient as described in **steps 11** and **12** of **Subheading 3.1.1.**
3. Resuspend pellet and store as described in **steps 13** and **14** of **Subheading 3.1.1.**

3.3. Assays for Endogenous HBV DDDP and RDDP Activity

3.3.1. Determination of Strand Specificity and Reaction Rate Linearity

1. Add Nonidet-P40 and DTT to HBV virion or core preparations (containing ≈10 ng/mL HBV DNA) to give final Nonidet-P40 and DTT concentrations of 0.4% (v/v) and 40 m*M*, respectively; mix and incubate overnight at 4°C.
2. Dispense 50 µL of freshly prepared polymerase reaction mixture into each of four microfuge tubes.
3. Add 50 µL of substrate solution (containing labeled and unlabeled dNTPs) to each tube.
4. Add 50 µL of water or 50 µL aqueous inhibitor solution (aphidicolin, phosphonoformic acid, or actinomycin D, each at 400 µg/mL) to successive tubes. Mix and briefly preincubate tubes to 37°C in a heating block.

5. Start the polymerase reaction by adding 50-μL aliquots of HBV virion or core preparation to each tube.
6. Withdraw 10-μL samples at 15–20 min intervals for 2–4 h and spot directly onto glass microfiber or DE81 paper disks prewet with 10% (w/v) TCA and 10 m*M* of sodium pyrophosphate.
7. Allow the disks to dry at room temperature, then wash once with cold 10% (w/v) TCA, 10 m*M* of sodium pyrophosphate, and then again at least five more times with cold 5% (w/v) TCA and 10 m*M* of sodium pyrophosphate and, finally, once with cold 95% ethanol.
8. Dry the disks and count in a liquid scintillation counter (*see* **Note 1**). The plot of radioactivity incorporated vs reaction time should be linear for at least 1.5–2 h and plateau after 3–4 h. Actinomycin D at a concentration of 100 μg/mL should inhibit DDDP activity by >80% and RDDP by <20%; phosphonoformic acid at 100 μg/mL should strongly inhibit both DDDP and RDDP activities, but neither should be affected by 100 μg/mL of aphidicolin.

3.3.2. Screening Assay for Inhibitors of Endogenous HBV DNA Polymerase Activity and Determination of 50% Inhibitory Concentrations (IC_{50}s)

This assay is essentially the assay described in **Subheading 3.3.1.** split into sets of miniassays and stopped at a single time point. Alternative methods of assaying incorporation of radioactivity from labeled dNTP into HBV DNA are described in **steps 1–5**. Incorporation of radiolabel can be monitored either by scintillation counting or, alternatively, by densitometric or computer-assisted image analysis of autoradiographs after separation of labeled products by agarose gel electrophoresis. The latter method is more tedious and time-consuming, but is useful for confirming that label is incorporated into HBV genome-sized products. For autoradiography, the label used must be [^{32}P].

1. Mix HBV virion or core preparation with Nonidet-P40 and DTT at final concentrations of 0.4% and 40 m*M*, respectively, and incubate overnight at 4°C (as in **step 1** of **Subheading 3.3.1.**).
2. Mix equal volumes of polymerase buffer and substrate solution and dispense 10-μL aliquots into sets of microfuge tubes. (If required, mixture or aliquots may be stored frozen for later use.)
3. To each tube, add 5 μL of water (control) or aqueous solution containing known or potential inhibitors of HBV DDDP or RDDP. For initial screening of potential inhibitors of RDDP and DDDP activities, a single high inhibitor concentration can be used (*see* **Note 2**). For determination of IC_{50}s of dNTP analogs, add 5 μL of serial-halving dilutions in the range 100–0.0097 μ*M* (final concentrations 25–0.0024 μ*M*, a range extending ≈200–500 times on either side of the estimated K_ms for natural dNTPS) to a series of microfuge tubes. (If required, tubes may also be stored frozen for later use at this stage.)

4. Preincubate to 37°C, then initiate the polymerase reaction by adding 5-μL aliquots of HBV virion or core preparation to each tube.
5. Stop the reaction after 2 h (or predetermined incubation time—*see* **Subheading 3.3.1.**) by spotting the entire reaction mix from each tube onto glass microfiber or DE81 paper disks wetted with 10 m*M* of sodium pyrophosphate, 10% (w/v) TCA. Continue processing the disks as described in **steps 7** and **8** of **Subheading 3.3.1.**

3.3.2.1. Screening Assay for Inhibitors of Endogenous HBV DNA Polymerase Activity: Assay by Agarose Gel Electrophoresis

1. Perform **steps 1–4** as described in **Subheading 3.3.2.**
2. Stop the reaction by adding 5 μL of 10% SDS, 10 μL of proteinase K, and 5 μL of 500 m*M* EDTA.
3. Digest the samples overnight at 37°C, and then dilute to 240 μL by adding 205 μL of 10 m*M* Tris-HCl, and 1 m*M* EDTA, pH 7.6. Mix and extract once with an equal volume of phenol:chloroform.
4. Remove the aqueous layer, add 10 μL of 5 *M* NaCl, and mix before adding 2 vol of absolute ethanol. Keep overnight at –20°C, and then pellet the precipitated DNA by centrifugation for 10 min at 12,000*g* in a microfuge.
5. Drain off the ethanol and redissolve pellets in water. Store at –80°C for subsequent electrophoresis.
6. Subject samples, together with suitable molecular size markers, to electrophoresis through 1.5% horizontal agarose slab gels in appropriate buffer. Gels should be fixed, dried, and autoradiographed. A radioactive product having apparent mol wt of ≈3.5 kb (corresponding to the relaxed circular form of HBV DNA) should be the main species detected. Autoradiographs can be analyzed using a scanning densitometer or computer-assisted image processor. Alternatively, gels may be analyzed for radioactvity directly by using a phosphorimager, if available. For extensive description of standard electrophoretic and autoradiographic techniques, *see* **ref.** *8*.

3.3.3. Determination of K_ms for dNTPs and K_is for dNTP Analogs or Other Inhibitors

K_ms and K_is may be determined using a modified assay of the type described in **Subheading 3.3.2.**

1. Mix HBV virion or core preparation with Nonidet-P40 and DTT at final concentrations of 0.4% and 40 m*M*, and incubate overnight at 4°C.
2. Mix equal volumes of polymerase buffer and kinetic substrate solution (containing only two cold dNTPs) and dispense 10-μL aliquots into a four separate sets of microfuge tubes. (If required, mixture or aliquots may be stored frozen for later use.)
3. Make up inhibitor solutions (dNTP analog or other inhibitor) at three or more different concentrations, each four times higher than the required final concentration. Prepare sets of serial-halving dilutions of the missing cold dNTP (suggested concentration range 100–0.0097 μ*M*, to give final concentrations of 25–0.0024 μ*M*) in these inhibitor solutions as well as a fourth set in water (*see* **Note 2**).

4. To each set of microfuge tubes set up in **step 2**, add 5 μL of one of the sets of dNTP ± inhibitor solutions prepared as described in **step 3** and mix. (If required, tubes may also be stored frozen for later use at this stage).
5. Preincubate all tubes to 37°C in a heating block, and then initiate the polymerase reaction by adding 5-μL aliquots of HBV virion or core preparation to each tube.
6. Stop the reaction after 2 h (or other predetermined incubation time), and then proceed as described in **Subheading 3.3.2.**
7. Alternatively, for assay using agarose gel electrophoresis, stop the reaction after 2 h (or other predetermined incubation time), and then proceed as described in **Subheading 3.3.2.1.**

3.4. Data Analysis

IC_{50}s can be easily estimated graphically from plots of incorporated radioactivity vs drug concentration; this can be done using any computer graphics program, many of which will also perform regression analyses and basic statistics (e.g., SigmaPlot from Jandel Scientific, San Rafael, CA). Kinetic data may be analyzed most easily with the aid of dedicated software programs, such as Enzyme Kinetics (Trinity Software, Campton, NH), or more sophisticated curve-fitting programs, such as TableCurve2D (Jandel Scientific), which are now readily available. Data analysis may be complicated because HBV polymerase assay reactions do not necessarily follow classical Michaelis-Menten kinetics (e.g., *see* **refs. *9*** and ***10***). For a detailed discussion of the principles and practice of enzyme assays and methods for determining kinetic parameters, *see* **ref. *1***.

4. Notes

1. Either [^{3}H]-dNTP (labeled on the purine or pyrimidine base) or α-[^{32}P]-dNTP may be used as the label. Both must be handled and disposed of appropriately. [^{3}H]-dNTP has the advantages of having a very long half-life and much less associated radiation hazard, but it requires liquid scintillation counting and is impractical for autoradiography. [^{3}H]-dNTPs are usually supplied as ethanolic solutions, and it is advisable to evaporate solvent by freeze drying immediately before use. Koch and Schlicht ***(12)*** correctly argue that the concentration of the labeled dNTP may be rate limiting or otherwise perturb kinetic measurements if a large excess of unlabeled dNTPs is used. They suggest using equimolar dNTP concentrations, but such a procedure has not been generally adopted, probably because it is impractical when α-[^{32}P] is used as the label.
2. Do not confuse dNTP "duo" and "trio" solutions. There is no generally accepted method for estimation of IC_{50}s, which may vary with dNTP concentration, even for inhibitors that are not dNTP analogs, and this conditions under which estimates are made need to be specified. For initial screening of dNTP analogs (final), concentrations 10- to 100-fold greater than that of the natural dNTP competitor are suggested. Some dNTP analogs (e.g., triphosphates of 2,6-diaminopurine and 5-methylcytosine derivatives) may have more than one natural competitor.

3. 2.2.15 cells can be adapted to grow in Dulbecco's modified Eagle's medium, which is more economical than RPMI. It is preferable to use efficient producers of HBV cores; different cell lines and different subclones of 2.2.15 cells vary widely in efficiency as producers of HBV cores. Geneticin (Gibco Life Technologies, Grand Island, NY; 500 μg/mL) may be added to the cell culture medium to select against the parent HepG2 cells *(7)*, which lack the HBV transfectant.
4. HBV virions and cores from infected sera and cells are potentially infectious for laboratory personnel, and samples should be handled according to prescribed institutional safety and containment guidelines and procedures. Similarly, precautions must be taken when handling phenol and chloroform, which are toxic.

References

1. Nassal, M. and Schaller, H. (1996) Hepatitis B virus replication—an update. *J. Viral Hepatitis* **3,** 217–226.
2. Shaw, T. and Locarnini, S. A. (1995) Hepatic purine and pyrimidine metabolism: implications for antiviral chemotherapy of viral hepatitis. *Liver* **15,** 169–184.
3. Oberhaus, S. M. and Newbold, J. E. (1996) In situ DNA polymerase and RNase H activity gel assays as applied to hepadnavirus particles. *Methods Enzymol.* **275,** 328–347.
4. Howe, A.Y. M., Elliott J. F., and Tyrrell, D. L. J. (1992) Duck hepatitis B virus polymerase produced by in vitro transcription and translation possesses DNA polymerase and reverse transcriptase activities. *Biochem. Biopyhs. Res. Commun.* **189,** 1170–1176.
5. Jeong, J. H., Kwak, D. S., Rho, H. M., and Jung, G. (1996) The catalytic properties of human hepatitis B virus polymerase. *Biochem. Biopyhs. Res. Commun.* **223,** 264–271.
6. Lanford, R. E., Notvall, L., and Beames, B. (1995) Nucleotide priming and reverse transcriptase activity of hepatitis B virus polymerase expressed in insect cells. *J. Virol.* **69,** 4431–4439.
7. Sells, M. A., Chen, M. L., and Acs, G. (1987) Production of hepatitis B virus particles in HepG2 cells transfected with cloned hepatitis B virus DNA. *Proc. Natl. Acad. Sci. USA* **75,** 4533–4537.
8. Moore, D. (1995) Preparation and analysis of DNA, in *Current Protocols in Molecular Biology,* vol. 1 (Absubel, F. M., Brent, R., Kingston, R. E., Moore, D. D., Siedman, J. G., Smith, J. A., and Struhl, K., eds.), Wiley, New York.
9. Shaw, T., Mok, S. S., and Locarnini, S. A. (1996) Inhibition of hepatitis B virus DNA polymerase by enantiomers of penciclovir triphosphate and metabolic basis for selective inhibition of HBV replication by penciclovir. *Hepatology* **24,** 996–1002.
10. Severini, A., Liu, X.-Y., Wilson, J. S., and Tyrrell, D. L. J. (1995) Mechanism of inhibition of duck hepatitis B virus polymerase by (–)-β-L-2',3'-dideoxy-3'-thiacytidine. *Antimicrob. Agents. Chemother.* **39,** 1430–1435.
11. Engel, P. C. (ed.) (1996) *Enzymology LABFAX.* Bios Scientific Publishers, Oxford, UK.
12. Kock, J. and Schlicht, H.-J. (1993) Analysis of the earliest steps of hepadnavirus replication: Genome repair after infectious entry into hepatocytes does not depend on viral polymerase activity. *J. Virol.* **67,** 4867–4874.

9

Development of a Hepatitis C Virus RNA Helicase High Throughput Assay

Ann D. Kwong and Christine Risano

1. Introduction

In this chapter, the development of a 96-well plate increasing signal helicase assay will be described. The authors have used this assay to detect inhibitors of hepatitis C virus (HCV) NS3/4A RNA helicase.

Detection of the unwound product (ssNA) in the high-throughput helicase assay is dependent on time, substrate, and enzyme concentration, and is prevented by the presence of an inhibitor. The assay format can utilize double-stranded DNA as well as RNA substrates, making the assay amenable to use with both DNA and RNA helicases. Traditional RNA or DNA helicase assays require separation of radiolabeled double-stranded substrate from unwound product by polyacrylamide gel electrophoresis (PAGE). Quantitation of a conventional helicase gel assay requires the use of a phosphorimager, or dissection of the radiolabeled separated substrate and displaced products from the dried gel and detection of associated cpm with a scintillation counter.

The 96-well plate helicase assay described in this method has several advantages over the traditional helicase assay: (1) the 96-well assay is a high-throughput assay—in a single afternoon, one person can easily screen (1–>1000) wells of compounds vs (1–<100) wells of compounds in a gel-based assay; and (2) the 96-well assay is easier and faster to quantitate than a conventional helicase assay.

1.2. Rationale for the Selection of HCV NS3 Helicase as a Target for Antiviral Drug Development

HCV is a positive-stranded RNA virus containing a linear RNA genome of approx 9.5 kb *(8)*. The HCV genome encodes a single large polyprotein of

From: *Methods in Molecular Medicine, vol. 24: Antiviral Methods and Protocols*
Edited by: D. Kinchington and R. F. Schinazi © Humana Press Inc., Totowa, NJ

approx 3010 amino acids. Proteolytic processing by both host signal peptidases and viral proteases results in at least 10 viral proteins in the following order: NH2-C-E1-E2-p7-NS2-NS3-NS4A-NS4B-NS5A-NS5B-COOH ***(2–4)***.

The NS3/4A protein complex is a multifunctional enzyme. The N-terminal domain of NS3 contains a serine protease that is required for polyprotein processing ***(5–7)***. The C-terminal ***(8,9)*** two-thirds of the NS3 protein contains both a helicase and a nucleic acid–stimulated NTPase activity ***(8,10–13)***. NS4A is a protein cofactor for protease activity and forms a tight, noncovalent complex with NS3. Interest in the HCV NS3as a target for antiviral drug development and structure-based drug design has been heightened by the recent descriptions of the structures of the NS3 serine protease domain in the absence ***(14)*** and presence ***(15)*** of a synthetic NS4A peptide activator and of the NS3 helicase domain ***(16)***.

The RNA helicase activity of the full-length NS3/4A enzyme ***(8)*** and of the NS3 C-terminal helicase domain has been demonstrated ***(10,11,17–19)*** by the unwinding of double-stranded RNA (dsRNA) molecules. The directionality of RNA helicase unwinding is 3' to 5' with respect to the template strand ***(8,19)***. Unlike most other helicases, the HCV NS3 helicase is capable of unwinding both RNA and DNA homoduplex and heteroduplex molecules ***(19)***. In common with other helicases, NS3 helicase requires divalent cations (Mg^{2+} or Mn^{2+}) in conjunction with the hydrolysis of nucleoside triphosphates (NTPs) to provide the energy source for unwinding ***(11,12)***.

For most viral helicases, not enough is known to define their role in the life cycle of the virus. The state of knowledge about virus-encoded RNA helicases has been recently reviewed ***(20)***. The essential genetic knockout mutants to test the essentiality of the HCV NS3 protease and helicase functions have not yet been reported. Until such experimental data become available, one can only speculate about possible roles for HCV NS3 helicase in viral replication. For example, RNA helicase activity may contribute to the efficiency of translation by denaturing secondary structure in the positive-strand RNA and increasing the efficiency of ribosome binding, similar to the mechanism of action proposed for eukaryotic initiation factors 4A and 4B ***(21)***. During RNA replication, RNA helicase may denature stable secondary structures in the HCV RNA genome such as the highly conserved 98 bp sequence (3'X tail) near the 3' end of the genome ***(22,23)*** and the internal ribosome entry site near the 5' nontranslated region of the genome ***(24,25)***. As shown in **Fig. 1,** we would expect at least two minimal enzymatic activities to be required for the replication of HCV RNA: (1) an RNA-dependent RNA polymerase, which catalyzes the formation of phosphodiester bonds between adjacent nucleotides; and (2) an RNA helicase, which separates the RNA strands of the intermediate negative-stranded RNA from the positive-stranded, genomic input RNA, and also

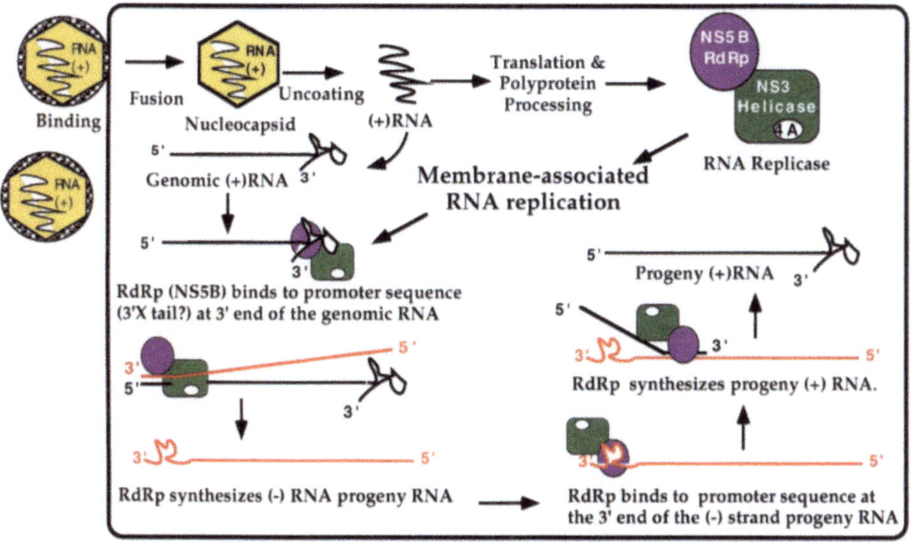

Fig. 1. Model for HCV RNA replication. The diagram shows the putative formation and function of the HCV replication complex that involves the RNA-dependent RNA polymerase (RdRp) together with the NS3/4A multifunctional enzyme. The RdRp catalyzes the formation of phosphodiester bonds between adjacent nucleotides, and the helicase separates the two RNA strands after synthesis.

separates the positive-stranded progeny RNA from the intermediate negative-stranded RNA template.

1.2. Helicase Assay Enzyme

The authors expressed and purified a *His*-tagged NS3/4A enzyme ***(26)*** for use in the helicase assay. Please note that the author's helicase assay is versatile and can be used be optimized for use with other DNA or RNA helicase enzymes.

1.3. Assay Concept and Design

Figure 2 is a schematic representation of the increasing signal high-throughput helicase assay. A substrate containing 3' single-stranded RNA (ssRNA) tails was chemically synthesized based on the sequence of the RNA helicase substrates produced by in vitro transcription reactions by Lee and Hurwitz ***(27)***. Large scale, reproducible chemical synthesis of RNA is restricted to oligonucleotides up to 36 nucleotides in length. Therefore, the 29-bp RNA duplex region in the standard RNA substrate of Lee and Hurwitz ***(27)*** was reduced to 21 bp, and the 41-nucleotide 3' overhang was reduced to 15 nucleotides, as shown in **Fig. 2**. The substrate was designed to be labeled in a strand-specific

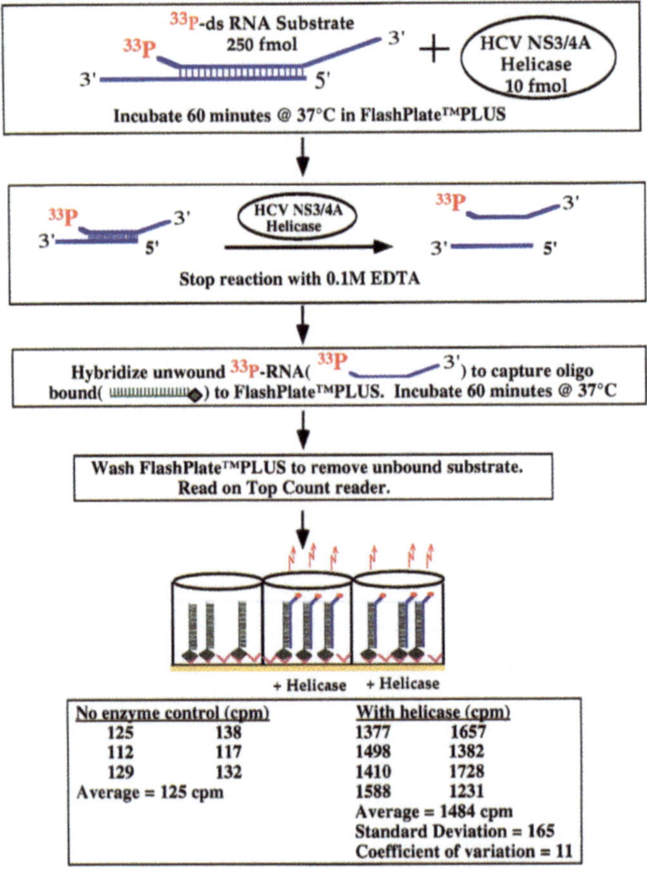

No enzyme control (cpm)		With helicase (cpm)	
125	138	1377	1657
112	117	1498	1382
129	132	1410	1728
Average = 125 cpm		1588	1231
		Average = 1484 cpm	
		Standard Deviation = 165	
		Coefficient of variation = 11	

Fig. 2. Flowchart of the HCV RNA helicase high-throughput assay. The diagram shows the major steps in the assay. A representative example of data obtained from the assay is shown at the bottom of the diagram.

manner so that only the 5' end of the upper strand can be end-labeled with ^{32}P or ^{33}P by the action of T4 polynucleotide kinase. The labeled ssRNA is released from the dsRNA substrate by the unwinding action of the HCV NS3/4A enzyme, or by boiling or heating the dsRNA at 95°C for 30 min. After the helicase reaction is stopped by chelating the Mg^{2+} in the reaction with ethylenediaminetetra-acetic acid (EDTA), the released radiolabeled ssRNA is hybridized to complementary biotinylated DNA oligonucleotides (capture oligo), which are bound to a 96-well plate (FlashPlate™PLUS, NEN Research Products, Boston, MA). The wells are washed to remove unbound substrate, and the signal is read on a TopCount (Packard, Meridan, CT) scintillation counter. In the absence of enzyme, the back

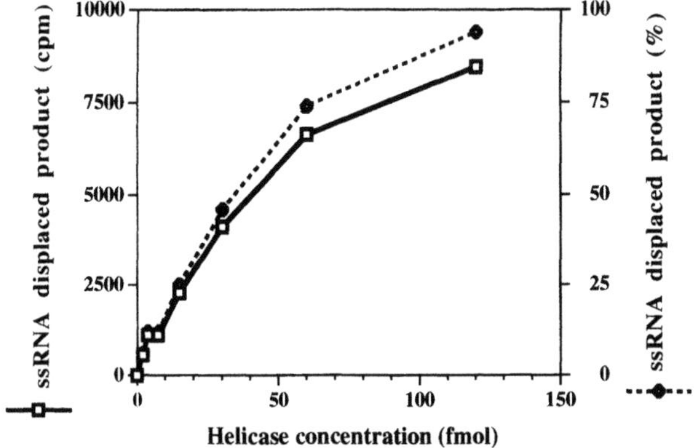

Fig. 3. Helicase titration. Enzyme was as described in **Subheading 3.** Triplicate values for each time point were averaged. Both cpm and percent displacement values are shown.

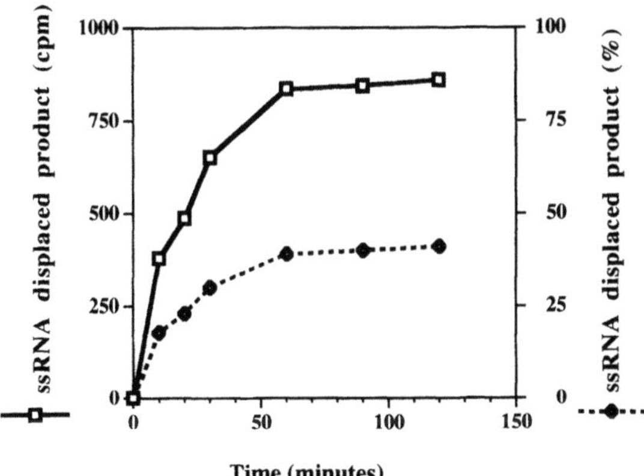

Fig. 4. Time course of the helicase reaction. Fifteen fmol of enzyme was incubated with 250 fmol of substrate for the periods of time indicated. Triplicate values for each time point were averaged. Both cpm and percent displacement values are shown.

ground cpm is low, but the addition of enzyme increases the signal to more than 10-fold above background.

The HCV helicase assay is linearly dependent on enzyme concentration up to 60 fmol with 250 fmol of dsRNA substrate (**Fig. 3**). The optimal time of incubation for the assay was determined by a time course experiment. Capture oligomer-coated FlashPlatePLUS wells containing 250 fmol of dsRNA and 10 fmol of helicase per reaction were incubated at 37°C, with stop solution being added at the time points shown in **Fig. 4**. The formation of ssRNA product as measured by cpm or graphed as percent of displaced ssRNA product was linearly dependent on time up to 60 min. Based on these data, 250 fmol of dsRNA substrate, 10 fmol of enzyme, and a 60-min incubation time were selected for use in the high-throughput assay.

Because the HCV RNA helicase has been shown to unwind various double-stranded nucleic acid (dsNA) substrates *(19)*, titrations of the enzyme were made utilizing RNA/RNA, RNA/DNA, DNA/RNA, and DNA/DNA standard substrates prepared as described by Lee and Hurwitz *(27)*. Helicase enzyme reactions were prepared in capture oligomer-coated FlashPlatePLUS wells, using 25 fmol of each substrate and a 60-min incubation time at 37°C. Following removal of the reaction mixes and wash buffers, the plates were read on a TopCount scintillation counter (Packard) (**Fig. 5E**). Replicate reactions were incubated in Eppendorf tubes for 60 min at 37°C, stopped with RNA loading buffer, and subjected to PAGE analysis (**Fig. 5A–D**). Similar results were obtained in both assays, indicating that the high-throughput helicase assay format is versatile enough to detect both DNA and RNA helicase activity and that can substitute for the traditional gel-based assay.

To assess the feasibility of using the FlashPlatePLUS system to detect inhibitors of helicase activity, several known known inhibitors of the helicase reaction were tested. These included ATP-γS, a nonhydrolyzable analog of ATP which prevents the ATPase function of the NS3 protein from providing energy for the unwinding of the duplex substrate (**Fig. 6A**); polyuridilic acid (poly U), which competes with the substrate for RNA binding (**Fig. 6B**); and EDTA, which chelates the divalent cation (Mg^{2+} or Mn^{2+}) required from in the reaction (**Fig. 6C**). All three compounds inhibited the helicase reaction in a dose-dependent fashion, demonstrating that this assay can be used to compare inhibitors quantitatively and thus derive IC_{50} measurements.

2. Materials

2.1. RNA and DNA Oligomers

1. The duplex RNA substrate is custom made by Oligos Etc. Inc. (Wilsonville, OR). The underlined portion of substrate sequences shows the area of duplex formation. Aliquot and store in RNA resuspension buffer (buffer I) at –80°C.

   Template: 5'PO4-<u>GCU CGC CCG GGG AUC CUC UAG</u> GAA UAC ACG UUC GAU-3'PO_4
   Primer: 5'HO-<u>CUA GAG GAU CCC CGG GCG AGC</u> CCU AUA GUG AGU CGU-3'PO_4

2. The capture DNA oligomer custom is made by Life Technologies (Gibco-BRL, Gaithersburg, MD). Resuspend oligo in 1 µg/µL of capture oligo binding buffer (buffer II) and store in aliquots at –20°C.
   Capture oligo: 5'-biotin-GCT CGC CCG GGG ATC CTC TAG-3'

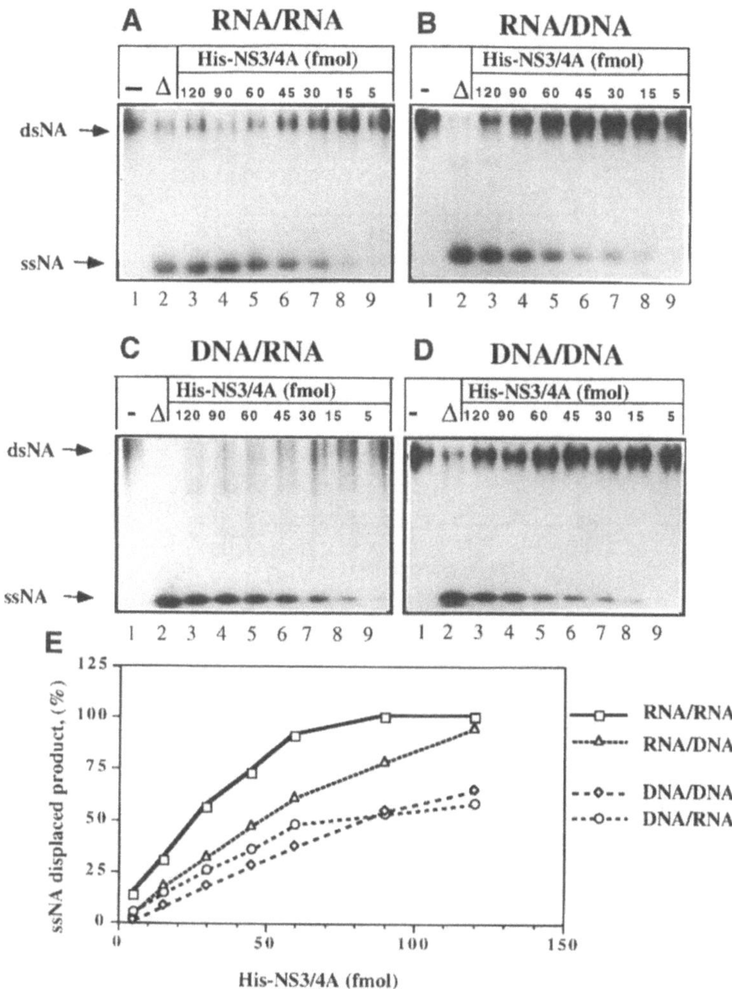

Fig. 5. The helicase high-throughput assay can detect both DNA and RNA unwinding activity and gives similar results to the traditional gel-based helicase assay. **(A–E)** Gel-based assay showing unwinding of RNA and DNA heteroduplex and homoduplex substrates by action of 5–120 fmol of HCV NS3/4A enzyme. The positions of the dsNA and ssNA are labeled.

2.2. Duplex Substrate Labeling and Purification

2.2.1. Duplex Substrate Labeling

1. dsRNA substrate (*see* **Subheading 2.1.**); store in buffer I at –80°C.
2. T4 polynucleotide kinase (T4 PNK) (Epicentre Technologies, Madison, WI); store at –20°C.

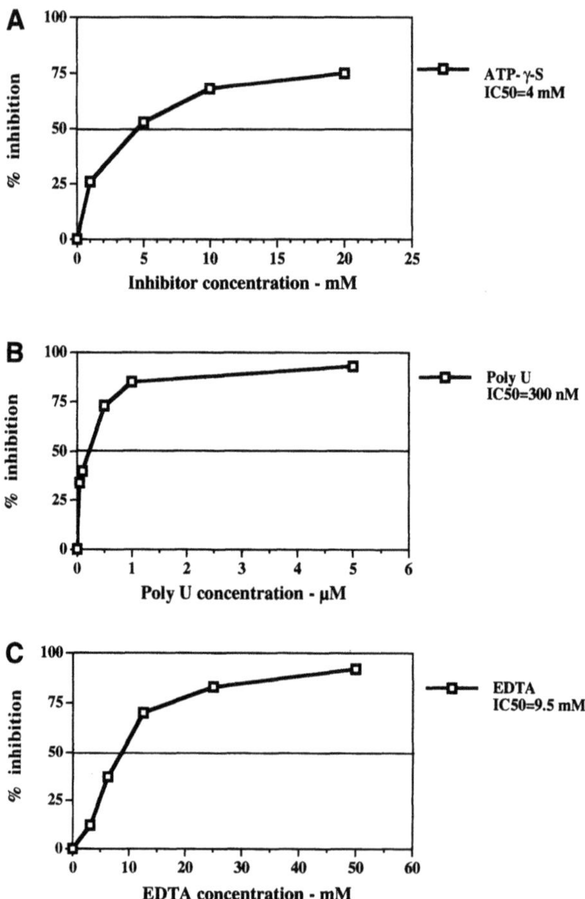

Fig. 6. Inhibitors of the helicase assay reaction. **(A)** ATP-γ-S, a nonhydrolyzable ATPase inhibitor; **(B)** poly U, which competes for RNA binding; **(C)** EDTA, which chelates Mg^{2+}. The assay was performed using 15 fmol of enzyme and 250 fmol of dsRNA substrate. Data from triplicate wells were averaged for all values.

3. 10X PNK buffer (330 m*M* Tris-acetate, pH 7.8, 660 m*M* K-acetate, 100 m*M* Mg-acetate, 5 m*M* dithiothreitol [DTT]) (Epicentre Technologies); store at –20°C.
4. [γ-^{32}P]-ATP (RediVue, NEN™ Life Science Products); store at 4°C.
5. [γ-^{33}P]-ATP (RediVue); store at 4°C.
6. 1 *M* $MgCl_2$ (molecular biology grade, Sigma, St. Louis, MO); store at room temperature.
7. Glycogen, 20 mg/mL (molecular biology grade, Boehringer Mannheim Biochemica, Indianapolis, IN); store at –20°C.
8. RNA precipitation buffer (buffer VII): 1 *M* NH_4-acetate, 0.2% sodium dodecyl sulfate (SDS), 2 m*M* EDTA. Warm at 37°C prior to use if the SDS precipitates; store at room temperature.

9. Buffered phenol (RNA molecular biology grade, Sigma); store at 4°C.
10. Chloroform: 2% isoamyl alcohol (24:1) (molecular biology grade, Sigma); store at room temperature.
11. 200-proof ethanol; store at –20°C.

2.2.2. Duplex Substrate Purification

1. dsRNA substrate (*see* **Subheading 2.1.**); store in buffer I at –80°C.
2. ^{32}P-labeled dsRNA; store in buffer I in acrylic-shielded, β radiation storage container at -80°C.
3. Polyacrylamide:bis solution (30:0.8), (30% solution, Owl Scientific, Woburn, MA); store at 4°C.
4. 5X TBE: 445 m*M* Tris, 445 m*M* boric acid, 10 m*M* EDTA, pH 8.0; store at room temperature.
5. NH_4 persulfate, 1 mg/mL (Bio-Rad, Hercules, CA); make up fresh as needed in H_2O.
6. TEMED (*N,N,N',N'*-tetramethylethylenediamine, Bio-Rad); store at room temperature.
7. 5X Native RNA loading buffer: 0.1 *M* Tris-HCl, pH 7.5, 5 m*M* EDTA, 0.1% bromophenol blue dye, 0.1% xylene cyanol dye, 0.1% Nonidet P-40, 50% glycerol; store at room temperature.
8. Gel electrophoresis apparatus (Owl Scientific or equivalent) and blank glass gel cassettes. Use 15 × 15-cm^2 gels and 1.5-mm-thick combs and spacers for large-scale purification. Otherwise, use 0.75-mm combs and spacers or smaller (the thinner the gel, the higher the yield of gel-purified RNA).
9. X-ray film for autoradiography.
10. Glycogen, 20 mg/mL (molecular biology grade, Boehringer Mannheim Biochemica); store at –20°C.
11. Disposable pestles for 1.5-mL microfuge tubes (Kontes, Vineland, NJ).
12. Bio-Rad Econo-Column™ (cat. no. 731-1550).
13. RNA extraction buffer (buffer VI): 500 m*M* NH_4OAc, 0.1% SDS, 10 m*M* EDTA; store at room temperature.
14. RNA resuspension buffer (buffer I): 20 m*M* HEPES, pH 7.3), 50 m*M* KCl, 0.1 m*M* EDTA, 0.05% Nonidet P-40. Add 0.4 U/μL RNase Block (Stratagene, La Jolla, CA) immediately prior to use.

2.3. Helicase Enzyme

1. Both RNA and DNA helicases can be used in this assay format.
2. In these studies, a *His*-tagged form of the HCV NS3/4A helicase was used ***(26)***. All enzyme aliquots in enzyme dilution buffer (buffer III) were stored at –80°C.

2.4. 96-Well Plates and Scintillation Reader

1. FlashPlatePLUS, store at 4°C.
2. TopCount scintillation reader (Packard A991200).

2.5. Buffers

Make all buffers with RNase-free H_2O.

1. Buffer I (RNA resuspension buffer): 20 m*M* HEPES (pH 7.3), 50 m*M* KCl, 0.1 m*M* EDTA, 0.05% Nonidet P-40; store at 4°C. Add 0.4 U/µL RNase Block immediately prior to use.
2. Buffer II (capture oligo binding buffer): 25 m*M* Tris-HCl (pH 8.0), 25 m*M* NaCl, 20% glycerol, 1 mg/mL bovine serum albumin (BSA) (Fraction V); store at 4°C.
3. Buffer III (enzyme dilution buffer): 20 m*M* HEPES (pH 7.3), 10% glycerol, 0.1% Nonidet P-40, 100 µg/mL BSA (FractionV); store at 4°C.
4. Buffer IV (helicase hybridization buffer): 40 m*M* HEPES (pH 7.3), 2 *M* NaCl, 2 mg/mL BSA (Fraction V); store at 4°C.
5. Buffer V (wash buffer): 20 m*M* HEPES (pH 7.3), 1.5 m*M* NaCl, 1.5 m*M* Na citrate, 0.05% SDS; store at room temperature.
6. Buffer VI (RNA extraction buffer): 500 m*M* NH_4OAc, 0.1% SDS, 10 m*M* EDTA; store at room temperature.
7. Buffer VII (RNA precipitation buffer): 1 *M* NH_4OAc, 0.2% SDS, 2 m*M* EDTA; store at room temperature if the SDS precipitates warm at 37°C before use.

2.6. Helicase Reaction Mix Stock Solutions

Make all solutions with RNase-free H_2O.

1. 500 m*M* PIPES (pH 6.0); store at room temperature.
2. 100 m*M* $MgCl_2$; store at room temperature.
3. 100 m*M* adenosine triphosphate (ATP), dissolve ATP (Boehringer Mannheim Biochemica) in 20 m*M* HEPES (pH 7.3) and neutralize the pH to 7.0 with NaOH; store at –20°C.
4. 100 m*M* DTT; store at –20°C.
5. 10 mg/mL BSA (Fraction V): Dissolve in 20 m*M* Tris (pH 8.0) and heat inactivate for 30 min at 55°C; store at 4°C.
6. 1 U/µL RNase Prime Inhibitor (5 Prime → 3 Prime, Inc., Boulder, CO); store at –20°C.

2.7. Miscellaneous Stocks and Solutions

1. RNase-free H_2O; store at room temperature.
2. 10% DMSO (make fresh).
3. 0.5 *M* EDTA (pH 8.0); store at room temperature.
4. 10% SDS; store at room temperature.
5. 5 *M* NaCl; store at room temperature.
6. Chloroform:2% isoamyl alcohol (24:1) (molecular biology grade); store at room temperature.
7. Dulbecco's phosphate-buffered saline (PBS); store at room temperature.
8. Buffered phenol (RNA molecular biology grade, Sigma); store at 4°C.
9. Nonidet P-40 (10% enzyme grade solution, Calbiochem, La Jolla, CA); store at –20°C.
10. 200-Proof ethanol; store at –20°C.

3. Methods

3.1. Overview of Radioactive Labeling, Gel Extraction, and RNA Substrate Preparation

The dsRNA substrate used in this high-throughput helicase assay is designed to be easily labeled in a strand-specific manner to a high specific activity with ^{32}P or ^{33}P. This is achieved by designing the RNA substrate so that only the RNA primer strand contains a 5'-OH that would be radiolabeled with [γ-^{32}P]. ATP or [γ-^{33}P]-ATP and T4 PNK. Any contaminating unannealed ssRNA primer in the RNA substrate mix is also labeled and anneals to the capture oligo in the assay plate, resulting in an unacceptably high level of background cpm. Despite the fact that contaminating template ssRNA does not lead to background noise in the assay, the ssRNA competes with the radiolabeled dsRNA substrate for RNA binding to the helicase, resulting in a lower efficiency of substrate unwinding. Therefore, the authors recommend gel purification of the annealed dsRNA substrate from contaminating ssRNA in the crude mixture.

Before gel purification, the percent of the mixture annealed (dsRNA substrate) should be determined. A small amount (usually 200 pmol by OD) of the crude unpurified substrate is end-labeled with ^{32}P and electrophoresed in a 15% polyacrylamide gel. The gel is dried onto Whatman DEAE paper, and the radiolabeled RNA bands are visualized by autoradiography. Determine the amount of label in the dsRNA and ssRNA bands using a phosphorimager, or cut the bands out of the dried gel using the autoradiograph as a template and measure the amount of label incorporated into each band with a scintillation counter. Use this data to calculate the percent of the mixture that is dsRNA. This number is used to determine the yield of purified dsRNA.

For gel purification, 200–400 pmol of ^{32}P-labeled RNA crude mixture is mixed as a tracer with 40,000 pmol of unlabeled crude substrate. Measure the radioactivity of a small aliquot of the mixture in a scintillation counter to calculate the specific activity of the RNA. The dsRNA and ssRNA in the crude mix are separated by electrophoresis in a preparative 8% polyacrylamide gel. After visualization by autoradiography, the region of the acrylamide gel containing the dsRNA is excised with a razor blade and the RNA is extracted from the gel. After gel purification, the dsRNA substrate is suspended in buffer I, and the radioactivity of an aliquot is measured on the scintillation counter. From the specific activity of the dsRNA, the amount of gel-extracted substrate can be determined. This is called the "cold" substrate because the specific activity is lower than that of the "hot" substrate, which is freshly labeled with ^{33}P for use in the assay. Since a small amount of the purified dsRNA is labeled with ^{32}P, aliquots of gel-purified "cold" substrate should be stored in an acrylic β-radiation storage container until they the radiation has decayed with time.

Gel-purified dsRNA is labeled with ^{33}P for use as a substrate in the high-throughput assay. ^{33}P-labeled substrate has a lower background and a longer half life than substrate labeled with ^{32}P. For secondary assays confirmation of "hits" in the high throughput, 96-well plate primary assay, gel-purified dsRNA substrate is labeled to a high specific activity with ^{32}P for use in a gel-based assay.

3.2. Radioactive Labeling of the RNA Substrate

1. The method in this section is used to label the crude, unpurified RNA mix-ture with ^{32}P prior to gel purification. To label the gel-purified dsRNA with for assay use, substitute the [γ-^{32}P]-ATP with [γ-^{33}P]-ATP in the T4 PNK labeling reaction.
2. Resuspend the annealed (template + primer) crude RNA substrate by OD to 200 pmol/mL in buffer I. Use siliconized Eppendorf tubes and keep all reagents and reactions on ice.
3. In a siliconized 1.5-mL Eppendorf tube, combine the following: 20 µL of 10X PNK buffer, 1 µL of 200 pmol dsRNA, (200 pmol/µL crude RNA stock), 100 µL of 1 mCi [γ-^{32}P]-ATP, 10 µL of T4 PNK, and 69 µL of RNase-free H_2O.
4. Mix and incubate the 200 mL reaction at 37°C for 90 min
5. Spin the reaction down briefly in a microfuge, and add: 3 µL of 1 *M* $MgCl_2$, 2 µL of glycogen (20 mg/mL), and 200 µL of buffer VII.
6. Vortex briefly, spin down in a microfuge and add: 200 µL of phenol and 200 µL chloroform:isoamyl alcohol (24:1).
7. Vortex briefly and spin in a microfuge. Note the color change of the lower organic layer from orange to pink. Transfer the yellow aqueous upper layer to a fresh siliconized Eppendorf tube. Discard the lower layer to radioactive phenol waste. Monitor with a Geiger counter; typically approx 0.1 mCi of the label is discarded in the waste.
8. Add 1.0 mL of ice-cold 200-proof EtOH to the aqueous yellow sample. Freeze in dry ice for 15 min, and spin for 30 min at 4°C in a microfuge. Aspirate the supernatant carefully, removing the liquid immediately above the white RNA precipitant with a 200-µL pipet tip.
9. Gently wash the pellet with 1 mL of ice-cold ethanol and repellet in the microfuge for 30 min at 4°C. Carefully remove the ethanol wash (the second pellet is usually very soft), and dry the pellet in a Speed-Vac (Savant Instruments, Inc., Holbrook, NY) at medium heat for 15 min.
10. Resuspend the crude RNA pellet in 25 µL of Buffer I. Use a Geiger counter to check that all of the labeled RNA has dissolved in solution by pulling up all the liquid into a pipet tip and comparing the counts in the tip with the counts remaining in the tube. Store in an appropriately shielded radioactive safety container at –80°C.
11. To make hot substrate for the assay, label 200-pmol aliquots of the gel-purified substrate with [γ-^{33}P]-ATP and T4 PNK. Resuspend the ^{33}P-labeled substrate in 200 µL of buffer I and store at –80°C.

3.3. Gel Purification of Duplex RNA Substrate

1. Pour an 8% polyacrylamide gel in 0.5X TBE buffer. For a 15 × 15 cm preparative gel with 1.5-mm spacers, mix 13.3 mL of 30% bis-polyacrylamide (0.8:30), 5.0 mL of 5X TBE, 20.7 mL of 1 mg/mL $(NH_4)_2SO_4$, and 31.0 mL of H_2O.
2. Remove 5.0 mL of the acrylamide mix, add 25 µL of TEMED and pour a plug at the bottom of the gel.
3. After the plug has hardened, add 50 µL of TEMED to the remainder of the acrylamide solution and pour the gel, inserting a 1.5-mm comb with 10 large wells.
4. Prepare the crude RNA substrate to load on the gel using 50 µL of 400 pmol ^{32}P-labeled crude RNA (8 pmol/µL), 400 µL of (2 labeling reactions) 80,000 pmol crude RNA substrate (200 pmol/µL), and 150 µL of 5X native RNA loading buffer.
5. Remove a 2-µL aliquot, and measure the radioactivity in a scintillation counter to determine the specific activity of the dsRNA substrate in the crude RNA mixture.
6. Rinse out the wells with 0.5X TBE electrophoresis buffer, and divide the crude RNA mixture between the 10 wells. Run the gel in 0.5X TBE buffer at 20 mA for 3 h. The dsRNA substrate usually runs between the xylene cyanol and bromophenol blue dye. Do not run the bromophenol blue out of the gel.
7. Stop the gel and separate the glass plates so that the gel adheres to one plate. Carefully cover the plate holding the gel with Saran Wrap and mark the location of the xylene cyanol and bromophenol blue markers with fluorescent markers. In a darkroom, develop 10–30-s autoradiographic exposures of the wrapped gel so that the RNA bands and the markers are clearly visible on the X-ray film.
8. Place an autoradiograph of the gel on a light box as a template. Position the wrapped gel plate over the template, lining up the markers. Outline the position of the dsRNA substrate in each lane of the gel on the Saran Wrap with a marker. Cut each lane of the dsRNA band from the gel, and place in a separate siliconized 1.5-mL Eppendorf tube.
9. Crush each gel slice with a Kontes 1.5-mL tube pestle, using a pipet tip to maneuver the ground acrylamide back to the bottom of the tube. Add 500 µL of buffer IV and crush the gel again with the pestle. Add 500 µL more of buffer IV, close the tube tightly, vortex for 2 min, and rotate end over end at room temperature overnight.
10. Transfer all the tubes of the acrylamide slurry to a disposable 5.0-mL Bio-Rad Econocolumn and collect the combined supernatants by gravity flow. Rinse the crushed gel in the tube with 1.0 mL of buffer IV. The crushed gel pieces should be clear, and the supernatant with the extracted RNA will be blue. Most of the radioactivity should be in the supernatant.
11. Add 100 µg of glycogen carrier to the supernatant, and distribute 0.75 mL into 2.0-mL siliconized microfuge tubes. Add 1 vol (0.75 mL) of ice-cold ethanol and mix. Freeze in dry ice for 15 min, and spin for 30 min at 4°C in a microfuge. Aspirate the supernatant carefully, removing the last bit with a 200-µL pipet tip. Dry the pellet in a Speed-Vac at medium heat for 15 min.

12. Resuspend the gel-purified dsRNA pellet in each tube with 100 µL of buffer I by vortexing for 2 min. Spin in the microfuge and use a Geiger counter to check that all of the labeled RNA has dissolved into solution, by pulling up the liquid into a pipet tip and comparing the counts in the tip with the counts remaining in the tube. Combine the RNA fractions and measure the radioactivity of a small aliquot in a scintillation counter. Use the specific activity of the RNA loaded on the gel to determine the concentration of purified dsRNA. Aliquot and store in an appropriately shielded radioactive safety container at –80°C.

3.4. High-Throughput Helicase Assay

3.4.1. Overview of Helicase Assay Setup

1. Prepare the assay plates at least 12 h before the assay is to be performed by binding the capture oligo to the FlashPlatePLUS wells.
2. The helicase reaction is set up in four parts: First, the RNA substrate hot mix is prepared. Second, 10-µL aliquots of the inhibitors to be tested are added to the capture oligo-coated FlashPlatePLUS wells. Third, 20 µL of reaction buffer containing the ^{33}P-dsRNA substrate is added to each well. Fourth, 20 µL of helicase in buffer III is added, and the reaction is incubated at 37°C.
3. After the helicase reaction is stopped by adding EDTA, buffer IV is added to promote annealing of the displaced ssRNA product to the capture oligo bound to the wells.
4. Finally, the wells are thoroughly washed to remove unbound substrate and the plates are read in a TopCount scintillation counter.

3.4.2. Binding of Capture Oligomer to FlashPlates

1. Dilute the capture oligomer to 50 pmol/mL in buffer II. Place 100 µL of this dilution (5 pmol) into each well of the 96-well FlashPlatePLUS. Return each plate to its Zip-Lock bag, and allow the capture oligo to bind overnight at 25°C. Store at 4°C until ready for use.
2. Immediately prior to use, remove the plate from the storage bag. Empty the wells by inversion, and wash three times with 200 µL of PBS per well. Thoroughly shake out the last wash, and pat the plate surface dry with a Kimwipe tissue.

3.4.3. Distribution of Inhibitor Test Samples

1. Place 10 µL of test inhibitor samples in FlashPlatePLUS wells to which capture oligo has been bound. Reserve wells for substrate alone, substrate plus enzyme, and positive controls. Add 10 µL of sample solvent, e.g., 10% DMSO, to the substrate and substrate plus enzyme control wells.

3.4.4. Preparation of RNA Substrate Hot Mix

1. The ratio of ^{33}P-labeled "hot" to "cold" dsRNA substrate in the RNA substrate hot mix in the assay is empirically determined and dependent on several factors. As a batch of hot substrate ages, more RNA substrate hot mix must be added to

Table 1
Preparation of Helicase Assay Mix

Final concentration (for a 50 µL-reaction)	Reaction mix stock solution	Volume (1 well/reaction)
100 m*M* PIPES, pH 6.0	500 m*M* PIPES, pH 6.0	10.0 µL
1 m*M* $MgCl_2$	100 m*M* $MgCl_2$	0.5 µL
1 m*M* ATP	100 m*M* ATP	0.5 µL
2 m*M* DTT	100 m*M* DTT	1.0 µL
1 U RNase inhibitor	1 U/mL prime RNase inhibitor	1.0 µL
5 mg BSA	10 mg/mL BSA	0.5 µL
250 fmol RNA substrate hot mix	1 fmol/µL ^{33}P-RNA substrate hot mix	2.5 µL
RNase-free H_2O	RNase-free H_2O	4.0 µL

the mixture owing to decay of the ^{33}P signal (half life = 25.4 d). Also, an assay designed to detect 10% displaced product will require a higher specific activity of substrate than an assay with a 50% displacement end point. The major factors affecting the product formation are the length of reaction time and enzyme concentration. With any given enzyme concentration and incubation time, the signal in the assay can be increased by increasing the amount of hot substrate in the mix. In this assay, the substrate ratio is adjusted so that a signal of 1000–1500 cpm can be detected over a background of 100–150 cpm using conditions resulting in 30% product formation. Depending on the age of the hot substrate, the ratio can range from 1:10 to 1:4, hot:cold in the 250-fmol substrate added to the reaction. The final concentration of the hot:cold mix of substrate is 100 fmol/µL.

3.4.5. Preparation of Helicase Assay Mix

1. The final volume of the helicase assay is 50 µL/well. Twenty microliters is contributed by the helicase assay mix, which is prepared as in **Table 1**.

3.4.6. Addition of Enzyme to Helicase Assay

1. Thaw and keep all enzyme dilutions on ice while setting up the assay reactions. Add enzyme as the last step in the assay.
2. The concentration of enzyme in the assay is empirically determined to obtain the best signal-to-noise ratio as well as the greatest sensitivity to inhibitors. Enzyme titrations are performed to determine the least amount of helicase that can unwind enough labeled ssRNA to give a signal (cpm) that is at least 10-fold over background. This corresponds to approx 10 fmol of His-NS3/4A enzyme. This enzyme concentration is able to displace ~20–30% of the ssRNA from the substrate. The signal (cpm) corresponding to 100% displacement is obtained by heating the substrate alone at 95°C for 30 min and processing it in the helicase assay.

3. The assay enzyme is prepared by diluting the concentrated enzyme stock to 500 fmol/mL in buffer III and adding 20 μL/reaction.
4. After adding the enzyme to the helicase assay, seal the wells of the FlashPlate-PLUS plates with the sealer tape that is provided with the plates. Mix gently and incubate at 37°C for 60 min.

3.4.7. Termination of the Helicase Assay and Hybridization of the Product to the Capture Oligo

1. Stop the reaction by adding 10 μL of 0.5 *M* EDTA to each well.
2. After stopping the reaction, add 60 μL of buffer IV per well to promote hybridization of the ssRNA product to the capture oligo bound to the FlashPlatePLUS plates. Reseal the plates, mix gently, and incubate at 37°C for 60 min.

3.4.8. Washing and Reading the Helicase Assay Plates

1. Remove the hybridized reaction mixtures and dispense into radioactive waste. Wash the wells three times with 200 μL of buffer V and reseal the plates.
2. Read the assay results with a TopCount scintillation counter that has been normalized for ^{33}P.
3. Calculate the percent displacement of a control reaction without inhibitor and the percent inhibition of the test compounds in the assay.

4. Notes

4.1. Radioactive Labeling of the RNA Substrate

1. Follow all appropriate radiation safety regulations when labeling and working with the substrate. Use a shield for ^{32}P β-radiation, and monitor gloves and all labeled reagent transfers with a Geiger counter. Change gloves frequently. The vacuum system for the aspirator and Speed-Vac should have two liquid traps to prevent radioactive contamination.
2. This protocol will label the 200 pmol of crude RNA substrate to a high specific activity: typically >99% of the label is incorporated. With this degree of radioactiviy, the audio signal on the Geiger counters will be overwhelmed if the tube is held too close to the detector. Hold the tubes at least 6 in. away from the detector to get a more accurate reading.
3. A good stopping point in the end-labeling reaction is the ethanol precipitation step after the phenol/chloroform extraction. The RNA precipitation can be left at –20°C from an hour to overnight.
4. The addition of glycogen to the ethanol precipitation step after labeling and gel purification increases the recovery of the precipitated RNA. After ethanol precipitation, the white RNA pellet is easily displaced from the bottom of the tube if the tube is jostled or allowed to stand. Remove the supernatant immediately after the microfuge centrifugation is completed. Take special care with the second pellet from the ethanol wash—it seems to stick less well to the tube and often floats loose. If this happens, use a pipet tip and carefully remove the supernatant without sucking up the pellet—do not use the aspirator.

5. It is critical to monitor the preparation of each batch of ^{33}P-labeled substrate by measuring the specific activity using a scintillation counter. A significant drop in specific activity is caused by a decrease in activity of the T4 PNK.

4.2. Gel Purification of Duplex RNA Substrate

6. High purity of the dsRNA substrate is essential. The presence of any contaminating ssRNA primer strands will result in high background readings. Because there is no way to measure the amount of unannealed ssRNA template in the crude mix, the annealing reaction for the dsRNA substrate should always have a slight excess of ssRNA primer to template.
7. After gel purification, the dsRNA substrate should be validated using a gel-based assay, as well as the 96-well plate assay. The gel-based assay requires ^{32}P-labeled substrate for autoradiography. When ^{32}P-labeled substrate is used in the 96-well assay, care must be taken to use low amounts of radioactivity or to leave blank wells around the reactions owing to "^{32}P cross talk" between wells.
8. To calculate the specific activity of the labeled RNA and the yield of the dsRNA after purification, use the following example:
   a. If the amount of dsRNA in the crude mix = 67% and if the total amount of RNA (by OD) for purification = 800,400 pmol, then the amount of dsRNA in the crude mix = 536,268 pmol.
   b. If the total amount of label in the crude mix = 548,777,775 cpm (this is the typical amount of cpm obtained from 400 pmol of crude substrate labeled with ^{32}P), then the specific activity of the RNA = 548,777,775 cpm/800,400 pmol = 686 cpm/pmol.
   c. If the amount of label in the gel-extracted dsRNA = 110,147,250 cpm, then the amount of purified dsRNA = 110,147,250 cpm/686 cpm/pmol = 160,565 pmol, and the recovery of the gel-purified dsRNA = 160,565 pmol/536,268 pmol = 30%.

4.3. Binding of Capture Oligomer to FlashPlates

9. NEN™ Life Science Products, the manufacturer of the FlashPlatesPLUS, provides information for each lot concerning the amount of biotin per well required for saturation. The authors have found that using the saturation amount of biotinylated capture oligomer, e.g., 9 pmol/well, gives a lower efficiency of capture for the ssRNA primer compared with using one-half to one-third of the saturated biotin concentration. To determine the optimal concentration of capture oligo to use, titrate each new batch of capture oligo against 5 pmol of 100% displaced labeled substrate.

4.4. Distribution of Test Sample

10. Primary screening of chemical files and natural product extracts can be performed with single or multiple compounds/well. The decision to perform the primary screen as a single or multiple point assay will depend on a number of considerations such as the number of compounds to be screened and the consequences of

getting false negatives or positives in the assay. The authors usually run the secondary assays and IC_{50} titrations in triplicate. It is critical that the control reactions of enzyme alone recieve the same buffer in which the compounds are dissolved, such as 10% DMSO.

4.5. Preparation of Helicase Assay Mix

11. A sufficient amount of substrate and enzyme should be prepared ahead of time so that the batch does not change midway through the run of compound screening. It is also prudent to order a sufficient amount of FlashPlatesPLUS plates because batch to batch variability has been observed. Always run a small-scale activity assay to check the new batches of substrate and enzyme before using the reagents in a large-scale assay.
12. The volumes of the helicase reaction in the assay were dictated in part by the requirements of multichannel pipets and robotic equipment for quick and reproducible handling. Calculate the total amount of helicase reaction mix needed for each run of the assay and prepare one large batch. Factor in extra reactions to account for loss of the mix on pipet tips, tubes, and so on.

4.6. Addition of Enzyme to Helicase Assay

13. To assure uniformity in the assay aliquot, use as large a stock of enzyme as possible at one time. Thaw and keep all enzyme dilutions on ice while setting up the assay reactions. Always add enzyme as the last step in the assay.
14. Stability studies should be performed on the assay enzyme to delineate the parameters for safe handling to preserve enzymatic activity.

4.7. Termination of the Helicase Assay and Hybridization of the Product to the Capture Oligo

15. Multichannel Titerteks, or the equivalent, may be used for the addition of stop solution and hybridization buffer. Care must be taken to change tips between sets of replicate wells to avoid well-to-well contamination.
16. To obtain numbers corresponding to 100% displacement, the substrate in control reactions is heated at 95°C for 30 min in helicase assay reaction mix in a siliconized 1.5-mL microfuge tube. After a brief spin in the microfuge, the substrate is hybridized to capture oligo bound to 96-well plates and processed in the same manner as the enzyme reactions. The data (cpm) from the heated substrate control reactions correspond to 100% displacement of the substrate.
17. To calculate percent displacement and percent inhibition, data from wells containing substrate alone are averaged for each plate, and that background value is subtracted from all remaining data on that plate. Percent displacement values are achieved by dividing the averaged data from the substrate plus enzyme wells by the data corresponding to 100% displacement of the substrate as calculated in **Note 16**.
    a. To calculate percent displacement, use the following formula: % displacement = [cpm of the enzyme control (substrate + enzyme)]/[cpm of the substrate control (Δ @ 95°C)] × 100.

b. To calculate % inhibition use the following formula:% inhibition = 100 – [cpm of the (substrate + enzyme + inhibitor) × 100]/[cpm of the enzyme control (substrate + enzyme)].

References

1. Kaito, M., Watanabe, S., Tsukiyama-Kohara, K., Yamaguchi, K., Kobayashi, Y., Konishi, M., Yokoi, M., Ishida, S., Suzuki, S., and Kohara, M. (1994) Hepatitis C virus particle detected by immunoelectron microscopic study. *J. Gen. Virol.* **75,** 1755–1760.
2. Grakoui, A., Wychowski, C., Lin, C., Feinstone, S. M., and Rice, C. M. (1993) Expression and identification of hepatitis C virus polyprotein cleavage products. *J. Virol.* **67,** 1385–1395.
3. Hijikata, M., Kato, N., Ootsuyama, Y., Nakagawa, M., and Shimotohno, K. (1991) Gene mapping of the putative structural region of the hepatitis C virus genome by in vitro processing analysis. *Proc. Natl. Acad. Sci. USA* **88,** 5547–5551.
4. Lin, C., Pragai, B. M., Grakoui, A., Xu, J., and Rice, C. M. (1994) Hepatitis C virus NS3 serine proteinase: trans-cleavage requirements and processing kinetics. *J. Virol.* **68,** 8147–8157.
5. Bartenschlager, R., Ahlborn-Laake, L., Mous, J., and Jacobsen, H. (1993) Nonstructural protein 3 of the hepatitis C virus encodes a serine-type proteinase required for cleavage at the NS3/4 and NS4/5 junctions. *J. Virol.* **67,** 3835–3844.
6. Grakoui, A., McCourt, D. W., Wychowski, C., Feinstone, S. M., and Rice, C. M. (1993) Characterization of the hepatitis C virus-encoded serine proteinase: determination of the proteinase-dependent polyprotein cleavage sites. *J. Virol.* **67,** 2832–2843.
7. Tomei, L., Failla, C., Santolini, E., de Francesco, R., and La Monica, N. (1993) NS3 is a serine protease required for processing of hepatitis C virus polyprotein. *J. Virol.* **67,** 4017–4026.
8. Hong, Z., Ferrari, E., Wright-Minogue, J., Chase, R., Risano, C., Seelig, G., Lee, C.-G., and Kwong, A. D. (1996) Enzymatic characterization of hepatitis C virus NS3/4A complexes expressed in mammalian cells using the herpes simplex virus amplicon system. *J. Virol.* **70,** 4261–4268.
9. Kim, D. W., Gwack, Y., Han, J. H., and Choe, J. (1995) C-terminal domain of hepatitis C virus NS3 protein contains an RNA helicase activity. *Biochem. Biophys. Res. Comm.* **215,** 160–166.
10. Morgenstern, K. A., Landro, J. A., Hsiao, K., Lin, C., Yong, G., Su, M. S.-S., and Thomson, J. A. (1997) Polynucleotide modulation of the protease, nucleoside triphosphatase, and helicase activities of a hepatitis C virus NS3-NS4A complex isolated from transfected COS cells. *J. Virol.* **71,** 3767–3775.
11. Preugschat, F., Averett, D. R., Clarke, B. E., and Porter, D. J. T. (1996) A steady-state and pre-steady-state kinetic analysis of the NTPase activity associated with the hepatitis C virus NS3 helicase domain. *J. Biol. Chem.* **271,** 24,449–24,457.
12. Suzich, J. A., Tamura, J. K., Palmer-Hill, F., Warrener, P., Grakoui, A., Rice, C. M., Feinstone, S. M., and Collett, M. S. (1993) Hepatitis C virus NS3 protein

polynucleotide-stimulated nucleoside triphosphatase and comparison with the related pestivirus and flavivirus enzymes. *J. Virol.* **67,** 6152–6158.
13. Tamura, J. K., Warrener, P., and Collett, M. S. (1993) RNA-stimulated NTPase activity associated with the p80 protein of the pestivirus bovine viral diarrhea virus. *Virology* **193,** 1–10.
14. Love, R. A., Parge, H. E., Wickersham, J. A., Hostomsky, Z., Habuka, N., Moomaw, E. W., Adachi, T., and Hostomska, Z. (1996) The crystal structure of hepatitis C virus NS3 proteinase reveals a trypsin-like fold and a structural zinc binding site. *Cell* **87,** 331–342.
15. Kim, J. L., Morgenstern, K. A., Lin, C., Fox, T., Dwyer, M. D., Landro, J. A., Chambers, S. P., Markland, W., Lepre, C. A., O'Malley, E. T., Harbeson, S. L., Rice, C. M., Murcko, M. A., Caron, P. R., and Thomson, J. A. (1996) Crystal structure of the hepatitis C virus NS3 protease domain omplexed with a synthetic NS4A cofactor peptide. *Cell* **87,** 343–355.
16. Yao, N., Hesson, T., Cable, M., Hong, Z., Kwong, A. D., Le, H. V., and Weber, P. C. (1997) Structure of the hepatitis C virus RNA helicase domain. *Nat. Struc. Biol.* **4,** 463–467.
17. Jin, L. and Peterson, D. L. (1995) Expression, isolation, and characterization of the hepatitis C virus ATPase/RNA helicase. *Arch. Biochem. Biophys.* **323,** 47–53.
18. Kim, D. W., Gwack, Y., Hang, J. H., and Choe, J. (1997) Towards defining a minimal functional domain for NTPase and RNA helicase activities of the hepatitis C virus NS3 protein. *Virus Res.* **49,** 17–25.
19. Tai, C.-L., Chi, W.-K., Chen, D.-S., and Hwang, L.-H. (1996) The helicase activity associated with hepatitis C virus nonstructural protein 3 (NS3). *J. Virol.* **70,** 8477–8484.
20. Kadare, G. and Haenni, A.-L. (1997) Minireview: virus-encoded RNA helicases. *J. Virol.* **71,** 2583–2590.
21. Rozen, F., Edery, I., Meerovitch, K., Dever, T. E., Merrick, W. C., and Sonnenberg, N. (1990) Bidirectional RNA helicase activity of eucaryotic translation initiation factors 4A and 4F. *Mol. Cell. Biol.* **10,** 1134–1144.
22. Kolykhalov, A., Feinstone, S. M., and Rice, C. M. (1996) Identification of a highly conserved sequence element at the 3' terminus of Hepatitis C Virus genome RNA. *J. Virol.* **70,** 3363–3371.
23. Tanaka, T., Kato, N., Cho, M.-J., Sugiyama, K., and Shimotohno, K. (1996) Structure of the 3' terminus of the hepatitis C virus genome. *J. Virol.* **70,** 3307–3312.
24. Tsukiyama-Kohara, K., Lizuka, N., Kohara, M., and Nomoto, A. (1992) Internal ribosome entry site within hepatitis C virs RNA. *J. Virol.* **66,** 1476–1483.
25. Wang, C., Sarnow, P., and Siddiqui, A. (1993) Translation oif human hepatits C virus RNA in cultured cells is mediated by an internal ribosome-binding mechanism. *J. Virol.* **66,** 3338–3344.
26. Sali, D. L., Ingram, R., Wendel, M., Gupta, D., McNemar, C., Tsarbopoulos, A., Chen, J. W., Hong, Z., Chase, R., Risano, C., Zhang, R., Yao, N., Kwong, A. D., Ramanathan, L., Le, H. V., and Weber, P. C. (1998) Serine protease of hepatitis C virus expressed in insect cells as the NS3/4A complex. *Biochemistry* **37,** 3392–3401.
27. Lee, C.-G. and Hurwitz, J. (1992) A new RNA helicase isolated from HeLa cells that catalytically translocates in the 3' to 5' direction. *J. Biol. Chem.* **267,** 4398–4407.

II

Herpesvirus

10

Determination of Viral Infectivity

HSV, VZV, and CMV

David R. Harper

1. Introduction

Compared to the wide range of antibiotics that are available, the number of antiviral drugs is limited. However, herpesviruses have always been a major target for antiviral drug design, and there are a wide range of drugs at various stages of development. All of the assays described in this chapter provide relatively simple methods for plaque reduction assay of herpesviruses. Clearly, it is not possible to perform such assays on those herpesviruses that do not grow in adherent cells, such as Epstein-Barr virus. These require a different approach and are discussed elsewhere in this volume.

2. Materials

2.1. Reagents

1. 199: Medium 199 with Hank's salts, without L-glutamine.
2. 199X10: 10X strength Medium 199 with Hank's salts, without L-glutamine.
3. Acyclovir: Prepared as stock solution at 1–5 m*M* in water, stored at –20°C; use intravenous (sodium salt) formulation to aid solubility.
4. Agarose: Stock solution of 3% type II agarose in water.
5. Antibiotics: 10,000 U/mL penicillin G sodium salt plus 10 mg/mL streptomycin, as sulfate 6 salt.
6. Bicarbonate: 44 g sodium hydrogen carbonate, 8 g sodium chloride/L in high purity water, autoclaved.
7. CMC: Carboxymethyl cellulose sodium salt, 1% in water, dissolved by boiling or gentle autoclaving.

From: *Methods in Molecular Medicine, vol. 24: Antiviral Methods and Protocols*
Edited by: D. Kinchington and R. F. Schinazi © Humana Press Inc., Totowa, NJ

8. Crystal violet: 0.5% (w/v) crystal violet, 50% (v/v) methanol, made up to volume with ddH_2O and filtered through a Whatmann No. 1 filter paper.
9. Fetal bovine serum: Australasian origin.
10. Formaldehyde: 10% (v/v) solution of 40% stock formaldehyde in PBS-A.
11. Ganciclovir: Prepared as stock solution at 1–20 m*M* in water, stored at –20°C.
12. Glutamine: 200 m*M* L-glutamine.
13. Hypochlorite: Concentrated hypochlorite solution, 11% (w/w) available chlorine.
14. MEM: Minimum Essential Medium Eagle with Earle's salts, without L-glutamine.
15. MEMX10: 10X strength Minimum Essential Medium Eagle with Earle's salts, without L-glutamine.
16. Methylene blue: 0.02% methylene blue in high purity water.
17. NEAA: Nonessential amino acid mixture for MEM, 100X.
18. PBS: Phosphate-buffered saline Dulbecco A.
19. PSGC: 5 g sucrose in 60 mL high-purity water, 0.1 g sodium glutamate in 20 mL high-purity water, 10 mL 10X PBS; All solutions autoclaved at 10 psi for 10 min, mixed after cooling, then 10 mL of heat-inactivated fetal bovine serum added *(1)*.

2.2. Cell Lines

1. Mewo human melanoma cells *(2)* (ECACC deposit no. 93082609).
2. MRC-5 human lung fibroblasts (ATCC deposit no. CCL-171; ECACC deposit no. 84101801).
3. Vero African Green Monkey kidney cells (ATCC deposit no. CCL-81; ECACC deposit no. 84113001).

2.3. Equipment

1. 32°C incubator, gassed with 5% CO_2 in air.
2. 37°C incubator, gassed with 5% CO_2 in air.
3. Binocular microscope.

3. Methods

All assays are performed in 24-well plates. Each drug dilution should be assayed in triplicate wells, and each drug tested at three or four concentrations, typically in a tenfold dilution series. Two drugs can be assayed on one plate. Include at least three uninfected control wells and at least nine control wells with virus but no drug (using half of a plate).

If the cytotoxicity of the drugs being tested has not been assayed, a duplicate set of plates should be prepared without virus to check for toxic drug effects. Make up drug stock solutions as required in water, ethanol, or dimethyl sulfoxide.

3.1. Herpes Simplex Virus 1 or 2

3.1.1. Preparation of Stock Virus

HSV (type 1 or 2) stock is prepared by infecting Vero cells (1 d after passage at 1:4) in plastic flasks at 37°C. Check by microscopy for cytopathic effect

(CPE). At 50–75% CPE, decant medium, add fetal calf serum to 20% and freeze at –70°C. After freezing, prepare tenfold dilution series down to 10^{-5} and assay plaque numbers as noted below. Note plaque forming unit titer and dilution to be used for assay.

3.1.2. Media

1. Vero growth medium: 500 mL 199, supplemented with 5 mL glutamine, 10 mL antibiotics and 25 mL fetal bovine serum.
2. Vero maintenance medium: 500 mL 199, supplemented with 5 mL glutamine, 10 mL antibiotics, and 10 mL fetal bovine serum.

3.1.3. Plaque Reduction Assay (Fig. 1)

1. Passage Vero cells into 24-well plates (1:4 split) 1 d before use.
2. Thaw stock HSV rapidly and prepare correct dilution in Vero maintenance medium. Add 100 mL of virus to all wells to be infected (do not tip off culture medium).
3. Allow virus to adsorb for 1 h at 37°C in 5% CO_2 in air.
4. Prepare CMC overlay medium:
   a. 100 mL 199 × 10, supplemented with 10 mL glutamine, 10 mL antibiotics, approx 40 mL sodium bicarbonate and 20 mL fetal bovine serum.
   b. Add 45 mL of CMC to 9 mL of the concentrated medium.
5. While virus is adsorbing, prepare drug dilutions in CMC overlay medium. Allow 1.5 mL per well.
6. After adsorption, remove medium and rinse each well with 1 mL PBS.
7. Add 1.5 mL drug-containing media to each well. Controls should include a set of wells with dilutions of a known effective drug (typically Acyclovir assayed at 0.1–100 μ*M*).
8. Incubate plates at 37°C in 5% CO_2 in air for 48 h.
9. Remove medium and fix cells with 1 mL per well formaldehyde for 10 min.
10. Stain cells with 1 mL per well of crystal violet solution for 20 min.
11. Remove stain and rinse gently three times with tap water. Allow to dry inverted overnight and count plaques. Autoclave all waste (including gloves).

3.2. Varicella-Zoster Virus

3.2.1. Preparation of Stock Virus

VZV stock is prepared by infecting Mewo cells (90% confluent) with cell-associated VZV at a ratio of 1:4, infected to uninfected cells in plastic flasks at 37°C. Check by microscopy for cytopathic effect (CPE). At 60–80% CPE, remove medium. Cell-free VZV is prepared by one of two methods:

1. Scrape VZV-infected Mewo cells into overlay medium when cytopathic effect is 60–80% (scraping ruptures syncytia and releases virus).
2. Centrifuge at 1500*g* for 15 min. Cell-free VZV is in supernatant and must be used immediately.

or

1. Remove medium, rinse with PBS, and scrape VZV-infected MRC5 fibroblasts into PSGC (1/10 vol of overlay medium).
2. Centrifuge at 1500*g* for 15 min. Cell-free VZV is in supernatant and can be stored by freezing at –70°C and transferring to gas-phase nitrogen storage at –142°C after 1 d. At the time of transfer, virus should be titrated as noted below. Typical yield is approx 1000–20,000 pfu/mL. Frozen virus is stable for at least 1 mo.

Cell-free VZV can be titrated using twofold dilution series (to 2^{-6}) and using 100 µL to infect each well as noted below. Fresh VZV cannot be titrated; use 100 µL (typically giving 20–60 PFU, but may be less).

3.2.2. Media

1. Mewo growth medium: 500 mL MEM, supplemented with 5 mL glutamine, 10 mL antibiotics, 10 mL bicarbonate, 50 mL fetal bovine serum, and 5 mL NEAA.
2. Mewo maintenance medium: 500 mL MEM, supplemented with 5 mL glutamine, 10 mL antibiotics, 10 mL sodium bicarbonate, 10 mL fetal bovine serum, and 5 mL NEAA.

3.2.3. Plaque Reduction Assay

1. Passage Mewo cells into 24-well plates 1 d before assay.
2. Dilute drug to twice the test concentrations to be assayed in Mewo maintenance medium.
3. Add virus in 100 µL of maintenance medium to the growth medium in each well and allow to adsorb for 1 h at 37°C.
4. After adsorption, remove virus and rinse monolayers with PBS.
5. Add 0.75 mL Mewo maintenance medium containing twice test concentrations of drugs, and 0.75 mL Mewo maintanance medium supplmeneted with 0.3% agarose (1/10 dilution of stock agarose). Controls should include a set of wells with dilutions of a known effective drug (typically acyclovir, assayed at 0.2–200 µ*M*).
6. Incubate cultures at 32°C in 5% CO_2 in air.
7. Remove overlay medium into hypochlorite. Fix cells with 1 mL per well of formaldehyde.
8. Stain cells with 1 mL per well of crystal violet for 20 min.
9. Remove stain and rinse gently three times with tap water. Allow to dry inverted overnight and count plaques (**Fig. 1**). Autoclave all waste (including gloves).

3.3. Cytomegalovirus

3.3.1. Preparation of Stock Virus

CMV stock is prepared by infecting confluent MRC-5 cells in plastic flasks at 37°C. Check by microscopy for CPE. At 50–75% CPE, decant medium, add fetal calf serum to 20%, and freeze at –70°C. After freezing, prepare tenfold

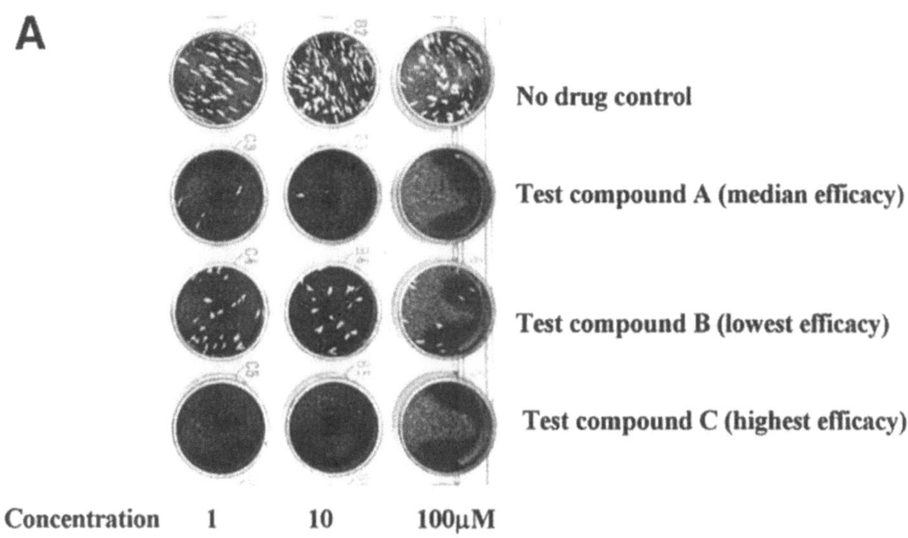

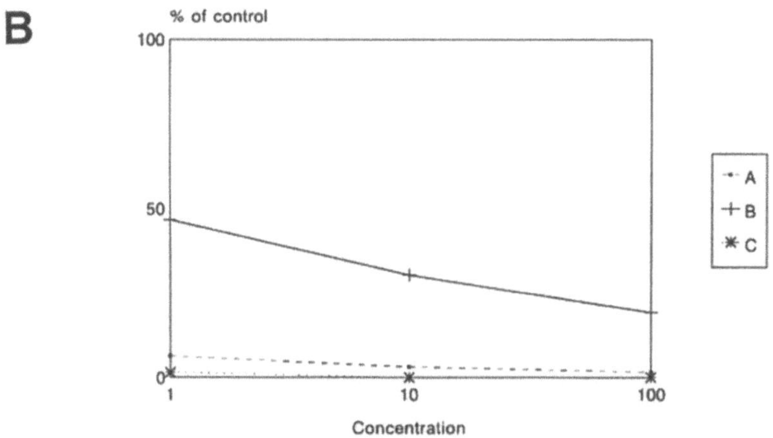

Fig. 1. Plaque reduction assay of varicella-zoster virus. **(A)** Varicella-zoster virus plaques in Mewo cell sheet. The upper row has no drug present. Note toxicity at 100 μ*M* for all compounds tested. **(B)** Efficacy of compounds A, B, and C. All have IC_{50} values of <1 μ*M*.

dilution series down to 10^{-5} and assay plaque numbers as noted below. Note pfu titer and dilution to be used for the assay.

3.3.2. Media

1. MRC-5 growth medium: 500 mL MEM, supplemented with 5 mL glutamine, 10 mL antibiotics, 10 mL bicarbonate, and 50 mL fetal bovine serum.

2. MRC-5 maintenance medium: 500mL MEM, supplemented with 5 mL glutamine, 10 mL antibiotics, 10 mL bicarbonate and 25 mL fetal bovine serum.

3.3.3. Plaque Reduction Assay

1. Passage MRC-5 cells into 24-well plates (1:3 split) and allow to grow to 90% confluency.
2. Thaw stock CMV rapidly and prepare the correct dilution in MRC-5 maintenance medium. Add 100 mL of virus to all wells to be infected (do not remove culture medium).
3. Allow virus to adsorb for 1 h at 37°C in 5% CO_2 in air.
4. Prepare CMC overlay medium:
   a. 100 mL MEMX10, supplemented with 10 mL glutamine, 10 mL antibiotics, approx 40 mL bicarbonate, and 20 mL fetal bovine serum.
   b. Add 45 mL of CMC to 9 mL of the concentrated medium.
5. While virus is adsorbing, prepare drug dilutions in CMC overlay medium. Allow 1.5 mL per well.
6. After adsorption, tip virus off into hypochlorite and rinse each well with 1 mL PBS.
7. Add 1.5 mL drug-containing media to each well. Controls should include a set of wells with dilutions of a known effective drug (typically ganciclovir, assayed at 0.1–100 μ*M*).
8. Incubate plates at 37°C in 5% CO_2 in air for 12 d.
9. Remove medium and fix cells with 1 mL per well of formaldehyde for 10 min.
10. Stain cells with 1 mL per well of methylene blue for 10 min.
11. Remove stain and rinse gently three times with tap water. Allow to dry inverted overnight and count plaques (dark areas) using low power magnification on a binocular microscope. Autoclave all waste (including gloves).

3.3.4. Calculation of Antiviral Effects

Antiviral effect is considered significant when a reduction in plaque numbers to 50% of the mean value seen without any drug present. This value is the IC_{50}, and is calculated from the graph using interpolation. In some cases it may also be possible to calculate an IC_{90} value for 90% reduction of plaque numbers.

3.4. Toxicity

When evaluating unknown drugs, it is essential to evaluate toxicity prior to determining antiviral efficiacy, since some of the drug concentrations to be assayed may destroy the cell monolayer, rendering the assay unusable.

Toxicity is evaluated by determining the level of stain uptake in wells treated with dilutions of test compound(s) covering the desired target range for antiviral assays. The assay should mirror the antiviral assay to be used in cell type, incubation temperature, overlay medium, and incubation time, but no virus should be used. For the evaluation of toxicity, a stain, such as crystal violet, should be used that provides strong contrast between live cells (purple) and damaged cells (clear). Wells in which no drug has been used provide the maximum stain uptake ("zero toxicity") control, whereas an unused plate is used for a minimum stain uptake ("zero stain") control.

Although it is possible to score toxicity crudely by eye, this will not be satisfactory for the purposes of publication. With assays like these, which are based on the use of adherent cell cultures in culture plates, densitometry provides the most direct method of determining toxicity. Older densitometers provide direct, simultaneous evaluation of density in the wells of multiwell plates, such as those used in these assays. This will provide the most direct method of evaluation.

The value for zero stain control is subtracted from the values obtained for all wells, and the corrected density is then plotted as a percentage of the zero toxicity control **(Fig. 2)**. The definitive value for toxicity is that at which stain uptake is reduced by 50% (the TC_{50}).

It is possible to count plaques when some general toxicity is present, but if stain uptake is reduced by more than 50% it will not be possible to obtain reliable values for plaque numbers. In many cases this will put an upper limit on the concentration of test compound for which antiviral efficacy may be determined.

The therapeutic index of a test compound is the TC_{50} divided by the IC_{50}. Although it is not possible to provide a generally acceptable value for the therapeutic index, a value in the range of 100–1000 is often considered a useful minimum.

4. Notes

1. The methods given may be adapted to the needs of the user. In particular, it is often possible to decrease the required incubation time by visualizing pre-plaques using immunostaining techniques; typically a monoclonal antibody to an immediate-early (IE) or early (E) antigen detected by a conjugated probe antibody. However, it is important to note that IE antigens are produced before DNA synthesis, and thus may be produced even in the presence of very high effective levels of drugs that work by inhibiting DNA synthesis, such as the nucleoside analogs acyclovir or ganciclovir.
2. When removing medium, it is simplest to tip from the plate into a bath of sodium hypochlorite. This avoids the damage to the monolayer, which can result from individual suction.
3. It should be noted that the solvent used may in some cases affect the drug efficacy *(3)*.
4. Use of magnification (e.g., a microfiche reader) makes reading crystal violet-stained plaques easier.
5. Although it is possible to perform assays using freshly prepared cell-free VZV, this results in at least half of all assays failing because of variations in virus titer. It is much better to use frozen, titrated stocks if possible because of the variability of VZV titer obtained.

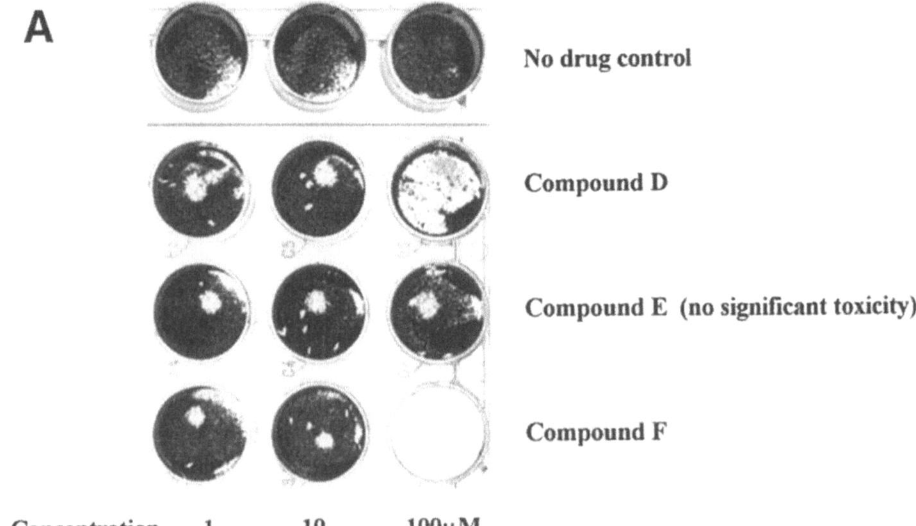

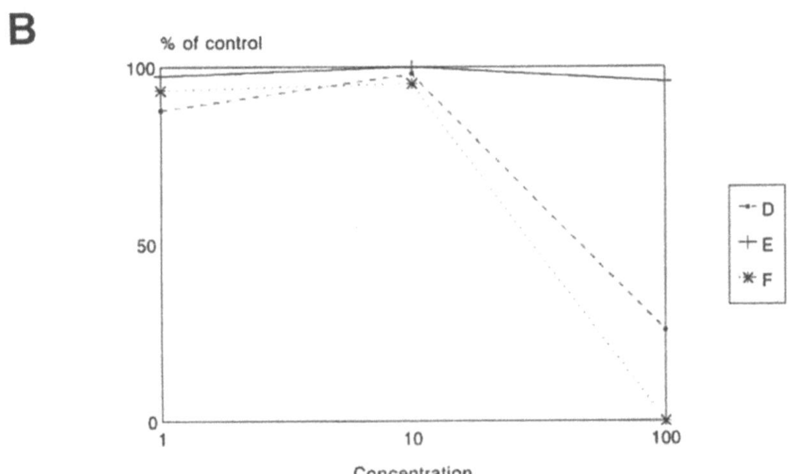

Fig. 2. Toxicity assay. **(A)** Toxicity of test compounds and uninfected cells stained with crystal violet. The densitometry of these wells allows quantitation of stain uptake, and thus of compound toxicity, expressed as a percentage of the density of the "no drug" control. **(B)** Toxicity of compounds D, E, and F. Compound E is not significantly toxic at any concentration tested. Compound D has a TC_{50} of 46 µ*M*; compound F has a TC_{50} of 30 µ*M* (interpolated values).

6. Cell-free VZV can be prepared from MRC-5 cells as for Mewo cells, with the of probe sonication for 3 × 15 s (with 15-s rests intervening) after scraping. Virus from MRC-5 cells may be more stable if preinfection incubation is required.

7. For VZV, Mewo cells give clear plaques, which are much easier to read than those obtained with MRC-5 cells as used by some workers.

References

1. Welsh, M. D. (1991) Studies on the neutralisation of VZV by two specific monoclonal antibodies. Honours thesis, Queens University of Belfast, Belfast, UK.
2. Grose, C. and Brunel, P. A. (1978) Varicella-zoster virus: isolation and propagation in human melanoma cells at 36 and 32 degrees C. *Infect. Immun.* **19,** 199–203.
3. Harper, D. R., Gilbert, R. L., O'Connor, T. J., Kinchington, D., Mahmood, N., McIlhinney, R. A. J., and Jeffries, D. J. (1996) Antiviral activity of 2-hydroxy fatty acids. *Antivir. Chem. Chemother.* **7,** 138–141.

11

Antiviral Screening Assays for Human Herpesviruses 6 and 7

Jodi B. Black and Philip E. Pellett

1. Introduction

Human herpesviruses 6 and 7 are ubiquitous herpesviruses that normally infect their hosts early in life. There are two variant groups of human herpesvirus 6 (HHV-6): variants A (HHV-6A) and B (HHV-6B). Variant A has not been unambiguously associated with a specific disease but may contribute to disease in immunocompromised patients; variant B is the major etiologic agent of roseola (roseola infantum or exanthem subitum) and other febrile illnesses of young children, and has been associated with disease in immunocompromised patients. HHV-6B is frequently present in plaque regions in the brains of multiple sclerosis patients, although an etiologic association has not been proven. Human herpesvirus 7 (HHV-7) has been associated with some cases of roseola. The clinical spectrum of these viruses remains to be completely defined. Braun et al. *(1)* recently described three clinical scenarios that might warrant the use of antivirals to treat HHV-6 infections: (1) transplant recipients with idiopathic pneumonitis (2), multiple sclerosis patients, and (3) patients with HHV-6-associated encephalitis. For HHV-7, cases of neurologic involvement during primary infection might warrant investigation *(2)*.

The literature on antiviral screening for HHV-6 and HHV-7 is sparse and has been reviewed elsewhere *(1,3–5)*. Cell systems for viral propagation have included primary human peripheral blood and cord blood lymphocytes (CBL), and T-cell lines. Methods for monitoring viral replication have included examining infected cultures for cytopathic effect, immunofluorescence analysis, quantitation of viral DNA, and focus-forming assays. Phosphonoformic acid (foscarnet), phosphonoacetic acid, and ganciclovir inhibit HHV-6 and HHV-7

From: *Methods in Molecular Medicine, vol. 24: Antiviral Methods and Protocols*
Edited by: D. Kinchington and R. F. Schinazi © Humana Press Inc., Totowa, NJ

infection in vitro. Acyclovir does not inhibit the growth of HHV-6A, HHV-6B, or HHV-7 at clinically achievable concentrations.

This chapter will describe systems for culturing HHV-6 and HHV-7 as well as assays for their replication that can be used to screen potential antiviral compounds.

2. Materials

1. Lymphocyte separation media (LSM) (Organon Teknika, Durham, NC).
2. Cell counting apparatus.
3. RPMI-1640 with L-glutamine (Gibco-BRL, Grand Island, NY).
4. Fetal bovine serum (FBS).
5. Penicillin/streptomycin solution (Gibco).
6. Phytohemagglutinin P (PHA) (Difco Laboratories, Detroit, MI).
7. Recombinant human IL-2 (Boehringer Mannheim, Indianapolis, IN).
8. Hydrocortisone: dissolve 1 g of hydrocortisone (Sigma, St. Louis, MO) in 100 mL of 95% EtOH. After dissolved, mix with 100 mL of sterile H_2O. Store at 4°C.
9. Cell media: 500 mL RPMI-1640 containing 10% FBS, 100 U/mL of penicillin, 100 g/mL of streptomycin, 0.29 mg/mL of L-glutamine.
10. Lymphocyte stimulation media: Cell media containing 0.01 mg/mL of hydrocortisone and 2 μg/mL of PHA.
11. Lymphocyte growth media: lymphocyte stimulation media but replacing the PHA with 0.1 U/mL of recombinant IL-2.
12. PBS/PS (phosphate-buffered saline [PBS] containing 100 U/mL of penicillin and 100 μg/mL streptomycin and filtered through a 0.22-μm filter).
13. 24-well tissue-culture plates.
14. Sterile 50-mL centrifuge tubes.
15. 10% sodium dodecyl sulfate (SDS) stock solution: Dissolve 100 g of SDS in 900 mL of H_2O. Heat to 68°C to assist dissolution. Adjust volume to 1 L with H_2O.
16. 20X SSC stock solution: Dissolve 175.3 g of NaCl and 88.2 g of sodium citrate in 800 mL of H_2O. Adjust the pH to 7.0 with a few drops of 10 *N* sodium hydroxide. Adjust volume to 1 L with H_2O.

3. Methods

3.1. Purification and Stimulation of Lymphocytes from Umbilical Cord Blood

A decrease in virus growth has been observed in mixed cultures, possibly resulting from mixed lymphocyte reactions. Thus, it is not advisable to not mix individual blood samples either before or after lymphocyte purification.

Collect cord blood into tubes containing an anticoagulant. The authors use 0.5 mL of a 1000 U/mL stock solution of heparin for 50 mL of blood. The blood should be processed within 24 h of collection for best results.

1. Centrifuge the blood for 10 min at 450*g*.
2. Remove most of the upper plasma layer (amber colored) using a 10-mL pipet and discard.

3. Collect the white buffy coat by removing 10 mL from the interface of the red blood cells and the plasma. The buffy coat may not be visible, or it may look like a gray paste covering the top of the red layer. Regardless of the appearance, collect 10 mL from the interface as just described.
4. Transfer the buffy coat to a sterile, 50-mL screw-cap centrifuge tube containing 10 mL of filtered PBS P/S and mix by swirling gently.
5. Aspirate 10 mL of LSM into a 10-mL pipet and insert the tip into the bottom of the tube containing the diluted buffy coat. Slowly pipet the LSM under the diluted cell layer.
6. Centrifuge for 20 min at 450*g*.
7. Remove and discard most of the top layer using a pipet and then collect approx 10 mL of the white opaque mononuclear fraction at the interface.
8. Transfer the cells to a sterile, 50-mL screw-cap centrifuge tube containing 10 mL PBS P/S, mix by swirling gently, and repeat **steps 5–7**.
9. Transfer the mononuclear cell fraction to a sterile 50-mL screw-cap centrifuge tube containing 35 mL of PBS P/S.
10. Centrifuge for 10 min at 450*g*.
11. Immediately decant the supernatant quickly.
12. Add 1.5 mL of PBS P/S to the tube for a total volume of approx 2 mL, and gently suspend the cell pellet by slowly pipeting up and down several times.
13. Measure the cell density and suspend them at 1×10^6 cells/mL in lymphocyte stimulation media in a tissue culture flask.
14. Incubate the flask upright and vented (capped loosely) for 2–3 d in a humidified chamber at 37°C under 5% CO_2.

3.2. Propagation and Passage of HHV-6 and HHV-7 in Human Umbilical CBLs

HHV-6 variants A and B and HHV-7 are passaged in CBL in the same manner. HHV-6A strain U1102 is commercially available (Advanced Biotechnologies, Columbia, MD, cat. no. 10-193-000). HHV-6B strain Z29 and HHV-7 strain SB are available from the American Type Culture Collection (VR-1348 and VR-1384, respectively).

1. Carefully remove most of the culture media from a flask of stimulated lymphocytes, using a pipet without disturbing the cell layer.
2. Infect the cells with either cell-free virus at the desired multiplicity of infection, or with an infected cell culture at a ratio of 1 part infected cell culture to 10 parts uninfected cell culture.
3. If cell-free virus is used as inoculum, adsorb for 2 h in the incubator, then pellet the cells at 450*g* to remove the inoculum, and suspend the cells at 1×10^6 cells/mL in infection medium. If cultures are inoculated with an infected culture, no adsorption period or inoculum removal is necessary. Typical cytopathic effect should be evident between 3 and 5 d postinfection **(Fig. 1)**.

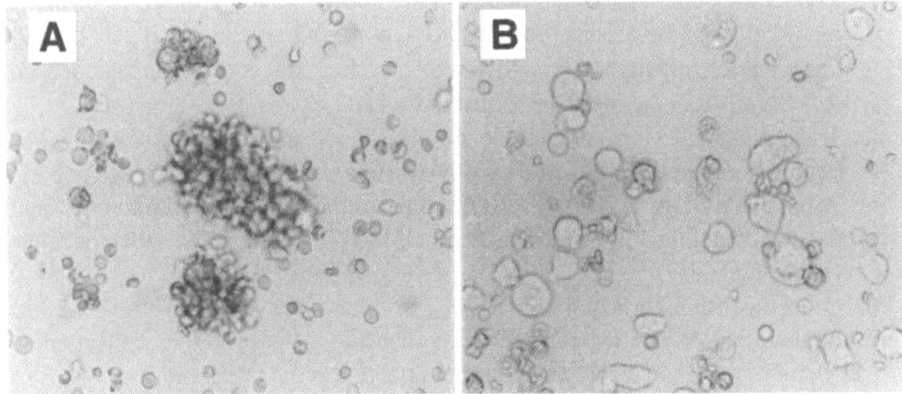

Fig. 1. **(A)** Uninfected stimulated CBL exhibiting typical clumping morphology. **(B)** HHV-6 (Z29)-infected CBL showing loss of cell clumping, enlarged single cells, and fused cells.

3.3. Propagation of HHV-6A, HHV-6B, and HHV-7 in Human T-Cell Lines

HHV-6A strain U1102 and HHV-6B strain Z29 have been adapted for growth in the T-cell lines JJhan and Molt-3, respectively (both available from ATCC) (reviewed in **ref. 5**). HHV-7 strain SB can be propagated in the T-cell line SupT1 (also available from the authors). All three cell lines are grown in cell media.

3.3.1. Propagation of HHV-6A Strain U1102 in JJhan Cells

1. Add one vial of thawed JJhan cells to 40 mL of cell media in a T-75 tissue culture flask (the proper technique for thawing frozen cells is described in **Subheading 3.4.1.**).
2. Incubate at 37°C for 1 wk.
3. Passage the cells by adding 1/10 of the cell culture (4 mL) into a new flask containing 36 mL of fresh cell media. Uninfected cells can continue to be passaged weekly in this manner.
4. To propagate the virus, add one vial of thawed, HHV-6A strain U1102-infected JJhan cells to a newly passaged uninfected cell flask.
5. To serially propagate virus-infected cells, add 4 mL of a 1-wk-old infected culture to 4 mL of a 1-wk-old uninfected culture, and bring up the volume to 40 mL with fresh cell media.

3.3.2. Propagation of HHV-6B Strain Z29 in Molt-3 Cells

1. Add one vial of thawed Molt-3 cells to 25 mL of cell media in a T-25 flask and incubate upright and vented at 37°C, 5% CO_2. (The proper technique for thawing frozen cells is described in **Subheading 3.4.1.**).

2. After 1 wk, remove most of the media without disturbing the cells, and transfer the remaining media and cells into a T-75 flask. Bring up the volume to 40 mL with fresh cell media.
3. Passage uninfected cells 1:5 weekly in the following manner. Remove 30 mL of the media without disturbing the cells. Add 2 mL of the remaining cells and media to each of five T-75 flasks, and bring the volume up to 40 mL with cell media.
4. To propagate HHV-6B strain Z29 in Molt-3 cells, thaw a vial of infected cells and infect an uninfected culture.
5. To serially propagate the virus, add 10 mL of a 1-wk-old infected cell culture to the 2 mL of a newly split uninfected culture described in **step 3**, and then bring up the volume to 40 mL with cell media.

3.3.3. Propagation of HHV-7 Strain SB in Sup T1 Cells

1. Uninfected SupT1 cells are cultured and passaged in a manner identical to the JJhan cells described in **Subheading 3.3.1**. However, the cell media contains only 5% FBS.
2. SupTl cells are infected with HHV-7 strain SB, and the infected cells are serially propagated in a manner identical to HHV-6A strain U1102 in JJhan cells described in **Subheading 3.3.1**.

3.4. Preparation of Frozen Virus Stocks

3.4.1. Virus and Cell Preservation

To preserve cells and virus-infected cells, freezing medium containing 10% dimethyl sulfoxide (DMSO) is used, along with a slow freezing process. DMSO is light sensitive, hazardous to handle, and toxic to cells. Use appropriate protection, sterile technique, and speed.

1. Pellet cells at 450*g* for 10 min.
2. Suspend the cell pellets in RPMI-1640 containing 20% serum and 10% DMSO (final concentration), so that the final cell density is 10^7 cells/mL.
3. Aliquot 1 mL/vial, labeled with cell and virus name, passage number, and date.
4. Freeze slowly by adding vials to either a standard freezer box that has been packed with cotton or a commercially available ethanol freezing container and leave it in a –70°C freezer overnight.
5. Move the frozen cells to liquid nitrogen the next day.

To revive live cells from frozen stock, thaw quickly by swirling in a 37°C water bath, add to 10 mL of cell medium in a T-25 flask, and then incubate the flasks vented and upright overnight. The next morning, pellet the cells and then suspend them in fresh medium to reduce the DMSO concentration. Infected cells are frozen in this manner for the purpose of virus preservation only; therefore, once thawed, the cells must be immediately added to a fresh culture of the appropriate cells.

3.4.2. Freezing in Skim Milk

This procedure is for preparing cell-free virus stocks that are useful for synchronous infections. The skim milk stock is prepared by dissolving a quart size package (90.7 g) of nonfat dry milk in 1 L of sterile, distilled, endotoxin-free water; autoclaving at 15 lb pressure for 15 min cooling overnight; and then repeating the autoclaving/cooling procedure twice more. Store the autoclaved milk at 4°C.

1. Pellet cells at 450*g* for 10 min.
2. Resuspend in a 1:1 solution of skim milk stock and RPMI medium containing 10% FBS, so that the final cell density is 10^7 cells/mL.
3. Aliquot 1 mL per vial, labeled with virus name, the letters SM (skim milk), passage number, and date.
4. Store the vials at –70°C.

3.5. Cell Cytotoxicity Assays

Before a compound can be tested for antiviral activity, it must first be assayed for cytotoxic effects on the uninfected cells at the same concentration.

1. Aliquot 2×10^6 cells in 2 mL of the appropriate media into the wells of a 24-well tissue-culture plate.
2. Add the appropriate dilution of the drug and incubate for 3 d. Do each dilution in duplicate for each drug used.
3. Assay for cell viability by staining an aliquot of the cells with trypan blue and counting the unstained viable cells, using a hemocytonrreter.
4. Calculate the 50% inhibitory concentration (IC_{50}).

3.6. Antiviral Screening Assays

Once the IC_{50} of the drug is known, the compound is ready to be tested for antiviral activity by using virus-infected cells.

1. Infect cells with cell-free virus. After the adsorption period, aliquot 2×10^6 cells in 2 mL of the appropriate media into the wells of a 24-well tissue-culture plate.
2. Immediately add the appropriate concentration of compound to duplicate wells.
3. Incubate for 5 d, removing aliquots every other day for immunofluorescence analysis (IFA).
4. On d 5, remove the remaining 1 mL and assay for evidence of viral DNA replication.

3.7. Viral Activity Assays

3.7.1. Indirect IFA

IFA is a method of assaying for infected cell proteins within individual cells and is useful for calculating the percentage of infected cells in a culture.

Because herpesviruses express proteins that are not dependent on viral DNA synthesis, caution must be taken when determining the efficacy of a compound by IFA. Inhibition of virus replication would be more directly reflected by measuring the concentration of viral DNA (*see* **Subheading 3.7.2.**). However, the IFA is useful when compounds are being evaluated for use in kinetic studies of virus gene expression. Infected cultures will usually become IFA-positive 3 d post infection, reaching a peak of virus-infected cells at approx 7 d post infection. The method consists of two steps: slide preparation and staining.

3.7.1.1. Slide Preparation

1. Add 0.3 mL of virus-infected cell suspension to 13 mL of 0.2-μm-filtered PBS in a 15-mL conical tube.
2. Centrifuge at 450*g* for 10 min.
3. Pour off the supernatant, leaving approx 0.3 mL of PBS.
4. Gently resuspend the cell pellet.
5. Apply a drop (approx 30 μL) of the cell suspension per well on a Teflon-coated slide.
6. Allow the slide to air-dry.
7. Fix the cells by submerging them in acetone that has been prechilled to –20°C for 5 min.
8. Remove the slide and allow to dry for approx 5 min. (The slides can be stored in a slide box at –20°C for at least 6 mo.)

3.7.1.2. Staining Procedure

Variant-specific and variant crossreactive monoclonal antibodies to HHV-6 are commercially available (Advanced Biotechnologies, Columbia, MD, and Chemicon, Temecula, CA). HHV-7 monoclonal antibodies are available from Advanced Biotechnologies.

1. Prepare a moist chamber (closed container with moistened paper towel on the bottom) and place the slides inside it.
2. Add antibody, diluted with PBS to a useful dilution (use PBS as a negative control).
3. Incubate inside the closed container at 37°C for 30 min.
4. Wash twice for 5 min in PBS.
5. Add the appropriately diluted fluorescein isothiocyanate-conjugated antimouse IgG to each well and repeat **steps 3** and **4**.
6. Dunk the slides in sterile water, air-dry in a dark place, and then mount a cover slip by adding three drops of buffered glycerol directly to the slide.
7. Store the slides in the dark.
8. Read at ×40 by picking three or four fields of 50–100 cells and counting infected vs uninfected cells. Infected IFA-positive cells will exhibit punctate or spotty fluorescence throughout the cell. Express the results as percent infected cells.

3.7.2. Quantitation of Viral DNA

DNA is purified from infected cells and then immobilized onto nitrocellulose sheets using a vacuum manifold apparatus (slot-blot). Viral DNA is detected by hybridization with a labeled (isotypically or nonisotypically) virus-specific probe, and then hybridization signal intensity is quantified.

3.7.2.1. DNA Purification

1. Aliquot 1 mL of cell suspension (approx 1×10^6 cells) into a screw-cap microcentrifuge tube.
2. Centrifuge the samples at 16,000*g* for 2 min.
3. Carefully remove all media without disturbing the cell pellet. The samples can be stored at –70°C or processed immediately.
4. Whole cell DNA is purified from virus-infected cells by using a commerically available kit according to the manufacturer's instructions (QiaAmp Blood Kit, Qiagen, Chatsworth, CA). The purified DNA can be stored at –20°C.

3.7.2.2. Slot Blotting

1. Denature the DNA by heating at 100°C for 10 min. Hold on ice.
2. Assemble the slot-blot apparatus with a suitable hybridization membrane, according to the manufacturer's instructions, and then add 200 µL from each sample to a well.
3. Add 200 µL 6X SSC to all wells that received no sample.
4. Apply vacuum gently until all liquid is removed.
5. Wash by adding 200 µL of 6X SSC to all wells and then repeating the vacuum procedure.
6. Remove the membrane from the apparatus and then submerge it in 6X SSC to wash off any debris.
7. Remove the membrane from the 6X SSC and blot to remove excess buffer.
8. Fix the DNA onto the membrane by either heat (20 min at 80°C in a vacuum) or ultraviolet crosslinking.

3.7.2.3. Prehybridization and Hybridization

1. Place filter in heat-sealable bag or hybridization tube.
2. Add 10 mL of hybridization solution: 4X SSC, 0.1% sodium pyrophosphate, 100 mg/mL of heparin, and 0.2% SDS. This can be prewarmed if it has precipitated.
3. Remove as many bubbles and air pockets from the bag as possible.
4. Seal the bag or close the tube.
5. Incubate the bag at 65°C with rocking for 2–5 h. For tubes, make sure that the rotation direction is correct (the opposite direction that the membrane was rolled to fit into the tube).
6. After prehybridization, pour off the hybridization solution.
7. Add 10 mL of hybridization solution that contains labeled probe ***(6–9)*** that has been boiled 5 min, and then cooled in ice for several minutes.
8. Seal bag or close tube.
9. Incubate at 65°C overnight with mild agitation.

3.7.2.4. Posthybridization Washes

Wash membranes twice for 5 min at room temperature vvith at least 50 mL of 2X SSC, 0.1% SDS (w/v)/100 cm^2. Then wash twice for 30 min at 65°C with 0.1X SSC, 0.1% SDS. Wash conditions (temperature and salt concentration) may need to be adjusted for the specific probe.

3.7.3. Virus Titration

1. Remove the test compound from the cells by pelleting the cells at 450*g*. Decant the supernatant and gently suspend the cells in PBS. Once again pellet the cells at 450*g* and discard the supernatant.
2. Inoculate serial dilutions of the washed cells into duplicate wells of a 24-well tissue-culture plate containing 2×10^6 cells in 2 mL of media per well.
3. Incubate the plates for 5 d and then monitor for virus growth by IFA or DNA quantitation.
4. Calculate the infectious particles/mL using the reciprocal of the last dilution showing evidence of virus growth as the end point titer.

4. Notes

1. Antimouse conjugates may vary between lots and should be titrated for appropriate dilution for each new lot. Filtering the conjugate dilution through a 0.45-µm filter prior to use helps decrease some background.
2. Always wear gloves when handling hybridization membranes, both before and after blotting.
3. Two milliliters of sterile PBS should be added to the unused wells of a 24-well plate to prevent media evaporation in the test wells. When all the wells are not necessary for an assay, it is best to confine the test wells to the internal wells of the plate.
4. Always wear a mask when handling SDS powder.

References

1. Braun, D. K., Dominguez, G., and Pellett, P. E. (1997) Human herpesvirus 6. *Clin. Microbiol. Rev.* **10,** 521–567.
2. Torigoe, S., Koide, W., Yamada, M., Miyashiro, E., Tanaka-Taya, K., and Yamanishi, K. (1996) Human herpesvirus 7 infection associated with central nervous system manifestations. *J. Pediatr.* **129,** 301–305.
3. Pellett, P. E., Black, J. B., and Yamamoto, M. (1992) Human herpesvirus 6: the virus and the search for its role as a human pathogen. *Adv. Virus Res.* **41,** 1–52.
4. Williams, M. V. (1992) HHV-6: response to antiviral agents, in *Human Herpesvirus-6: Epidemiology, Molecular Biology, and Clinical Pathology* (Ablashi, D. V., Krueger, G. R. F., and Salabuddin, S. Z., eds.), Elsevier, Amsterdam, pp. 317–335.
5. Pellett, P. E. and Black, J. B. (1996) Human herpesvirus 6, in *Fields Virology*, 3rd ed., vol. 2 (Fields, B. N., Knipe, D. M., Howley, P. M., Channock, R. M., Melnick, J. L., Monath, T. P., Roizman, B., and Straus, S. E., eds.), Lippincott-Raven, Philadelphia, PA, pp. 2587–2608.

6. Martin, M. E. D., Thomson, B. J., Honess, R. W., Craxton, M. A., Gompels, U. A., Liu, M. Y., Littler, E., Arrand, J. R., Teo, I., and Jones, M. D. (1991) The genome of human herpesvirus 6: maps of unit-length and concatemeric genomes for nine restriction endonucleases. *J. Gen. Virol.* **72,** 157–168.
7. Lindquester, G. J., Inoue, N., Allen, R. D., Castelli, J. W., Stamey, F. R., Dambaugh, T. R., O'Brian, J. J., Danovich, R. M., Frenkel, N., and Pellett, P. E. (1996) Restriction endonuclease mapping and molecular cloning of the human herpesvirus 6 variant B strain Z29 genome. *Arch. Virol.* **141,** 367–379.
8. Dominguez, G., Black, J. B., Stamey, F. R., Inoue, N., and Pellett, P. E. (1996) Physical and genetic maps of the human herpesvirus 7 strain SB genome. *Arch. Virol.* **141,** 2387–2409.
9. Nicholas, J. (1996) Determination and analysis of the complete nucleotide sequence of human herpesvirus 7. *J. Virol.* **70,** 5975–5989.

12

Strategies for Evaluation of Antiviral Agents Against Epstein-Barr Virus in Culture

Jung-Chung Lin

1. Introduction

Evaluation of antiviral agents against Epstein-Barr virus (EBV) has been hampered by the lack of a permissive cell system for the replication of this virus. The extent of EBV replication detected in producer cell lines (P3HR-1 and B95-8) is limited: only a small fraction (<10%) of the cell population spontaneously produces virus at any given time. Attempts to increase the virus yield by manipulation of the culture conditions, such as temperature shifts, exposure to halogenated pyrimidines, such as BUdR and IUdR, and X-ray, have not been very successful. Superinfection of Raji (a nonvirus-producer line) cells with P3HR-1 virus enhances EBV replication and provides a more efficient system for evaluation of antiviral drugs. However, this method requires infection with virus isolated from a large quantity of culture fluids of P3HR-1 cells The virus yield varies from preparation to preparation. In addition, the system is not practical for large-scale drug screening.

zur Hausen et al. *(1)* reported a very efficient induction of EBV antigen synthesis in virus-producing cell lines by a potent tumor promoter, 12-*O*-tetradecanoyl-phorbol-13-acetate (TPA). Subsequently, Lin et al. *(2)* showed that treatment of the P3HR-1 cells with TPA results in a dramatic increase in EBV DNA replication, paralleling the appearance of viral antigen synthesis. EBV genome copy number per P3HR-1 cell is approx 230 and increases more than 10-fold after TPA induction *(2)*. As shown by *in situ* cytohybridization *(2)*, this increase is not caused by the contribution of a small proportion of the cell population, as demonstrated by the marked increase in percentage of cells participating in the virus-productive cycle (from 6% in the

From: *Methods in Molecular Medicine, vol. 24: Antiviral Methods and Protocols*
Edited by: D. Kinchington and R. F. Schinazi © Humana Press Inc., Totowa, NJ

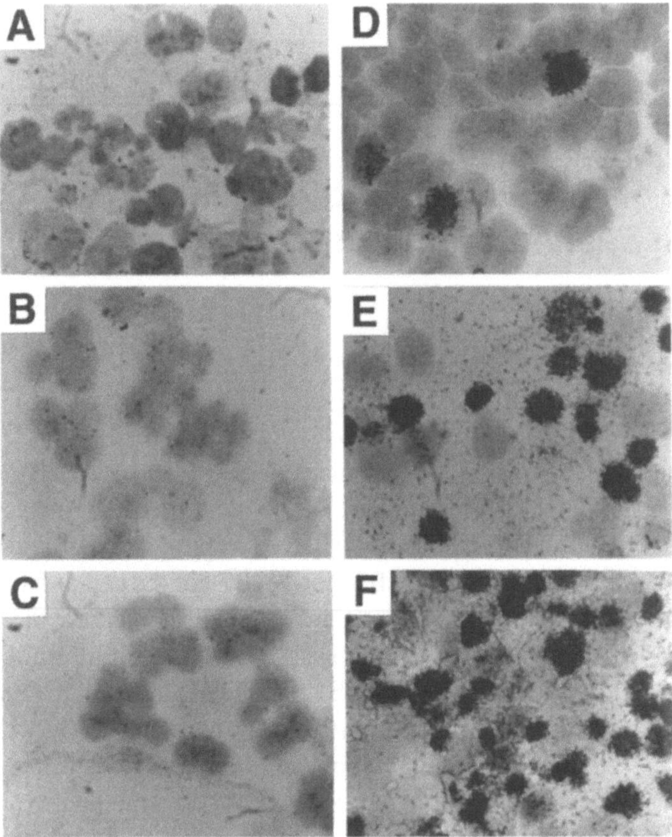

Fig. 1. The effect of TPA on EBV DNA replication. *In situ* cytohybridization of P3HR-1 and Raji cells with EBV cRNA. **(A, D)** Raji and P3HR-1 control, respectively; **(B, E)** and **(C, F)** Raji and P3HR-1 cells exposed to TPA for 4 and 6 d, respectively. (Reproduced with permission **ref. *2***).

control to as much as 95% in TPA-treated cultures, **Fig. 1**). These effects, however, are not observed in Raji cells similarly exposed to TPA, despite a marked induction of early antigen synthesis *(2)*. The practical consequences of these findings for evaluating antiviral agents in an EBV system are obvious and important.

Although TPA induction is an efficient system for anti-EBV drug screening, TPA itself is a potent carcinogen and may create biohazards. In addition to a TPA induction system, the author has developed two alternative cell culture systems for evaluation of anti-EBV drugs. Optimization of each system will be fully described herein.

2. Materials

1. 12-*O*-tetradecanoyl-phorbol-13-acetate (phorbol 12-myristate 13-acetate) (Sigma, St. Louis, MO). Stock solution is prepared by dissolving the powder in ethanol/acetone (50/50), or in dimethyl sulfoxide. The solution is stable for 6 mo at –20°C.
2. RPMI-1640 medium containing 10% fetal calf serum (FCS), 2 m*M* L-glutamine, 100 IU/mL penicillin, and 100 µg/mL streptomycin.
3. Human lymphoblastoid cell lines carrying EBV genome: P3HR-1, B95-8, and Raji (American Type Culture Collection, Rockville, MD).
4. Phosphate-buffered saline (PBS) (Dulbecco A).
5. Trypan blue 0.1%.
6. Sarkosyl-97, proteinase K, phenol, chloroform, RNase A, and ethylenediamine-tetra-acetic acid (EDTA).
7. Nitrocellulose filters and Hybond-N paper (Amersham, Arlington Heights, IL).
8. Refrigerated benchtop centrifuge.
9. Water bath.
10. CO_2 incubator.
11. Cell culture T-flask (Costar, Cambridge, MA).
12. Inverted light microscope.
13. Biosafety cell culture hood.

3. Methods

3.1. Optimization of TPA Induction and Antiviral Drug Effect

The effect of TPA on P3HR-1 cell growth and replication of EBV DNA was assessed *(3)*. The results indicated that (1) cell proliferation is reversibly inhibited on exposure to TPA; (2) noncycling cells are more sensitive to the antiproliferative effect of TPA than cycling cells; (3) inhibition in cell proliferation may be associated with the effect of TPA in viral induction; and (4) transient exposure to TPA is sufficient to trigger the cells to enter the EBV replicative cycle.

Although TPA is able to induce replication of EBV genomes in P3HR-1 cells in all phases of growth, the greatest increase in viral genome copies per cell (15-fold above the control level) occurred in cells in the stationary phase, as opposed to only a sixfold increase in cells growing exponentially *(4)*. **Figure 2** shows the effect of growth phase on the induction of EBV genome replication in TPA-treated P3HR-1 cells.

On the basis of these findings, the author examined three protocols for evaluating the effect of antiviral drugs under the TPA induction system *(5)*. First, when P3HR-1 cells were treated with an effective dose of acyclovir [9-(2-hydroxyethoxymethyl)guanine] and TPA for 7 d, a 90% inhibition of EBV genome copy numbers was observed. Because of prolonged exposure to TPA, cell numbers decreased after 7 d of treatment, making determination of EBV genome copy numbers difficult. Second, when cells were transiently

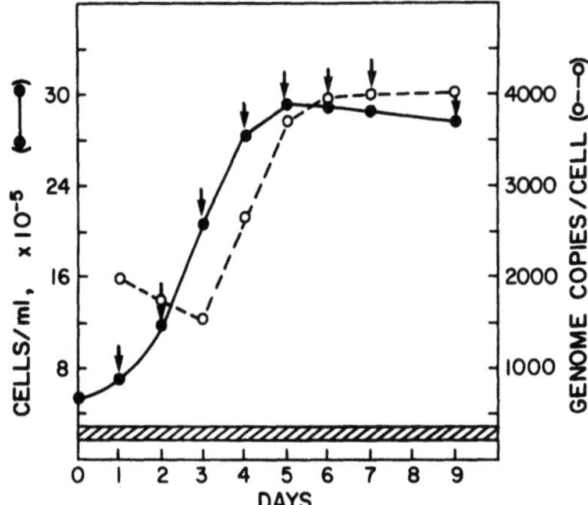

Fig. 2. Effect of growth phase on the induction of EBV genome replication in TPA-treated P3HR-1 cells. Exponentially growing cells were seeded at a density of 6 $\times 10^5$ cells/mL. At different phases of growing (indicated by arrows), samples of viable cells were harvested and incubated in fresh medium containing TPA for 7 d. At the end of TPA induction, DNA was isolated, and EBV genome copies/cell were determined by cRNA–DNA hybridization. (●) Growth curve of P3HR-1 cells in culture, (○) EBV genome copies/cell; the hatched horizontal bar represents the range of EBV genome copies/cell in nontreated cells during the experimental period. (Reproduced with permission **ref. *4***).

exposed to TPA for 1 d, washed, and resuspended in fresh medium plus drug for 7 d, a partial inhibition (40–50% by acyclovir) was observed, although cells proliferated under these conditions. Third, when cells were cotreated with acyclovir and TPA for 1 d, washed, and refed with fresh medium plus drug for 7 d, a similar degree of inhibition (95%) as in the first protocol was observed. However, cell growth was not affected.

Based on these observations, the author developed an optimized protocol for effective evaluation of antiviral drugs against EBV replication, detailed as follows:

1. Grow P3HR-1 cells in tissue culture flasks (max. 100 mL for 75-cm^2 T-flask and 200 mL for 162-cm^2 T-flask) in RPMI-1640 medium containing 10% FCS supplemented with 2 m*M* L-glutamine, 100 IU/mL penicillin, and 100 µg/mL of streptomycin.
2. Maintain the cells in exponential growth by seeding at a density of 4×10^5–6×10^5 cells/mL, and count daily until a density of 2×10^6 cells/mL is reached. During this interval the cells are growing in a strict exponential fashion. In practice, the cells are subcultured and maintained with fresh medium containing 10% serum every 3 d. The cell viability should be maintained at approx 90–95%, as determined by the trypan blue exclusion method.

3. For each concentration of drug, harvest 2×10^7 viable cells from the exponentially growing culture by centrifugation at 800*g* for 5 min and suspend in 20 mL of fresh medium. Also, harvest two sets of cells as controls (*see* **step 6**).
4. Grow the cells at 37°C in a humidified 5% CO_2/95% air incubator for 5–6 d without additional medium. Count the cell number and check the viability. If the cell viability is <85%, do not start the experiments.
5. Harvest the cells by spinning in a benchtop centrifuge at 800*g* for 5 min.
6. Resuspend the cells in 20 mL of fresh medium containing TPA (30 ng/mL) and the appropriate concentration of the testing drug.
7. Set up two control cultures (from **step 3**). Control 1: no TPA or testing drug; control 2: TPA (30 ng/mL) only.
8. Incubate the three sets of cultures from **steps 6** and **7** at 37°C for 24 h in a humidified 5% CO_2/95% air incubator.
9. Harvest the cells by centrifugation at 800*g* for 5 min.
10. Gently wash the cells twice with warm medium, and resuspend in 40 mL of fresh medium plus the appropriate concentration of the testing drug, but without TPA, in the experimental group. For controls 1 and 2, resuspend the cells in 40 mL of fresh medium.
11. Incubate at 37°C in a humidified 5% CO_2/95% air incubator for 7 d without additional medium or testing drug.
12. Harvest the cells and wash three times with cold (4°C) PBS.
13. Take small alicluots of cells to prepare cell smears on the slide for detection of viral antigens. Air-dry the cells, fix the cells in cold acetone for 10 min, air-dry, and then perform indirect immunofluorescent assay (*see* **Appendix 1**).
14. The remaining cells are used to isolate genomic DNA for filter membrane hybridization to determine EBV genome copy numbers per cell (*see* **Appendices 2** and **4**).

3.2. Low Serum Selection of P3HR-1 Cells

P3HR-1 cells contain a mixture of virus-productive and non- or less-virus-productive populations. By analogy to the transformed cells, one hypothesizes that the virus-productive population does not require as much serum as the nonvirus-productive or less productive population. Consequently, as the serum concentration in the medium is gradually reduced, the nonproductive or less productive population will be eliminated from the culture. The procedures of low serum selection for highly virus-productive population from P3HR-1 cells are detailed as follows:

1. P3HR-1 cells grown in RPMI-1640 medium containing 10% FCS are gradually adapted to grow in medium containing 1.5% serum by the stepwise reduction of 1% serum in every third feeding interval (feed twice a week).
2. When the cells are adapted to 3% serum, reduce the serum to 1.5%, and maintain the cells at this concentration for an additional 7 d before using in the experiments. This adaptation takes 8 wk. The selected cell line can be propagated in 1.5% serum. However, it cannot survive in medium containing <1.5% serum.

3. Under the low serum (1.5%) conditions, approx 20–50% of the cells are spontaneously activated to produce virus.
4. Such cell lines, designated P3HR-1(LS), maintain a highly virus-productive state for about 8–12 mo. The EBV genome copy numbers normally maintain approx 600–1500 copies per cell as opposed to approx 200 copies in the parental P3HR-1 cells. The cells can be used for subsequent antiviral drug screening.

3.2.1. Antiviral Drug Screening Using P3HR-1(LS) Cells

EBV-infected cells contain two forms of viral DNA: linear and episomal. The linear form of viral DNA is synthesized by EBV-specified DNA polymerase and is sensitive to nucleoside analogs, whereas the episomal form of EBV DNA is synthesized by the cell polymerase and is not sensitive to any nucleoside analogs tested so far. In a study comparing the kinetics of inhibition and reversibility of EBV DNA replication in P3HR-1(LS) cells treated with acyclovir and DHPG [9-(1,3-dihydroxy-2-propoxymethyl)guanine], the author found that a drug exposure of 14 d was needed to reduce the EBV genome copy number to the residual episome level (30 copies per cell) ***(6)***. Thus, it is imperative to treat the cells with a drug for 14 d to accurately estimate the viral 50 and 90% effective doses (ED_{50} and ED_{90}) of inhibition. To screen, proceed as follows.

1. Grow P3HR-1(LS) cells in tissue-culture flasks in RPMI-1640 medium containing 1.5% FCS supplemented with 2 m*M* of L-glutamine, 100 IU/mL of penicillin and 100 μg/mL of streptomycin.
2. Maintain the cells at exponential growth by seeding at a density of 4×10^5 -6×10^5 cells/mL, and count daily until a density of 2×10^5 cells/mL is reached. In practice, the cells are subcultured and fed with fresh medium containing 1.5% serum every 3 d. The cell viability should be maintained at approx 90% or higher.
3. For each concentration of drug to be tested, harvest 2×10^7 viable cells by centrifugation (800*g*, 5 min) from the exponentially growing culture, and resuspend in 20 mL of fresh medium containing 1.5% serum and the test drug. Also harvest one set of cells as no-drug controls.
4. Incubate the cells at 37°C in a humidified 5% CO_2/95% air incubator.
5. Every 3 d remove half of the medium and replace with fresh medium containing 1.5% serum and the same concentration of the test drug. The amount of fresh medium to be added at the time of feeding depends on the culture cell density. Most nucleoside analogs exert cytotoxic or cytostatic effect at high concentration.
6. The cells are continuously treated with the drug for 14 d.
7. Harvest the cells by spinning at 800*g* for 5 min, and wash the cells three times with cold (4°C) PBS.
8. The washed cells are ready to process for immunofluorescent assay and determination of EBV genome copy numbers as described (*see* **Appendices 1** and **4**).

3.3. Umbilical Cord Blood Lymphocyte Transformation

Among the diseases with which EBV is prominently associated are African endemic Burkitt's lymphoma, nasopharyngeal carcinoma, and immunoblastic B-cell lymphomas in immunosuppressed persons, especially in patients with AIDS. This is thought to reflect the lymphotropic phase of this infection. After initial infection of epithelial cells, the crucial step in the development of these diseases, as well as of infectious mononucleosis, is the immortalization of B lymphocytes, which thus acquire the capability for unlimited growth. The cord-lymphocyte immortalization assay provides a means of gaging the effects of agents *(7)* that might inhibit EBV-induced lymphoproliferation in immunodeficiency states.

3.3.1. Separation of Lymphocytes from Human Umbilical Cord Blood Using Ficoll Hypaque Gradients

1. Collect cord blood into heparinized tubes.
2. Dilute blood 1:2 in serum-free RPMI-1640 medium.
3. Carefully layer the diluted blood onto Ficoll-Hypaque gradients (1:3 ratio) in a 15-mL conical culture tube (3 mL blood onto 9 mL Ficoll-Hypaque).
4. Centrifuge at 800*g* for 30 min at room temperature.
5. Collect the white opaque mononuclear cells from the interface using a Pasteur pipet.
6. Wash the cells with serum-free medium five times.
7. Count the cell numbers and determine the viability by Trypan blue exclusion method.

3.3.2. Effect of Cell Numbers on Formation of Transformed Foci

1. Perform the transformation assay in a flat-bottomed, 96-well microtiter plate.
2. Determine the optimal cell concentration per well for the formation of transformed foci by distributing various numbers (10^3–10^6) of infected cells (*see* **Subheading 3.3.3.**) to wells. For each cell concentration, use 10 replicate wells.
3. Grow the cells in 200 µL of RPMI-1640 medium containing 20% heat-inactivated FCS supplemented with 2 m*M* L-glutamine, 50 IU/mL penicillin, and 50 µg/mL streptomycin.
4. Incubate at 37°C in a humidified 5% CO_2/95% air incubator.
5. Score the numbers of transformed foci after 5–6 wk, and determine which cell concentration produces maximal transformed foci. In general, cell numbers between 3×10^5 and 10^6 per well give uniform results; 5×10^5 cells per well is recommended.

3.3.3. Transformation Assay and Effect of Drug

1. For each drug concentration, take 5×10^6 cells (for 10 replicates) and infect with 0.5 mL of virus stock prepared from B95-8 cells (*see* **Appendix 3**).
2. Incubate at 37°C for 2 h with periodic gentle agitation. Cells incubated with virus-free medium serve as controls.

3. Centrifuge at 800*g* for 5 min, and resuspend the cells in 2 mL RPMI-1640 medium containing 20% heat-inactivated FCS supplemented with 2 m*M* L-glutamine, 50 IU/mL penicillin, and 50 μg/mL streptomycin.
4. Distribute 5×10^5 cells (200 μL) into each well of a 96-well microtiter plate.
5. Add appropriate concentrations of the test drug into each well. Ten replicate wells are prepared for each drug concentration.
6. Incubate at 37°C in a humidified 5% CO_2/95% air incubator.
7. Gently remove the medium and replenish with fresh drug medium twice a week.
8. Count by microscopic examination the number of transformed foci weekly. Normally, the transformed foci are visible between 4 and 6 wk after infection.

4. Notes

1. Cell viability of the cultures should be maintained at approx 90% or higher. If the cell viability is <85%, do not not start the experiments.
2. For maximal production of extracellular virus by TPA induction of B95-8 or P3HR-1 cells (*see* **Appendix 3**), harvest cells at the stationary phase of growth by centrifugation, resuspend in the same volume of fresh medium containing TPA, and incubate for 10 d without additional medium.
3. For best drug effect using P3HR-1(LS) cells, the culture should be kept in an exponential growth state (1×10^6–2.7×10^6 cells/mL) during experiments.

Appendix 1: Indirect Immunofluorescent Assay

1. Wash printed microscope slides (Cell-Line Associates, Newfield, NJ) in methanol:acetone (1:1) and air-dry the slides.
2. Resuspend a small aliquot (10^6 cells) of PBS-washed cells in approx 50 μL of PBS.
3. Place a monolayer of cells in each well and air-dry the slides.
4. Fix the cells in cold (–20°C) acetone for 10 min and air-dry the slides. Slides can be stored at –20°C until use.
5. Soak the slides in PBS for 5 min and air-dry.
6. Layer appropriately diluted monoclonal antibody or humna serum containing antibodies against EBV early antigen and viral capsid antigen over the cells.
7. Incubate at 37°C for 30 min in a moist chamber.
8. Wash slides three times (5 min each) with PBS and air-dry slides.
9. Layer fluorescein isothiocyanate-conjugated antimouse (or antihuman) IgG (1:10 in PBS) over cells.
10. Incubate at 37°C for 30 min in a moist chamber.
11. Wash slides three times (5 min each) with PBS and air-dry slides.
12. Place a drop of 50% glycerol (in PBS) over wells and seal wells with coverelip.
13. Read the slides under the fluorescence microscope.

Appendix 2: Isolation of Genomic DNA

1. Resuspend cell pellet in digestion buffer (0.5 mL for 10^7 cells) containing 10 m*M* of Tris-HCl, pH 8.0, 100 m*M* of NaCl, 25 m*M* of EDTA, 0.5% Sarkosyl, and proteinase K (0.1 mg/mL).

2. Incubate at 55°C overnight and 95°C for 10 min.
3. Extract with an equal volume of phenol-chloroform twice, and dialyze against 10 m*M* Tris-HCl, pH 8.0, and 1 m*M* EDTA.
4. Add RNase A (100 µg/mL) to the dialyzed sample and incubate at 37°C for 2 h.
5. Extract with an equal volume of phenol-chloroform twice, and dialyze against 10 m*M* Tris-HCl, pH 8.0, and 1 m*M* EDTA.
6. Determine the concentration of DNA by spectrophotometry.

Appendix 3: Preparation of Virus Stock from B95-8 Cells

1. Grow 2 L of B95-8 cells in RPMI-1640 medium containing 10% FCS supplemented with 2 m*M* L-glutamine, 100 IU/mL penicillin, and 100 µg/mL streptomycin.
2. When cells reach a stationary phase of growth (6 d after subculture without additional medium), spin down the cells at 800*g* for 5 min and resuspend in the same volume of fresh medium containing TPA (30 ng/mL).
3. Incubate at 37°C in a humidified 5% CO_2/95% air incubator for 10 d without additional medium.
4. Spin cell suspension at 8400*g* for 10 min at 4°C in a GS-3 rotor.
5. Pour the supernatant into new bottles and spin at 10,650*g* rpm for 90 min at 4°C in a GS-3 rotor.
6. Carefully pour off supernatant (pellet will be loose) and wipe off the residual medium (keep on ice).
7. Resuspend virus pellets in 8 mL RPMI-1640 medium with 1.5% FCS. This virus preparation represents a 250-fold concentration.
8. Sterilize and clarify (to remove cellular debris) the virus suspension by consecutive filtrations through 1.2-, 0.8-, and 0.45-µm filters.
9. Aliquot and store at –70°C for 1 yr or at 4°C for approx 3 mo.
10. Determine the transforming titers of the virus preparation by end-point titration on human umbilical cord blood lymphocytes (*see* **Subheading 3.3.2.**), and calculate by the method of Reed and Muench *(8)*.

Appendix 4: Determination of EBV Genome Copy Numbers

The purpose of this appendix is to deal with methods for the labeling, detection, and quantitation of viral DNA. Two methods, cRNA–DNA and DNA–DNA hybridization, which have been routinely used in the author's laboratory for assessing the drug efficacy in the EBV system, are discussed.

Method 1: cRNA–DNA Hybridization on Nitrocellulose Filters

1. Denature 50 µg DNA by heating at 80°C for 10 min in 200 µL 0.025 *M* NaOH and 0.5 m*M* EDTA, and then rapidly chill it in an ice bath.
2. Add an equal volume of neutralization buffer (1 *M* Tris-HCl, pH 7.4) and filter through presoaked (in water) nitrocellulose disk filters (25 mm in diameter) (Schleicher & Schuell, Keene, NH) set up on a suction manifold (Millipore Corp., Bedford, MA).
3. Wash the filters with 6X SSC (1X SSC is 0.15 *M* NaCl, 0.015 *M* sodium citrate) twice and air-dry.

4. Heat the filters at 80°C for 4 h in a vaccuum oven.
5. Wet the filters with 6X SSC and put into vials containing 0.8 mL 6X SSC, 100 μg yeast RNA, 0.1% sodium dodecyl sulfate (SDS), and 10^5 cpm [^{3}H] EBV cRNA (specific activity 10^7 cpm/μg). cRNA is prepared according to the method described previously ***(9)***.
6. Incubate in a 66°C water bath for 22–24 h.
7. Wash the filters three times with 2X SSC.
8. Incubate the filters in 2X SSC containing RNase (30 μg/mL) at 37°C for 30 min.
9. Wash the filters twice with 2X SSC, dry, and count in a liquid scintillation counter.
10. Remove the filters from the scintillation fluid, wash in toluene, and dry.
11. Determine the amount of DNA attached to the filters by the diphenylamine method of Burton ***(10)***.

Calculation of EBV Genome Copy Numbers

I. Reconstruction Curve

1. Mix graded amounts (0.001–0.5 μg) of EBV DNA with 50 μg HEp-2 or HeLa cell DNA.
2. Denature the DNA mixture by heating at 80°C for 10 min in the presence of 0.025 *M* NaOH and 0.5 m*M* EDTA and rapidly chill in an ice bath.
3. Follow **steps 2–12** under **Method 1**.
4. Subtract the background hybridized counts (50 μg HEp-2 DNA alone) from each value.
5. Plot the hybridized counts (cpm) vs amounts of EBV DNA (μg) added; a linear curve should be obtained. These data provide the basis for calculation of the number of viral genome equivalents detected by hybridization.
   a. The molecular weights of EBV DNA (linear, doubled-stranded) and diploid human cell DNA are 117×10^6 (172×10^3 bp) and 4×10^{12} Daltons, respectively; thus, 0.1 μg of EBV DNA in 50 μg of human tissue DNA is equivalent to 68 EBV genomes per cell.
   b. Assuming the hybridized counts for 0.1 μg EBV DNA to be 4000 cpm, this represents 59 cpm/copy/cell. EBV genome copy numbers in 50 μg genomic DNA from drug-treated P3HR-1(LS) cells can then be calculated by dividing the net hybridized counts (subtract the cpm from 50 μg HEp-2 cell DNA) by 59 cpm.

II. Standardization Based on Raji Cell DNA

Raji cells, a latently infected cell line derived from Burkitt's lymphoma, contain constant EBV genome copy numbers (60 copies/cell). One can construct a standard linear curve by using various amounts of Raji cell DNA attached to nitrocellulose filters and hybridizing to the EBV cRNA probe as described above. EBV genome copy numbers can then be calculated, based on the net hybridized counts from the same amount of itaji DNA and drug-treated P3HR-1(LS) DNA.

Method 2: DNA-DNA Hybridization on Nitrocellulose Filters

The classic cRNA-DNA hybridization has proved to be valuable in determining EBV genome copy numbers, but it presents a number of problems, which curtailed its wide use in nonviral laboratories. As noted above, the difficulty of attaining sufficient amounts of pure EBV DNA is the first problem encountered. Although DNA–DNA hybridization requires relatively large amounts of probe DNA, the availability of EBV clones makes this approach feasible.

1. Prepare genomic DNA following steps described in **Appendix 2**.
2. Digest 20 µg DNA with 40 U *Bam*HI restriction enzyme at 37°C for 16 h. Use Raji DNA as a standard reference (60 copies/cell).
3. Electrophorese the digested DNA fragments in 0.8% agarose gel.
4. Southern blot onto Hybond-N paper.
5. Crosslink the DNA attached to Hybond-N paper by irradiation using a UV Stratalinker (Stratagene, La Jolla, CA).
6. Bake the Hybond-N paper in a vacuum oven at 80°C for 30 min.
7. Prehybridize at 65°C for 2 h in buffer containing 6X SSC, 20 m*M* NaH_2PO_4, 0.4% SDS, and 500 µg/mL denatured, sonicated salmon sperm DNA.
8. Hybridize for 16–20 h at 65°C in fresh prehybridization buffer containing EBV *Bam*HI-W fragment labeled with ^{32}P by random primer kit (Stratagene).
9. Wash the paper three times in 2X SSC containing 0.5% SDS at 65°C with shaking.
10. Air-dry the paper and expose to Kodak XAR-5 film (Eastman Kodak, Rochester, NY).
11. Quantitate the radioactivity by densitometry, and calculate the EBV genome copy numbers using Raji DNA as a standard reference of 60 copies/cell. The radioactivity on the blot can also be quantitated by using Bio Image Whole Band Analyzer (Millipore, Bedford, MA).

References

1. zur Hausen, H., O'Neill, F. J., and Freeze, J. K. (1978) Persisting oncogenic herpesvirus induced by the tumor promoter TPA. *Nature (London)* **272,** 373–375.
2. Lin, J.C., Shaw, J. E., Smith, M. C., and Pagano, J. S. (1979) Effect of 12-O-tetradecanoyl-phorbol-13-acetate on the replication of Epstein-Barr virus. I. Characterization of viral DNA. *Virology* **99,** 183–187.
3. Lin, J. C., Smith, M. C., and Pagano, J. S. (1982) Effects of 12-O-tetradecanoyl-phorbol-13-acetate on cell proliferation and Epstein-Barr virus DNA replication. *Virology* **117,** 186–194.
4. Lin, J. C., Smith, M. C., and Pagano, J. S. (1983) Activation of latent Epstein-Barr virus genomes: selective stimulation of synthesis of chromosomal proteins by a tumor promoter. *J. Virol.* **45,** 985–991.
5. Mar, E. C. and Lin, J. C. (1996) Effects of temporal treatments of nucleoside analogs on replication of Epstein-Barr virus. Ninth International Conference on Antiviral Research, Fukushima, Japan, May 19–24.

6. Lin, J. C., Smith, M. C., and Pagano, J. S. (1984) Prolonged inhibitory effect of 9-(1,3)-dihydroxy-2-propoxymethyl)guanine against replication of Epstein-Barr virus. *J. Virol.* **50,** 50–55.
7. Lin, J. C., Zhang, Z. X., Chao, T. C., Sim, I., and Pagano, J. S. (1989) Synergistic inhibition of Epstein-Barr virus transformation of B lymphocytes by a and r interferon and by 3'-azido-3'-deoxythymidine. *J. Infect. Dis.* **159,** 248–254.
8. Reed, L. J. and Muench, H. (1938) A simple method of estimating fifty percent endpoints. *Am. J. Hygiene* **27,** 493–497.
9. Nonoyama, M. and Pagano, J. S. (1971) Detection of Epstein-Barr viral genome in nonproductive cells. *Nature (London) New Biol.* **233,** 103–106.
10. Burton, K. (1956) A study of the conditions and mechanism of the diphenylamine reaction for the colorimetric estimation of DNA. *Biochem. J.* **62,** 315–319.

13

Monitoring Drug Resistance for Herpesviruses

Graciela Andrei, Pierre Fiten, Erik De Clercq, Robert Snoeck, and Ghislain Opdenakker

1. Introduction

Herpes simplex type 1 (HSV-1) and type 2 (HSV-2), varicella-zoster virus (VZV) and human cytomegalovirus (CMV) cause diseases that are usually self-limiting in the immunocompetent host. However, HSV-1, HSV-2, VZV, and CMV are major causes of morbidity and mortality in the immunocompromised patient. Prolonged antiviral treatment is often required for the clinical management of herpesvirus infections in the immunocompromised patient, and this favors the emergence of drug-resistant strains. The isolation of acyclovir-resistant (ACV^r) HSV-1, HSV-2, and VZV strains as well as ganciclovir-resistant (GCV^r) CMV strains has been reported with increasing frequency and is a major concern ***(1–3)***. Resistance to foscarnet (phosphonoformic acid [PFA]), the drug of choice when ACV or GCV fails, has also been described in the clinic ***(4,5)***. Furthermore, double resistance to both GCV and PFA (for CMV) and to both ACV and PFA (for HSV) has been observed in immunocompromised patients after sequential and concomitant treatment with either or both drugs.

Alternative antiviral agents for the treatment of drug-resistant herpesviruses are the acyclic nucleoside phosphonate analogs. The lead compound of this new series of antiviral molecules is cidofovir [*(S)*-1-(3-hydroxy-2-phosphonylmethoxypropyl)cytosine] (HPMPC), which has a broad-spectrum antiviral activity in vitro and in vivo against several DNA viruses. Cidofovir has been approved for the treatment of CMV retinitis in AIDS patients, and it has also been shown to be effective in the treatment of persistent mucocutaneous infections caused by ACV^r HSV and ACV^r/PFA^r HSV ***(6,7)***.

From: *Methods in Molecular Medicine vol. 24: Antiviral Methods and Protocols*
Edited by: D. Kinchington and R. F. Schinazi © Humana Press Inc., Totowa, NJ

Mutations in two specific CMV genes (UL97 and DNA polymerase) have been associated with resistance to antiviral drugs *(2)*. The gene product of UL97 is a phosphotransferase enzyme that is responsible for the initial phosphorylation of GCV. CMV mutants resistant to GCV that do not exhibit crossresistance to other DNA polymerase inhibitors contain mutations in the UL97 open-reading frame, which results in a reduced ability of the UL97 virus-encoded enzyme to phosphorylate the drug in CMV-infected cells. GCV kinase activity of the UL97 gene is not required for the anti-CMV activity of HPMPC and its congener HPMPA [*(S)*-9-(3-hydroxy-2-phosphonylmethoxypropyl)adenine]. This explains the fact that the GCV^r strains containing mutations in the UL97 gene remain sensitive to HPMPC and HPMPA. By contrast, GCV^r strains containing mutations in the DNA polymerase gene show crossresistance to HPMPC and HPMPA. Although mutations in the UL97 and DNA polymerase genes may generate resistance to GCV in vitro, lack of phosphorylation seems to be the mechanism of resistance occurring most frequently in vivo.

For HSV at least three mechanisms have been described that generate resistance to ACV: deficiency or loss of viral TK activity, alteration in substrate specificity of the virus-encoded TK, and alteration in the substrate specificity of the viral DNA polymerase *(1,8)*. Most of the ACV^r mutants that have been isolated in vitro and recovered from clinical specimens are TK-deficient (TK$^-$). However, resistant clinical mutants that have an altered TK or altered DNA polymerase activity have occasionally been described too. Although TK mutants are crossresistant with drugs that also depend on viral TK for their activation (i.e., GCV, penciclovir and brivudin (BVDU), they remain sensitive to agents, such as PFA, vidarabine (Ara-A), and the acyclic nucleoside phosphonate (ANP) analogs. PFA, a pyrophosphate analog, is a direct inhibitor of the viral DNA poly-merase in which it binds to the site involved in releasing the pyrophosphate product of DNA synthesis. Phosphorylation of Ara-A to Ara-A triphosphate is carried out by cellular enzymes; phosphorylation of ANP derivatives to their mono- and diphosphoryl derivatives is also carried out by cellular enzymes.

Resistance of HSV and CMV strains to PFA are owing to mutations in the DNA polymerase gene. The authors have shown a significant degree of crossresistance between PFA and the phosphonylmethoxyethyl (PME) derivatives of adenine (PMEA) and 2,6-diaminopurine (PMEDAP) on the one hand, and between HPMPC and HPMPA on the other *(9,10)*. Although observed in the laboratory, resistance to cidofovir has not yet been documented in the clinic following treatment of CMV or HSV infections.

The isolation of drug-resistant virus mutants in the laboratory and the determination of their patterns of crossresistance may be useful to clarify the mechanisms of selective drug action. Indeed, one of the best ways to determine the overall mechanism of action of an antiviral drug is via drug resistance. The fact that it is possible to isolate virus mutants resistant to a drug implies that the drug selectively interferes with a virus-specific process. Once a drug-resistant virus mutant is isolated, the gene in which the mutation that is responsible for the resistant phenotype can be identified, and the drug target in the viral replicative cycle that contributes to antiviral selectivity can be defined. Compounds can be classified according to their patterns of crossresistance ***(9,10)***, which is important for the management of drug-resistant virus infections in the clinic.

In addition, the evaluation of the drug susceptibility profile of clinical strains to estimate the incidence and prevalence of drug resistance in immunocompromised patients is mandatory. Phenotyping studies, i.e., determination of antiviral drug susceptibilities, should be correlated with genotyping, i.e., characterization of mutations in the target genes. Surveillance of the patterns of drug susceptibilities of clinical strains is a prerequisite for the clinical management of drug-resistant herpesvirus infections.

This chapter presents in detail the procedure, used for the in vitro selection of drug-resistant herpesvirus mutants, the determination of the patterns of drug susceptibility, and the characterization of mutations in the drug-target gene.

2. Materials

2.1. Selection of Drug-Resistant Strains

1. Monolayers or African green monkey kidney (Vero) cells (for HSV) and human embryonic lung (HEL) fibroblasts (for VZV and CMV), grown in 25-cm^2 tissue-culture flasks.
2. MEM 10%: Minimum essential medium (MEM, Life Technologies) supplemented with 10% inactivated fetal calf serum (FCS), 1% L-glutamine, and 0.3% sodium bicarbonate.
3. MEM 2%: MEM supplemented with 2% FCS, 1% L-glutamine and 0.3% sodium bicarbonate.
4. Wild-type strain of HSV, VZV, and CMV.
5. Stocks of antiviral compounds prepared at a concentration of 20 mg/mL in dimethyl sulfoxide (DMSO) or 2 mg/mL in phosphate-buffered saline: 170 m*M* NaCl, 3.4 m*M* KCl, 10 m*M* Na_2HPO_4, 1.8 m*M* KH_2PO_4 (pH 7.2) according to their solubility.
6. Trypsin (Life Technologies).
7. DMSO (Merck).

2.2. Virus Titration

1. MEM 10% and MEM 2%.
2. Monolayers of HEL cells grown in 96-well microplates (Falcon).
3. Stock of HSV, CMV, or VZV.
4. Ethanol.
5. 2.5% Giemsa solution in distilled water.

2.3. Determination of the Drug-Susceptibility Profile of the Drug-Resistant Strains by Cytopathic Effect (CPE) Reduction Assay or Plaque Reduction Assay

1. MEM 10% and MEM 2%.
2. Monolayers of HEL cells grown in 96-well microplates.
3. Stocks of previously titrated wild-type virus and drug-resistant virus.
4. Serial dilutions of the antiviral compounds in MEM 2% with inclusion of test compounds and reference compounds, i.e., ACV (Glaxo-Wellcome), GCV (Syntex), BVDU (Rega Institute), foscarnet (Sigma), and cidofovir (Gilead Sciences).
5. Ethanol.
6. 2.5% Giemsa solution in distilled water.

2.4. Preparation of Plaque-Purified Virus

2.4.1. Plaque Purification Assay

1. MEM 10% and MEM 2%.
2. Monolayers of Vero cells (for HSV) or HEL cells (for CMV and VZV) grown in 6-well tissue culture plates.
3. 1.6% (w/v) autoclaved agarose.
4. FCS/MEM 2X: 4% inactivated FCS, 2% L-glutamine, and 0.6% sodium bicarbonate in 2X MEM.
5. 1% Neutral red stain (Sigma).
6. Stocks of drug-resistant strains.

2.4.2. Selection and Growth of Individual Plaques

1. MEM 10% and MEM 2%.
2. Monolayers of Vero cells (for HSV) or HEL cells (for CMV and VZV) grown in 25-cm^2 tissue culture flasks.
3. Sterile Pasteur pipets or plastic tips.

2.5. Determination of the Pathogenicity of the Plaque-Purified Drug-Resistant Strain

1. Stock of plaque-purified virus.
2. Monolayers of HEL cells grown in 96-well microplates.
3. MEM 10% and MEM 2%.
4. Adult mice.

2.6. Subcloning of the Viral Gene Responsible for the Resistant Phenotype: HSV-1 DNA Polymerase Gene

2.6.1. Large-Scale Preparations of Virus

1. Plaque-purified virus.
2. MEM 10% and MEM 2%.
3. Monolayers of Vero cells grown in 175-cm^2 tissue culture flasks (Falcon).

2.6.2. Preparation of Viral DNA

1. Virus pellet from **Subheading 3.7.1.**
2. Proteinase K (Sigma): 50 mg/mL in H_2O, freshly prepared or stored aliquoted at –20°C.
3. Proteinase K buffer: 0.01 *M* Tris (pH 7.8), 0.005 *M* ethylenediaminetetra-acetic acid (EDTA), 0.5% sodium dodecyl sulfate.
4. 10 mg/mL RNase A (Sigma) in TE (10 m*M* Tris-HCl, pH 8.0, 1 m*M* EDTA): heat to 100°C for 15 min to remove DNase activity; store in aliquots at –20°C.
5. Buffer-saturated phenol: ultrapure (Life Technologies).
6. Chloroform (Merck).
7. Phenol:chloroform (1:1, v/v).
8. 4 *M* NaCl.
9. Ethanol (Merck).
10. 70% Ethanol, room temperature.

2.6.3. Purification of Viral DNA Fragments Containing the DNA Polymerase Gene

1. Purified viral DNA from **Subheading 3.7.2.**
2. *Bam*HI restriction enzyme (Boehringer).
3. *Sac*I restriction enzyme (Boehringer).
4. Ultrapure agarose for electrophoresis of nucleic acids (Life Technologies).
5. 50X TBE: 242 g Tris base/L, 57.1 mL glacial acetic acid/L, 100 mL 0.5 *M* EDTA (pH 8.0)/L.
6. 6X gel-loading buffer: 0.25% bromophenol blue, 0.25% xylene cyanol FF, 30% glycerol in water.
7. Ethidium bromide: 10 mg/mL in water, stored at room temperature in light-shielded bottles.
8. DNA molecular marker (Boehringer).
9. QIAquick gel extraction kit (Qiagen).

2.6.4. Preparation of Plasmid Vector

1. Plasmid pUC18 (Pharmacia Biotech).
2. *Bam*HI restriction enzyme (Boehringer).
3. *Sac*I restriction enzyme (Boehringer).
4. Calf intestinal alkaline phosphatase (Boehringer).
5. Dephosphorylation buffer: 0.5 *M* Tris-HCl, 1 m*M* EDTA, pH 8.5.
6. 20% SDS.
7. 200 m*M* EDTA.
8. Buffer-saturated phenol: ultrapure (Life Technologies).
9. Chloroform.
10. Phenol:chloroform (1:1, v/v).
11. 4 *M* NaCl.
12. Ethanol.
13. 70% Ethanol.

2.6.5. Ligation Procedure

1. Purified viral DNA fragments prepared as described in **Subheading 3.7.3.**
2. Plasmid vector prepared as described in **Subheading 3.7.4.**
3. T4 DNA ligase (Boehringer).
4. 10X ligation buffer: 50 m*M* Tris-HCl (pH 7.5), 100 m*M* $MgCl_2$, 100 m*M* dithiothreitol, 10 m*M* adenosine triphosphate.

2.6.6. Preparation of Competent Bacterial Cells

1. *Eschericha coli*, strain DH5α (Life Technologies).
2. L-broth: 10 g/L Difco Bacto tryptone, 5 g/L Difco Bacto yeast extract, 5 g/L NaCl; autoclave.
3. 0.1 *M* $CaCl_2$. Sterilize the solution by filtration through a Nalgene filter (0.45-μ pore size). It is convenient to store a 1 *M* stock solution of $CaCl_2$ (made in Milli-Q water) in 10-mL aliquots at –20°C. When preparing competent cells, thaw an aliquot and dilute it to 100 mL with pure water.
4. Glycerol, autoclave.

2.6.7. Transformation Procedure

1. Competent bacterial cells prepared as described in **Subheading 3.6.6.**
2. DNA from ligation reactions (**Subheading 3.6.5.**).
3. Control plasmid pUC18.
4. X-gal (5-bromo-4-chloro-3-indolyl (-galactopyranoside) (Life Technologies) 20 mg/mL in dimethyl-formamide. Use a glass or polypropylene tube. Wrap the tube containing the solution in aluminium foil to prevent damage by light and store at –20°C. It is not necessary to sterilize X-gal solutions by filtration.
5. Isopropyl β-3-thiogalactopyranoside (IPTG) (Life Technologies) 100 mg/mL in water. Sterilize by filtration through a 0.22-μ disposable filter. Store in aliquots at –20°C.
6. L-broth.
7. L-broth 1.6% agar: L-broth containing 1.6 g/0.1 L Difco agar. Autoclave.
8. Top agar: L-broth containing 0.8 g/0.1 L Difco agar. Autoclave.
9. Ampicillin 50 mg/mL. Store at –20°C.

2.6.8. Identification and Screening of Recombinant Plasmids

1. L-broth.
2. Ampicillin 50 mg/mL (Life Technologies).
3. Nucleobond AX (Macherey-Nagel).
4. *Bam*HI and *Sac*I restriction enzymes.
5. 0.8% Agarose gel.
6. TBE.
7. 30% Glycerol, sterile.

2.6.9. Large-Scale Preparation of Plasmid DNA for Sequencing

1. L-broth ampicillin plates.
2. L-broth.

3. Ampicillin 50 mg/mL.
4. Nucleobond AX.

2.7. DNA Sequencing

1. Plasmid DNA.
2. Autoread Sequencing Kit (Pharmacia Biotech).
3. Cycle sequencing kit (Amersham Life Science).
4. Specific fluoresceine isothiocyanate (FITC) or Cy5-labeled primers designed according to the DNA-sequence of the wild-type strain.
5. Fluorescence DNA sequencer.

2.8. Screening of Identified Mutations in Various Plaque-Purified Virus Clones

1. Total viral DNA or the 3.4 kb *Bam*HI fragment from different plaque-purified virus strains, prepared as described in **Subheadings 3.6.2.** and **3.6.3.**
2. Cycle sequencing kit.
3. Specific FITC or Cy5-labeled primers that will allow the determination of the nucleotide sequence of the region of the viral DNA polymerase gene in which the mutation has been previously identified.

3. Methods

3.1. Selection of Drug-Resistant Strains

Drug-resistant virus strains are obtained by serial passage of a reference strain in cell culture in the presence of increasing concentrations of the compounds. For HSV and CMV, the passages of the virus are done with cell-free virus; for VZV, all the passages must be done with infected cells because the virus remains associated to the cells.

1. Grow Vero cells (for HSV) or HEL cells (for VZV and CMV) in MEM 10% in 25-cm^2 tissue culture flasks.
2. Remove the medium and add a virus inoculum at a multiplicity of infection (moi) of 0.002 plaque forming units (PFU)/cell.
3. Incubate the infected cell cultures at 37°C in a 5% CO_2 atmosphere for 2 h.
4. Remove residual virus and add MEM 2% containing a concentration of the antiviral drug that corresponds to its 50% inhibitory concentration (IC_{50}).

3.1.1. HSV

1. Incubate at 37°C until virus-induced cytopathicity is maximal.
2. Once 100% cytopathic effect (CPE) is observed, freeze the flasks and their contents at –80°C and thaw them at room temperature. Transfer the content in a sterile plastic tube and centrifuge at 1500*g* for 10 min to remove cell debris. Store at –80°C.
3. Dilute the virus stock in order to do the next passage at a higher concentration of the compound. Repeat **Subheading 3.1.** and **steps 1** and **2**. With every passage of

the virus, the drug concentration is usually increased twofold. After reaching the highest possible concentration for a given compound, a last passage in drug-free medium is done to obtain the virus stock that will be used in the drug-susceptibility profile test.

3.1.2. CMV

1. Incubate at 37°C until virus-induced cytopathicity is maximal.
2. Once 100% CPE is observed, harvest the supernatant and clarify by centrifugation at 1500*g* for 10 min. Store at –80°C in aliquots.
3. Harvest the infected cells by trypsinization and freeze them in MEM 10% containing 10% DMSO.
4. Dilute the virus supernatant to do the next passage of the virus. Repeat **Subheading 3.1.** and **steps 1–3**. Grow the virus for two consecutive passages with the same concentration of compound, and then increase the drug concentration twofold for each passage. When viral CPE does not develop, it is convenient to do a passage with the infected cells obtained from the previous passage. When the highest possible concentration for a given compound is reached, a last passage in drug-free medium is done. This viral stock is then used in the drug-susceptibility assay.

3.1.3. VZV

1. Incubate at 37°C until approx 70% of the cells are infected.
2. When approx 70% CPE is observed, harvest the infected cells by trypsinization. Prepare 1-mL aliquots of the infected cells in MEM 10% containing 10% DMSO. Store at –80°C.
3. To do a next passage of the virus, thaw the cells, centrifuge at 800*g* for 10 min, discard the supernatant, and resuspend the cells in 1 mL of MEM 2%. Dilute the infected cells and repeat **Subheading 3.1.** and **steps 1 and 2**. Grow the virus for two consecutive passages with the same concentration of compound, and then double the drug concentration. When the highest possible concentration for a given compound is reached, a last passage in drug-free medium is done to obtain the virus stock that will be used in the drug-susceptibility assays.

3.2. Virus Titration

Once a drug-resistant virus strain is obtained, a titration of the viral stock must be done before evaluating its drug-susceptibility profile.

1. Prepare 10-fold dilutions of the virus stock in MEM 2%. Dilutions in the range of 10^{-2}–10^{-7} (for HSV) and in the range 10^{-1}–10^{-4} (for CMV and VZV) are appropriate for most virus stocks. Use a fresh pipet or tip for each dilution to prevent carryover of virus (which might otherwise result in an anomalously high virus titer).
2. Remove the medium from the plates and apply 100 µL of diluted virus per well; use six wells per dilution.
3. Incubate the cell cultures at 37°C in a 5% CO_2 atmosphere for 2 h.

4. Remove the inoculum and add MEM 2%.
5. Incubate the cells at 37°C in a 5% CO_2 atmosphere for 3 (for HSV), 5 (for VZV), and 7 d (for CMV).
6. For HSV, evaluate CPE or plaque formation microscopically.
7. For CMV and VZV, fix the microplates with ethanol and stain them with 2.5% Giemsa solution for 2 h; then monitor viral plaque formation or viral CPE.
8. Determine the $CCID_{50}$, with 1 $CCID_{50}$ being the virus dose that is infective for 50% of the cell cultures, or calculate the titer of the virus stock in PFU/mL.

3.3. Determination of the Drug-Susceptibility Profile of the Drug-Resistant Strains by CPE Reduction Assay or Plaque Reduction Assay

Different assays are available to detect and measure antiviral drug susceptibility of HSV. The most commonly used methods are the CPE and plaque reduction assays, the neutral red dye uptake assay, and a DNA hybridization assay *(5)*. The CPE and plaque reduction assays measure viral efficiency in inducing CPE or in forming plaques in the presence of different concentrations of the antiviral compound. The difference between these two assays is determined by the viral inoculum used, allowing evaluation of viral-induced CPE or enumeration of the number of plaques. The dye uptake assay uses a semiautomated method to quantify spectrophotometrically the uptake of neutral red by viable cells. Drug activity is then measured as a reduction in HSV-induced cell death. The DNA hybridization assay quantifies viral DNA after exposure to an antiviral agent using a radiolabeled DNA probe specific for HSV-1 and HSV-2. A specific DNA hybridization assay exists also for CMV and VZV. Commercially available hybridization assays (Hybriwix assay; Diagnostic Hybrids, Athens, OH) for HSV-1, HSV-2, and CMV are relatively widely used. Calculation of IC_{50} values is made by plotting DNA reduction curves against drug concentration.

The CPE or plaque reduction assays can be performed faster, have less variability than the DNA hybridization assay, do not need special materials and equipment, and avoid the need to handle radioisotopes and nuclear waste. The DNA hybridization technique may be quite useful for confirmatory purposes but not for large-scale evaluation of clinically or in vitro isolated drug-resistant strains. The CPE reduction assay and the plaque reduction assay are the most commonly used tests to evaluate the drug-susceptibility profile of drug-resistant strains, for HSV, VZV, or CMV.

1. Dilute the virus stocks in MEM 2% to a final concentration of 100 $CCID_{50}$/0.1 mL (for HSV), 20 PFU (for VZV), and 100 PFU (for CMV). Ten milliliters of virus preparation are needed per microtiter plate.
2. Remove the medium from the microplate-grown cells and inoculate these with 0.1 mL of the diluted virus per well. Always change the tips when you infect the

cells with a different strain. It is advisable to include only one viral strain per microplate.

3. Incubate the infected cells at 37°C in a 5% CO_2 atmosphere for 2 h.
4. Remove the virus inoculum.
5. Add the serial dilutions of the test compounds in duplicate.
6. Incubate the infected cells at 37°C in a 5% CO_2 atmosphere for 2–3 (for HSV), 5–6 (for VZV), and 7–8 d (for CMV). A longer time of incubation may be necessary for some mutants.
7. For HSV CPE can be monitored easier without fixing and staining the cells. For CMV and VZV fix the cells with ethanol and stain with 2.5% Giemsa solution for 2 h.
8. Virus plaque formation (VZV) or viral CPE (HSV and CMV) is evaluated microscopically. Evaluate CPE microscopically using a scale from 0 to 5, with 0 indicating an absence of CPE and 5 being 100% CPE (comparable to the untreated controls), or count the number of plaques in treated and untreated cultures.
9. Express the minimal antiviral inhibitory concentration as the IC_{50}, or the concentration required to inhibit virus-induced CPE or plaque formation by 50%. IC_{50}s are estimated from (semilogarithmic) graphic plots of the number of plaques (percentage of control) or percentage of CPE as a function of the concentration of the test compound.

3.4. Preparation of Plaque-Purified Virus

3.4.1. Plaque Purification Assay

It is possible that the virus mutant selected under the pressure of a certain drug is a mixture of two or more populations of virus. It has been found that the HSV-1 mutants arising under the selective pressure of HPMPC or HPMPA are not pure populations. Thus, plaque-purified virus must be prepared, and the drug-susceptibility profile of a few classes of compounds should be determined as well as the mutations in the drug-targeted viral gene that are associated with the resistant phenotype.

1. Prepare 10-fold dilutions of the virus stocks in MEM 2%.
2. Inoculate confluent monolayers of Vero cells (for HSV) or HEL cells (for CMV and VZV) grown in 6-well tissue culture plates with 0.5 mL of the virus dilution per well.
3. Incubate at 37°C in a 5% CO_2 atmosphere for 2 h, gently shaking the plates periodically.
4. While the plates are incubating, melt the agarose in a microwave oven.
5. Cool the agarose to 45°C in a water bath.
6. Mix the agarose with an equal volume of FCS/MEM 2X that has been warmed at 37°C; 18 mL of overlay medium/plate are needed.
7. Remove the virus inoculum.
8. Add 3 mL of overlay medium per well. Leave at room temperature until agarose solidifies.

9. Incubate the cultures at 37°C in inverted orientation in a 5% CO_2 atmosphere for 2–3 (HSV), 5 (VZV), or 7 d (CMV), at which time the plaques are usually visible.
10. Stain the monolayers by adding a further 1 mL of agarose-FCS/MEM 2X containing 0.08% neutral red stain per well. Plaques can normally be visualized 16–24 h later.

3.4.2. Selection and Growth of Individual Plaques

1. Allow the plaques to grow to a reasonable size to facilitate selection.
2. Select plaques from wells containing a small number of well-separated plaques. Use a sterile Pasteur pipet or plastic tip for each plaque and carefully withdraw the overlay from the area of the plaque and transfer it to a 4-mL plastic tube containing 1 mL of MEM 2%.
3. Rinse a few times the Pasteur pipet or the plastic tip in the medium and vortex the tube in order to disaggregate the overlay.
4. Inoculate confluent Vero cells (for HSV) or HEL cells (for VZV and CMV) grown in 25-cm^2 flasks with the selected plaque isolates.
5. Incubate at 37°C in a CO_2 atmosphere for 2 h, remove the inoculum, and add 5 mL MEM 2%.
6. Incubate at 37°C until full CPE is observed (for HSV and CMV) or until 70% of the cells are infected (for VZV).
7. For HSV and CMV freeze the flasks and their contents at –80°C and thaw at room temperature. Decant the contents into sterile plastic tubes and centrifuge at 1500*g* for 10 min to remove cell debris. Store aliquots of the virus at –80°C.
8. For VZV, prepare the stocks as virus-infected cells and freeze at –80°C.
9. Each plaque-purified virus needs to be titrated (as described in **Subheading 2.**) and evaluated for its drug-susceptibility profile (as described in **Subheading 3.**).

3.5. Determination of the Pathogenicity of the Plaque-Purified Drug-Resistant Strains

Once a drug-resistant HSV strain is obtained, it is important to determine its pathogenicity in a mouse model of HSV disease. The neurovirulence assay involves lethal infection of the central nervous system using immunocompetent mice. Almost all drug-resistant HSV mutants exhibit some degree of pathogenicity. This is particularly true for the TK^- mutants. TK-altered and DNA polymerase mutants tend to be less virulent than wild-type strains but more virulent than TK^- mutants in neurovirulence assays. Obviously, one must be cautious in extrapolating neurovirulence results to humans.

1. Prepare 10-fold dilutions of the stock of the plaque-purified drug-resistant strain in MEM 2%.
2. Titrate the virus stock in cell culture as described in **Subheading 3.2.**
3. Express the titer in PFU/mL.
4. In parallel, inoculate intracerebrally adult mice with 50 µL of each viral dilution. Use five mice/dilution.

5. Record mortality over a period of 20 d.
6. Express the virus titer in lethal dose 50 (LD_{50})/mL.
7. Calculate the pathogenicity index as the log PFU/LD_{50}. The higher the index, the less neurovirulent the viral strain.

3.6. Subcloning of the Viral Gene Responsible for the Resistant Phenotype: HSV-1 DNA Polymerase Gene

Once some drug-resistant clones have been studied for their drug-susceptibility profile, the mutation(s) in the drug-target viral gene that are associated with the resistant phenotype should be determined. To identify new mutations, the authors do not recommend the use of polymerase chain reaction amplification techniques to avoid problems of infidelity of the various *taq* polymerases. Although the recommended procedure is more laborious, the authors prefer to subclone the drug-target viral gene and to determine its nucleotide sequence. The subcloning of the HSV-1 DNA polymerase gene will be described here as an example. This is a general procedure that can be adapted to subclone other herpesvirus genes. To subclone the DNA polymerase gene, a 3.4-kb fragment obtained after digestion of the viral DNA with *Bam*HI is isolated. The 3.4-kb fragment, which contains about 87% of the HSV-1 DNA polymerase gene coding region, is further digested with *Sac*I. The two resulting fragments of 2.0 and 1.4 kb are purified and ligated to pUC18 cleaved with *Bam*HI and *Sac*I. The ligation mixtures are used to transform competent *E. coli*. Ampicillin-resistant colonies are identified and screened for plasmids containing the appropriate fragments of 2.0 and 1.4 kb. Plasmid DNA is prepared and the inserts are sequenced by the dideoxynucleotide chain termination method with T7 DNA polymerase and *taq* DNA polymerase. Universal forward and reverse M13 primers and specific oligonucleotide primers designed on the basis of the wild-type HSV-1 KOS strain are used for sequencing; analysis is on an automated laser fluorescent DNA sequencer.

3.6.1. Large-Scale Preparations of Virus

1. Use 8–10 tissue culture flasks (175-cm^2) of Vero cells grown to confluence.
2. Remove the medium and add a virus inoculum at an moi of 0.002 PFU/cell in 40–50 mL of MEM 2%
3. Incubate at 37°C for 3 d, by which time all the cells should have rounded and will have detached from the bottle or can be removed by gently shaking the medium.
4. After shaking off the cells, decant the mixture of cells and medium into 50-mL centrifuge tubes, freeze at –80°C, and thaw at room temperature. Separate the cell debris from the cells by centrifugation at 1500*g* for 15 min at 4°C.
5. Decant the medium into bottles without disturbing the pellet. The medium contains virus that has been released from the cells and is a good source of virions.
6. Pellet the virus by centrifuging at 120,000*g* for 3 h at 4°C. Discard the supernatant.

3.6.2. Preparation of Viral DNA

1. Resuspend the virus pellet for each 25 mL of original culture in 500 μL of proteinase K buffer. Transfer the suspension to a 1.5-mL microcentrifuge tube and add RNase to a final concentration of 100 μg/mL. Incubate at 37°C for 1 h.
2. Add proteinase K to a final concentration of 250 μg/mL. Incubate at 37°C overnight.
3. Add an equal volume of phenol:chloroform.
4. Mix the contents of the tube until an emulsion forms.
5. Centrifuge the mixture at 13,000*g* for 20 min in a microfuge at room temperature.
6. Transfer the upper aqueous phase to a fresh tube.
7. Repeat **steps 3–6** until no protein is visible at the interface of the organic and aqueous phases.
8. Add an equal volume of chloroform and repeat **steps 3–6.**
9. Add NaCl to a final concentration of 0.2 *M*.
10. Add 2 vol of ice-cold ethanol and gently mix the solution.
11. Allow the DNA to precipitate by incubating for 2 h at –80°C or overnight at –20°C.
12. Recover the DNA by centrifugation at 13,000*g* for 30 min in a microfuge.
13. Carefully remove the supernatant without disturbing the DNA pellet.
14. Add 1 mL of 70% ethanol to the DNA pellet.
15. Microcentrifuge at 13,000*g* for 10 min, and carefully discard the supernatant.
16. Store the open tube on the bench at room temperature until the ethanol has evaporated.
17. Dissolve the DNA pellet in the desired volume of distilled water.

3.6.3. Purification of Viral DNA Fragments Containing the DNA Polymerase Gene

1. Digest 3–5 μg of viral DNA with an excess of *Bam*HI in a volume of 10–15 μL at 37°C for 2 h. Approximately 20–40 μg viral DNA is necessary as starting material for the subcloning of the DNA polymerase gene.
2. Prepare a 0.8% agarose gel in 1X TBE.
3. Add 6X gel-loading buffer to the DNA samples. Prepare a DNA size marker.
4. Load the samples into the gel slots and carry out the electrophoresis overnight at 20–25 V to ensure a good resolution.
5. Stain the gel with ethidium bromide (0.5 μg/mL) for 30 min.
6. Examine the gel by ultraviolet (UV) light illumination and photograph it.
7. Using a sharp scalpel, cut out a slide of agarose containing the band of interest (3.4 kb) and transfer it to a clean tube.
8. After cutting out the band, photograph the gel so that there is a record of which band was eluted.
9. Recover the DNA from the agarose gel using the QIAquick gel extraction kit protocol.
10. Digest the 3.4 kb DNA fragment with *Sac*I.
11. Prepare a 0.8% agarose gel in 1X TAE.
12. Add 6X gel-loading buffer to the DNA samples. Include a DNA size marker.

13. Load the samples on the gel, and electrophorese at 75–80 V until the bromophenol blue and xylene cyanol FF markers have migrated through the gel.
14. Stain the gel with ethidium bromide, locate the bands of interest by using a UV lamp, and photograph the gel.
15. Recover the bands of 2.0 and 1.4 kb as described in **steps 7–9**.
16. Store the DNA at –20°C until the ligation reactions are performed.

3.6.4. Preparation of the Plasmid Vector

1. Digest 5 µg of plasmid with 10 uL of *Bam*HI in a volume of 40 µL at 37°C for 3–4 h. Use the restriction buffer that gives 100%, or nearly 100%, activity for both *Bam*HI and *Sac*I restriction enzymes, e.g., Boehringer's buffer A.
2. Add 10 U of *Sac*I and continue the incubation for another 3–4 h.
3. To dephosphorylate the plasmid, incubate it with 20 U of calf intestinal phosphatase alkaline at 37°C for 15 min.
4. Add 20% SDS and 200 m*M* EDTA to a final concentration of 1% and 25 m*M*, respectively.
5. Extract twice with phenol:chloroform (1:1, v/v), once with chloroform; precipitate with ethanol and resuspend in distilled water as described in **Subheading 3.6.2.**
6. Store the plasmid vector at –20°C until use in the ligation reactions.
7. Estimate by electrophoresis in agarose gel the concentration of DNA; verify that the plasmid vector runs as the relaxed (digested) form.

3.6.5. Ligation Procedure

1. Ligate approx 50 ng of each viral DNA fragment to 100 ng vector DNA in a total volume of 20 µL of 1X ligation buffer containing 1 U of T4 DNA ligase.
2. In a separate tube, set up an additional ligation reaction as control, containing the plasmid vector alone.
3. Incubate at 15°C overnight.
4. Heat-inactivate the ligase at 70°C for 10 min.
5. Use 10 µL of the ligation reactions to transform competent *E.coli* using the methods described in **Subheading 3.6.6.** Store the remaining 10 µL of ligation mixture at –20°C in case the transformation needs to be repeated.

3.6.6. Preparation of Competent Bacterial Cells (11)

1. Inoculate a single colony of *E. coli* strain DH5α into 5 mL of L-broth and incubate at 37°C overnight while shaking.
2. Add 2 mL of the overnight culture to 200 mL of L-broth. Continue incubation at 37°C with vigorous shaking (300 cycles/min in a rotary shaker) until the culture has reached the logarithmic phase of growth. This normally takes 3 h.
3. Transfer the cells to sterile, disposable, ice-cold 50-mL polypropylene tubes. Cool the cultures at 0°C by storing the tubes on ice for 10 min.
4. Harvest the cells by centrifugation at 4000 rpm for 10 min at 4°C in a Sorvall GS3 rotor (or equivalent).
5. Decant the supernatant from the cell pellets. Leave the tubes in a inverted position for 1 min to allow the last traces of media to drain away.

6. Resuspend each pellet in 10 mL of ice-cold 0.1 *M* $CaCl_2$ and store on ice.
7. Recover the cells by centrifugation at 4000 rpm or 10 min at 4°C in a Sorvall GS3 rotor (or its equivalent).
8. Decant the fluid from the cell pellets, and position the tubes inverted to allow the culture of fluid to drain away.
9. Resuspend each pellet in 2 mL of ice-cold 0.1 *M* $CaCl_2$ for each 50 mL of original culture.
10. Divide the cells into aliquots and freeze at –80°C with 30% glycerol.

3.6.7. Transformation Procedure

1. Melt L-broth 1.6% agar and incubate it in a water bath at 55°C. When cooled to 55°C, add ampicillin to a final concentration of 50–100 µg/mL and prepare the L-broth ampicillin plates.
2. Remove competent cells from –80°C freezer; thaw on ice. Place required number of 17 × 100 mm polypropylene tubes (Falcon 2059) on ice.
3. Gently mix the cells, then aliquot 100 mL of competent cells into chilled polypropylene tubes.
4. Immediately add 10 µL of each of the ligation reactions (1–10 mg) to separate tubes. Two controls should be included, one containing 10 ng of pUC18 and the other without plasmid DNA. Mix the DNAs with the bacteria by tapping the sides of the tubes gently.
5. Incubate the cells on ice for 30 min.
6. Melt the L-broth top agar. Store at 55°C until used.
7. Transfer the tubes containing the competent bacteria and DNA to a water bath at 37°C. Incubate for 30 s. Do not shake.
8. Place the tubes on ice for 30 s.
9. Repeat the heat-shock twice more.
10. Make a 10-fold dilution for each sample.
11. Add 0.9 mL of room temperature L-broth medium to each tube.
12. Shake at 225 rpm (37°C) for 1 h.
13. Add 40 µL of a solution of X-gal 20 mg/mL and 10 µL of a solution of IPTG 100 mg/mL to each tube on different sites of the tube.
14. Add 3 mL of top agar to each tube and mix.
15. Poor the mixture onto L-broth ampicillin plates. Swing the plate gently to ensure an even distribution of bacteria and top agar. Leave the plates open for X min in a laminar flow hood to evaporate excess water.
16. Close the plates and allow the top agar to solidify for 5 min at room temperature.
17. Invert the plates and incubate at 37°C overnight.
18. Screen recombinant plasmids.

3.6.8. Identification and Screening of Recombinant Plasmids

The pUC vectors contain an ampicillin-resistance gene and a multiple cloning site at the 5'-end of the *lac*Z gene. Insertional inactivation of *lac*Z allows color detection of recombinants using X-gal. Colonies formed by bacteria transformed by wild-type pUC18 will be deep blue; those transformed by recombinant pUC18 will be colorless owing to inactivation of the β-galactosidase. To analyze the foreign DNA sequences in the colorless plaques, stocks of putative recombinant plasmids from single plaques are prepared.

1. Fill 4 mL L-broth 10-mL bacterial cultures tubes.
2. Touch the surface of a colorless colony using a sterile toothpick.
3. Wash the end of the stick in the medium.
4. Incubate the infected cultures overnight with constant agitation.
5. Use a part of the culture (3 mL) to prepare plasmid DNA using Nucleobond AX-20. The rest of the bacterial culture is kept at 4°C until the results of the screening are known. If the clone has the desired insert, the bacterial cultures are cryopreserved at –20°C.
6. Digest an aliquot of the plasmid DNA that has been prepared using Nucleobond AX-20 with *Bam*HI and *Sac*I with the buffer that gives 100% activity for both enzymes (e.g., buffer A, Boehringer) for 1–2 h at 37°C. Include as control undigested pUC18 and pUC18 digested with the restriction enzymes.
7. Separate the samples by electrophoresis in 0.8% agarose gel in TBE as described in **Subheading 3.6.3.**
8. After electrophoresis, examine the gel by UV light illumination of ethidium bromide stained DNA and photograph the gel. Detect the clones that have the insert of 2.0 and 1.4 kb.
9. Screen the recombinant clones by sequencing with reverse and forward primers as described in **Subheading 3.7.** to verify the presence of the viral sequences.
10. Freeze the bacterial cultures (that were kept at 4°C) from which recombinant clones were observed at –20°C in 30% glycerol.

3.6.9. Large-Scale Preparation of Plasmid DNA for Sequencing

1. Select one recombinant clone for the 2.0-kb insert and one for the 1.4-kb insert for each drug-resistant mutant and plate them in ampicillin L-broth plates.
2. Incubate overnight at 37°C.
3. To prepare enough plasmid DNA for sequencing, inoculate a single colony in ampicillin L-broth and incubate at 37°C overnight with shaking.
4. Prepare plasmid DNA using Nucleobond AX100 or Nucleobond AX20.

3.7. DNA Sequencing

1. Aliquots from the plasmid DNA of 6 μg for T7 DNA polymerase sequencing or 500 ng for cycle sequencing were prepared.
2. The total insert of the plasmid DNAs were sequenced starting with fluorescent universal forward and reverse M13 primers, followed by primer walking using internal fluorescent primers (Pharmacia Biotech). The sequencing reactions were done according to the manufacturer's protocols. For T7 DNA polymerase sequencing the AutoRead Sequencing Kit was used and for cycle sequencing, the Thermo Sequenase fluorescent-labeled primer cycle sequencing kit was used.

3. The sequencing reaction products were run on automated DNA sequencers using standard sequencing gel conditions, on the ALF DNA sequencer (Pharmacia Biotech) for the FITC-labeled primers, and on the ALF express (Pharmacia Biotech) for the CY5-labeled primers.
4. The sequencing data were collected and processed by the ALF manager software (Pharmacia Biotech). Assembly of the processed sequence fragments was done with the ASSEMGEL, sequence gels assembly program (PCGENE, IntelliGenetics).

3.8. Screening of Identified Mutations in Various Plaque-Purified Virus Clones

Once a mutation that confers resistance to an antiviral drug has been identified, it is important to establish if this is the only resistant genotype that is selected for. For this purpose several clones should be screened for the presence of a given mutation.

1. Cycle sequencing on the total viral DNA or on the 3.4-kb *Bam*HI fragment, prepared as described in **Subheadings 3.6.2.** and **3.6.3.,** is performed.
2. Specific primers that allow the determination of the nucleotide sequence of the region of the viral DNA polymerase in which the mutation has been identified are used.
3. If the identified mutation is not found in some phenotypic-resistant viral clones, then it is worthwhile to determine the whole nucleotide sequence of the DNA polymerase after subcloning the viral gene (to find new mutations).

4. Notes

1. During the process of selection of drug-resistant strains, it is possible that virus-induced CPE appears very slowly under the selective pressure of a given compound; in this case it is recommended that the medium be replaced with medium without compound or eventually that a passage of the virus in the absence of the compound be done.
2. The number of passages in increasing concentrations of a drug that are necessary to select mutant virus depends on several factors, such as the type of virus, the antiviral drug, and the cell line used. Thus, drug resistance for HSV appears more rapidly than for CMV or VZV, probably owing to the shorter replicative cycle of HSV compared with that of CMV and VZV. With some antiviral drugs (i.e., ACV and BVDU), resistant virus appears even after a single passage of HSV under the selective pressure of these drugs *(12)*. By contrast, with other antiviral compounds like HPMPC and HPMPA, the virus needs to be grown over several months (HSV) or years (CMV and VZV) in the presence of these compounds before drug-resistant virus can be selected. In addition, the authors have shown that for HSV, the selection of drug-resistant virus can be accelerated in certain cell lines *(13)*. CMV and VZV, owing to their cell-type specificity, can only be propagated efficiently in human embryonic fibroblasts.

3. The use of an appropriate virus inoculum in the CPE reduction assay is extremely important, because either a large or a small virus inoculum may give misleading results in the drug-susceptibility profile.
4. Drug resistance should be defined as a function of the nature of each class of antiherpetic compound. For example, the authors have defined drug resistance as an IC_{50} value increase of 100-fold for drugs that depend on virus-induced TK for their activation, of 8- to 10-fold for HPMP derivatives (HPMPA, HPMPC) and of fivefold for pyrophosphate analogs and PME derivatives (PMEA, PMEDAP) *(9)*.
5. In the determination of the drug-susceptibility profile of drug-resistant strains, the reference wild-type virus strain needs to be included in each experiment. The assays should be repeated at least in three independent experiments to calculate the mean IC_{50} value standard deviation for each drug and each viral mutant, and these values should be compared with those obtained for the wild-type reference strain.
6. In the plaque purification assay, it should be ensured that the agarose is at 45°C and that the FCS/MEM 2X is at 37°C before mixing. Do not allow them to cool, and dispense them as quickly as possible.
7. Cell-associated virus is a useful source of virus, but it is heavily contaminated with cellular debris. It should be ascertained that the supernatant containing the free virus is well clarified before ultracentrifuging the virus. Sometimes it is convenient to repeat the centrifugation at 1500*g* for 15 min at 4°C.
8. To prevent self-ligation of the vector without an insert and to increase the efficiency of insertion of the viral DNA fragments, the vector is dephosphorylated prior to ligation, even if two restriction sites with incompatible termini for cleavage of the vector DNA and the viral fragments are used.

Acknowledgments

The authors thank Christiane Callebaut and Inge Aerts for dedicated editorial help.

References

1. Field, A. K. and Biron, K. K. (1994) "The end of innocence" revisited: resistance of herpesviruses to antiviral drugs. *Clin. Microbiol. Rev.* **7,** 1–13.
2. Anonymous (1996) Drug resistance in cytomegalovirus: current knowledge and implications for patient management. *J. Acquir. Immune Defic. Syndr. Hum. Retrovir.* **12,** S1–SS22.
3. Coen, D. M. (1991) The implicatons of resistance to antiviral agents for herpesvirus drug targets and drug therapy. *Antiviral Res.* **15,** 287–300.
4. Coen, D. M. (1995) Nucleosides and foscarnet—mechanisms, in *Antiviral Drug Resistance* (Richman, D. D., ed.), Wiley, Chichester, pp. 81–102.
5. Safrin, S. (1995) Nucleosides and foscarnet—clinical aspects, in *Antiviral Drug Resistance* (Richman, D. D., ed.), Wiley, Chichester, pp. 103–122.
6. Snoeck, R., Andrei, G., Girard, M., Silverman, A., Hedderman, A., Balzarini, J., Sadzot-Delvaux, C., Tricot, G., Clumeck, N., and De Clercq, E. (1994) Successful treatment of progressive mucocutaneous infection due to acyclovir- and

foscarnet-resistant herpes simplex virus with (S)-1-(3-hydroxy-2-phosphonyl-methoxypropyl)cytosine (HPMPC). *Clin. Infect. Dis.* **18,** 570–578.

7. Hitchcock, M. J. M., Jaffe, H. S., Martin, J. C., and Stagg, R. J. (1996) Cidofovir, a new agent with potent anti-herpesvirus activity. *Antiviral Res.* **7,** 115–127.
8. Collins, P. and Darby, G. (1991) Laboratory studies of herpes simplex virus strains resistant to acyclovir. *Rev. Med. Virol.* **1,** 19–28.
9. Andrei, G., Snoeck, R., and De Clercq, E. (1995) Susceptibilities of several drug-resistant herpes simplex virus type 1 strains to alternative antiviral compounds. *Antimicrob. Agents Chemother.* **39,** 1632–1635.
10. Snoeck, R., Andrei, G., and De Clercq, E. (1996) Patterns of resistance and sensitivity to antiviral compounds of drug-resistant strains of human cytomegalovirus selected in vitro. *Eur. J. Clin. Microbiol. Infect. Dis.* **15,** 574–579.
11. Sambrook, J., Fritsch, E. F., and Maniatis, T. (eds.) (1989) *Molecular Cloning. A Laboratory Manual,* 2nd ed., Cold Spring Harbor Laboratory, Cold Spring Harbor, NY.
12. Morfin, F., Snoeck, R., Andrei, G., and De Clercq, E. (1996) Phenotypic resistance of herpes simplex virus type 1 strains selected in vitro with antiviral compounds and combinations thereof. *Antiviral Chem. Chemother.* **7,** 270–275.
13. Andrei, G., Snoeck, R., and De Clercq, E. (1994) Human brain tumour cell lines as cell substrate to demonstrate sensitivity/resistance of herpes simplex virus types 1 and 2 to nucleoside analogues. *Antiviral Chem. Chemother.* **5,** 263–270.

14

Herpesvirus Protease Assays

Peter Ertl, Linda Russell, and Jane Angier

1. Introduction

Herpesviruses encode a serine protease that is essential for the maturation of viral capsids *(1,2)*. The protease is expressed as part of a polyprotein. The catalytic domain is contained within the N-terminal third of the protein, and the remainder comprises a structural "scaffold" protein. The scaffold protein is independently expressed in excess to the polyprotein from an internal initiation codon. The protease cleaves the polyprotein at two sites: one at the c-terminus of the protease catalytic domain, the release or R-site, and the other close to the c-terminus of the scaffold protein, the maturation or M-site (**Fig. 1**). Cleavage of the M-site follows assembly of the viral procapsids and precedes packaging of the viral DNA. The M-site sequence is conserved among the herpesviruses and has a consensus sequence (V/L)-X-A-S, with cleavage between A-S *(3)*. Structural studies have shown that the herpesvirus proteases have a novel structure, and their essential role in capsid maturation makes them a potential target for antiviral intervention.

The first step in identification of herpesvirus inhibitors that act via this mechanism is the evaluation of compounds for their ability to inhibit the protease enzyme. A number of assay formats have been used to examine the effect of herpesvirus protease inhibitors. This chapter describes four of these assays, and their relative merits and problems are discussed. In particular, the conditions for HCMV protease are described, with reference to modifications for other herpesvirus proteases where possible in the notes. A source of purified recombinant enzyme will be assumed, because a number of studies have described the use of *Escherichia coli* to express active herpesvirus proteases from a number of viruses, along with suitable purification methods *(4–6)*.

From: *Methods in Molecular Medicine, vol. 24: Antiviral Methods and Protocols*
Edited by: D. Kinchington and R. F. Schinazi © Humana Press Inc., Totowa, NJ

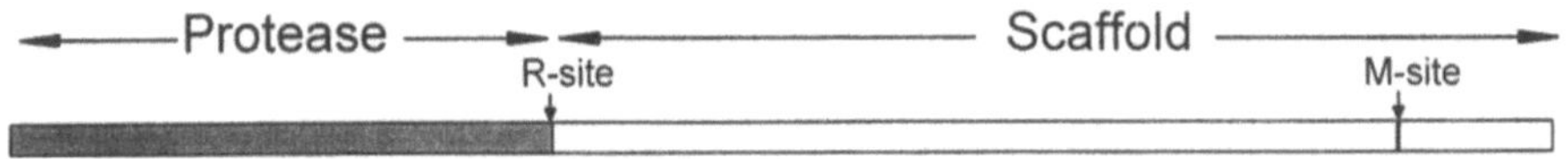

Fig. 1. Cartoon illustration of the structure of the herpesvirus protease/scaffold polyprotein showing the position of the protease catalytic domain, the scafold protein, and the release and maturation cleavage sites.

2. Materials

2.1. High-Pressure Liquid Chromatography (HPLC) Peptide Assay

1. Substrate peptide: RGVVNASSRLAK, 10 m*M* in dimethyl sulfoxide (DMSO) (store at –20°C).
2. Assay buffer: 30% glycerol, 100 m*M* HEPES pH 7.7, 2 m*M* dithiothreitol (DTT) (prepare fresh).
3. Stop reagent: 0.2% trifluoroacetic acid (TFA) in water.
4. 0.2 µm PVDF filters (Whatman [Maidstone, UK] 6792-0402).
5. HPLC C18 reverse phase column (ABI Brownlee [San Jose, CA] [10 × 4.6] No. 0711 002]).
6. HPLC grade acetonitrile (ACN) + 0.1% TFA.
7. HPLC grade water + 0.1 % TFA.

2.2. Scintillation Proximity Assay (SPA)

1. Substrate: Biotin-Aha-RGVVNASSRL(^{3}H)G (Amersham, [Little Chalfont, UK] 125 Ci/mmol, 1 mCi/mL) (store at +4°C).
2. Assay buffer: 30% glycerol, 100 m*M* HEPES, pH 7.7, 5 m*M* DTT (prepare fresh).
3. Streptavidin coated SPA beads (Amersham NK8972).
4. 3 m*M* $ZnCl_2$.
5. SPA plates.
6. Microbeta counter (WALLAC, Milton Keynes, UK).

2.3. Chromogenic Assay

1. Substrate: RGVVNA-paranitroanilide (pNA), 100 m*M* in DMSO (store at –20°C).
2. Assay buffer: 30% glycerol, 100 m*M* HEPES, pH 7.7, 5 m*M* DTT (prepare fresh).
3. 10 m*M* $ZnCl_2$.
4. Spectrophotometer/plate reader with 405 nm filter.

2.4. Quenched Fluorescence Assay

1. Substrate: Dabcyl-Arg-Arg-Val-Val-Asn-Ala-Ser-Aba-Arg-Leu-Asp(Edans)NH_2, dissolve to 1 m*M* in DMSO, dilute 1 in 10 in H_2O. Store at 4°C for 7 d.
2. Assay buffer: 50 m*M* Tris-HCl, pH 7.5, 1 m*M* EDTA, 1 m*M* DTT, and 30% glycerol (prepare fresh).
3. 96-well fluorimeter (e.g., Fluostar) with excitation at 355 nm and emission at 538 nm.
4. 96-well, black-walled fluorescence plates.

3. Methods

3.1. HPLC Assay

HPLC provides a simple method of evaluating protease activity using a standard peptide substrate and equipment available in most laboratories. The method is suitable for inhibitor evaluation and may be used for screening small to moderate numbers of compounds.

3.1.1. Determination of Appropriate Enzyme Concentration

1. Prepare dilutions of protease in assay buffer to give concentrations from 0.3 to 30 μ*M* (~9–900 μg/mL).
2. Dilute substrate peptide to 600 μ*M* in assay buffer.
3. Mix 10 μL of each enzyme concentration with 10 μL of assay buffer in a round-bottomed microtiter plate in duplicate.
4. Incubate at 25°C for 15 min.
5. Add 10 μL of substrate and mix well.
6. Incubate at 25°C for 60 min.
7. Add 30 μL of 0.2% TFA in water to stop the reaction.
8. Monitor cleavage by HPLC (*see* **Subheading 3.1.4.**).
9. Determine the concentration of enzyme required to achieve 30–50% substrate cleavage. This typically corresponds to a final concentration of approx 0.5 μ*M* for HCMV protease.

3.1.2. Primary Screen

1. Prepare compounds as 10 m*M* stocks in DMSO.
2. Dilute 3 μL of compound in 100 μL of assay buffer to give 300 μ*M* stock.
3. Dilute enzyme appropriately in assay buffer.
4. Dilute substrate peptide to 600 μ*M* in assay buffer.
5. Mix 10 μL of enzyme with 10 μL of each compound in a round-bottomed microtiter plate in duplicate. In addition, include two wells with assay buffer instead of compound as enzyme controls (EC), and two without enzyme as substrate controls (SC). Zinc chloride 3 m*M* may also be included as a positive control compound.
6. Incubate at 25°C for 15 min.
7. Add 10 μL of substrate.
8. Incubate at 25°C for 60 min.
9. Add 30 μL of 0.2% TFA in water to stop the reaction.
10. Monitor cleavage by HPLC (*see* **Subheading 3.1.4.**).

3.1.3. IC_{50} Determination

An IC_{50} value provides a simple way of ranking the potency of hits from the primary screen.

1. From 10 m*M* compound stocks in DMSO prepare twofold dilution series to give compound concentrations over the range 300, 150, 75, 37.5, 18.75, 9.38, and

4.69 μ*M* in assay buffer. Note: these are diluted threefold in the assay to give a range of 100–1.56 μ*M*.
2. Proceed as for the primary screen from **step 3, Subheading 3.1.2.**
3. The IC_{50} value should be determined by regression analysis of the concentration-dependent percent inhibition values determined following HPLC analysis.

3.1.4. HPLC Analysis

1. Place 0.2-μm filters into 0.5-mL centrifuge tubes. Load with 50 μL of sample. Spin sample through the filters at low speed (~2000 rpm).
2. Install C18 column on HPLC unit and equilibrate with 10 mL of 5% ACN/water + 0.1% TFA.
3. Program HPLC protocol:
   a. Flow rate 2 mL/min.
   b. Inject 20 μL of sample.
   c. Gradient 5–30% ACN over 3.5 mL.
   d. Gradient 30–100% ACN over 0.5 mL.
   e. ACN for 1.5 mL.
   f. Gradient 100–5% ACN over 0.5 mL.
   g. Re-equilibrate column with 3 mL 5% ACN.
4. Cleavage products should elute at approx 2.7 mL (P1) and 3.1 mL (P2), and the substrate at 3.3 mL (S).
5. Peak areas should be integrated and used to calculate the percent of cleavage in each reaction from the formula 100 × [(Pl + P2)/(P1 + P2 + S)].
6. The percent of inhibition by compounds may be calculated using the formula 100 × [1 – (cleavage in sample/cleavage in enzyme control)]. Compounds giving >50% inhibition would be considered "hits."

3.2. Scintillation Proximity Assay

The SPA is ideally suited to high-throughput screening of compounds as it uses small amounts of substrate and is easily automated. It may be used to determine IC_{50} values, but is not well suited to detailed kinetic analysis. A similar assay has also been described by Baum et al. *(7)*.

3.2.1. Determination of Appropriate Enzyme Concentration

1. Prepare dilutions of protease in assay buffer to give concentrations from 0.3 to 30 μ*M* (~9–900 μg/mL).
2. Dilute substrate 1/600 in assay buffer (13.3 n*M*).
3. Prepare SPA beads at 0.23 mg/mL in 3 m*M* $ZnCl_2$.
4. Mix 10 μL of each enzyme concentration with 10 μL of assay buffer in an SPA plate in duplicate. Prepare two extra wells with 10 μL of assay buffer instead of enzyme as SC.
5. Incubate at 25°C for 15 min.
6. Add 10 μL of substrate.
7. Incubate at 25°C for 60 min.

8. Add 170 µL of SPA beads in 3 m*M* $ZnCl_2$ to stop the reaction.
9. Leave to stand for 60 min.
10. Count on a Microbeta counter, tritium protocol.
11. Determine the concentration of enzyme required to achieve 50–70% substrate cleavage. This can be calculated from the formula % cleavage = 100 × $(SC_{cpm} - sample_{cpm})/(SC_{cpm})$ assuming that the substrate is fully cleavable. A suitable enzyme concentration typically corresponds to a final concentration of approx 0.5 µ*M* for HCMV protease.

3.2.2. Primary Screen

1. Prepare compounds as 10 m*M* stocks in DMSO.
2. Dilute 3 µL of compound in 100 µL of assay buffer to give 300 µ*M* stock
3. Dilute enzyme appropriately in assay buffer.
4. Dilute substrate 1/600 in assay buffer (13.3 n*M*).
5. Prepare SPA beads at 0.23 mg/mL in 3 m*M* $ZnCl_2$.
6. Mix 10 µL of enzyme with 10 µL of each compound in a round bottomed microtiter plate in duplicate. In addition include two wells with assay buffer instead of compound as enzyme controls, and two without enzyme as substrate controls. Zinc chloride 3 m*M* may also be included as a positive control compound.
7. Incubate at 25°C for 15 min.
8. Add 10 µL of substrate.
9. Incubate at 25°C for 60 min.
10. Add 170 µL of SPA beads in 3 m*M* $ZnCl_2$ to stop the reaction.
11. Leave to stand for 60 min.
12. Count on a Microbeta counter, tritium protocol.
13. The percent of inhibition by compounds may be calculated using the formula 100 × $[(sample_{cpm} - EC_{cpm})/(SC_{cpm} - EC_{cpm})]$. Compounds giving >50% inhibition would be considered "hits."

3.2.3. IC_{50} Determination

An IC_{50} value provides a simple way of ranking the potency of hits from the primary screen.

1. From 10 m*M* compound stocks in DMSO, prepare twofold dilution series to give compound concentrations over the range 300, 150, 75., 37.5, 18.75, 9.38, and 4.69 µ*M* in assay buffer. **Note:** These are diluted threefold in the assay to give a range of 100–1.56 µ*M*.
2. Proceed as for the primary screen from **step 3, Subheading 3.2.2.**
3. The IC_{50} value should be determined by regression analysis of the concentration-dependent percent of inhibition values determined following counting. Further compound dilutions may be required if the IC_{50} is out of range.

3.3. Chromogenic Assay

The chromogenic assay may be used as a screen for inhibitors in the end-point format described here, although relatively high substrate costs may limit its practical capacity. However, it is well suited to kinetic analysis of inhibitors using real-time measurements.

3.3.1. Determination of Appropriate Enzyme Concentration

1. Prepare dilutions of protease in assay buffer to give concentrations from 0.3 to 30 μ*M* (~9–900 μg/mL).
2. Dilute substrate 1/33 in assay buffer.
3. Mix 30 μL of each enzyme concentration with 30 μL of assay buffer in a 96-well flat-bottomed plate in duplicate. Prepare two extra wells with 30 μL of assay buffer instead of enzyme as blanks.
4. Incubate at 25°C for 15 min.
5. Add 30 μL of substrate and mix.
6. Incubate at 25°C for 60 min.
7. Stop reactions with 10 μL of 10 m*M* $ZnCl_2$.
8. Measure OD_{405} in a microplate spectrophotometer.
9. Determine the concentration of enzyme required to achieve an OD_{405} of approx 0.2 after blank subtraction. A suitable enzyme concentration typically corresponds to a final concentration of approx 1.0 μ*M* for HCMV protease.

3.3.2. Primary Screen

1. Prepare compounds as 10 m*M* stocks in DMSO.
2. Dilute 3 μL of compound in 100 μL of assay buffer to give 300 μ*M* stock.
3. Dilute enzyme appropriately in assay buffer.
4. Dilute substrate 1/33 in assay buffer.
5. Mix 30 μL of enzyme with 30 μL of each compound in a 96 well flat-bottomed plate in duplicate. In addition include two wells with assay buffer instead of compound as EC, and two without enzyme as blanks. Zinc chloride 3 m*M* may also be included as a positive control compound.
6. Incubate at 25°C for 15 min.
7. Add 30 μL of substrate.
8. Incubate at 25°C for 60 min.
9. Add 10 μL of 10 m*M* $ZnCl_2$ to stop the reaction.
10. Measure OD_{405} in a microplate spectrophotorneter.
11. The percent of inhibition by compounds may be calculated using the formula $100 \times [1 - (\text{sample } OD_{405}/\text{EC } OD_{405})]$ after blank subtraction. Compounds giving >50% inhibition would be considered "hits."

3.3.3. IC_{50} Determination

An IC_{50} value provides a simple way of ranking the potency of hits from the primary screen.

1. From 10 m*M* compound stocks in DMSO prepare twofold dilution series to give compound concentrations over the range 300, 150, 75, 37.5, 18.75, 9.38, and 4.69 μ*M* in assay buffer. Note: these are diluted threefold in the assay to give a range of 100–1.56 μ*M*.

2. Proceed as for the primary screen from **step 3, Subheading 3.3.2.**
3. The IC_{50} value should be determined by regression analysis of the concentration-dependent percent of inhibition values determined following OD_{405} measurement. Further compound dilutions may be required if the IC_{50} is out of range.

3.4. Quenched Fluorogenic Assay

This assay may be used for primary screening and for kinetic analysis, with the advantage that the high signal produced by this substrate allows lower concentrations of protease enzyme to be used than in the other systems. Similar assays have also been described ***(8,9)***.

3.4.1. Determination of Appropriate Enzyme Concentration

1. Prepare dilutions of protease in assay buffer to give concentrations from 0.1 to 10 μ*M* (~3–300 μg/mL). These will be diluted a further 10-fold in the assay.
2. Mix 10 μL of each enzyme concentration with 70 μL of assay buffer in a 96-well, black-walled fluorescence plate in duplicate. Prepare two extra wells with 10 μL of assay buffer instead of enzyme as blanks.
3. Incubate at 25°C for 15 min.
4. Add 10 μL of substrate and mix thoroughly.
5. Place the plate in a fluorescence reader and read immediately at an excitation wavelength of 35.5 nm emission wavelength of 538 nm.
6. Incubate at 25°C for 40 min.
7. Place the plate in the fluorescence reader and read again.
8. Subtract readings at time 0 from 40-min readings to get the change in fluorescence.
9. Determine the concentration of enzyme required to achieve a reliable, measurable change in fluorescence. This corresponds to around 14 fluorescence units (FU) after blank subtraction at a gain setting of 22 on the instrument described, but may vary with instrumentation. A suitable enzyme concentration typically corresponds to a final concentration of approx 25 n*M* for HCMV protease.

3.4.2. Primary Screen

1. Prepare compounds as 10 m*M* stocks in DMSO.
2. Dilute 10 μL of compound with 90 μL of assay buffer to give 1 m*M* stock.
3. Dilute enzyme appropriately in assay buffer.
4. Mix 10 μL of each enzyme concentration with 10 μL of compound and 70 μL of assay buffer in a 96-well, black-walled fluorescence plate in duplicate. In addition include two wells with assay buffer instead of compound as EC, and two without enzyme as blanks. Zinc chloride 3 m*M* may also be included as a positive control compound.
5. Incubate at 25°C for 15 min.
6. Add 10 μL of substrate and mix thoroughly.
7. Place the plate in a fluorescence reader and read immediately at an excitation wavelength of 355 nm, emission wavelength of 538 nm.

8. Incubate at 25°C for 40 min.
9. Place the plate in the fluorecence reader and read again.
10. Subtract readings at time 0 from 40-min readings to get the change in fluorescence.
11. The percent of inhibition by compounds may be calculated using the formula 100 × [1 – (sample FU/EC FU)] after 0 time subtraction. Compounds giving greater that 50% inhibition would be considered "hits."

3.4.3. IC_{50} Determination

1. From 10 m*M* compound stocks in DMSO prepare twofold dilution series to give compound concentrations over the range 1000, 500, 250, 125, 62.5, 31.25, and 15.6 µ*M* in assay buffer. **Note:** these are diluted 10-fold in the assay to give a range of 100–1.56 µ*M*.
2. Proceed as for the primary screen from **step 3, Subheading 3.4.2.**
3. The IC_{50} value should be determined by regression analysis of the concentration-dependent percent of inhibition values determined following Fluorescence measurement. Further compound dilutions may be required if the IC_{50} is out of range.

4. Notes

The four methods described in this chapter provide some different advantages and disadvantages. Choice of an appropriate method will depend on factors including available equipment, screening capacity required, and whether further detailed kinetic analysis will be needed. The following notes describe some of the differences in the methods and the problems that may be encountered when using these methods.

1. Substrate concentration: A major difference among the four protease assays described is the level of substrate used in the reaction mix, which ranges from 1 m*M* in the PNA assay through 200 µ*M* in the HPLC assay, 10 µ*M* in the quenched fluorescence assay to 14 n*M* in the SPA. The high substrate concentration in the HPLC and PNA assays reflects the high K_m for these substrates under the assay conditions described, and allows easy detection of cleavage products without exhaustion of the substrate. The quenched fluorescence assay affords much higher sensitivity of product detection, and also allows use of much lower enzyme concentrations in. the assay. However, in this assay the substrate concentration must be kept low to avoid internal quenching by the high concentration of EDANS groups in solution. The low level of substrate used in the SPA is facilitated by the high specific activity of the substrate, which minimizes cost and the amount of SPA beads that must be used to bind the substrate for detection. Despite the wide range of substrate concentrations used, little difference in the potency of inhibitors is observed in the different assays because the substrate concentration is always kept at or below the K_m.
2. Compound concentration: The initial concentration of compounds in the assay must be decided before screening. Use of high compound concentration maximizes the possibility of identifying weak inhibitors, which may provide a lead to

a chemical series that can be improved for potency. It will also maximize the number of false positives and occurrences of compound interference. Use of low concentrations will only allow identification of more potent inhibitors, but minimizes interference. A level of approx 100 μ*M* has been suggested as a reasonable starting point.

3. Interference by compounds: All the methods described are subject to interference by compounds. The HPLC assay, although least affected by colored or insoluble compounds, may experience anomalous results if the compounds interact with the peptide substrate or elute from the column at a position that interferes with one of the substrates or product peaks. In the latter case, it may be possible to estimate the size of the missing peak from the other two peaks, if measurable. The SPA may be affected by highly colored or turbid compound solutions that "quench" the signal. Quench may be minimized by using a counting protocol with quench correction as described in the operating instructions for the microbeta counter. The chromogenic assay may also be affected by highly colored, fluorescent, or turbid compounds. These can be corrected, in some cases, by generation of "compound blanks" by addition of compound at assay concentration to both enzyme control and background wells following the assay, so that the effect of compound can be subtracted from all readings. In the fluorogenic assay, the subtraction of a 0-time reading from the 40-min reading will facilitate correction for many of these problems. When operating a screen, it is normally accepted that some compounds will be missed or registered as false positives owing to anomalous results, although these must be kept at acceptable levels.
4. Effect of DTT: DTT is normally included in the assay buffer to provide reducing conditions, which are found in living cells. Reducing conditions may also provide a slight increase in the activity of the protease in some assays. In the absence of DTT in the assay buffer, it has been found that it is possible to identify large numbers of thiotropic HCMV protease inhibitors that target the reduced cysteines of the protease. Such molecules are not generally consiclered to be viable antiviral compounds.
5. DMSO: Compounds and peptides are commonly dissolved in DMSO as the most "universal" solvent. HCMV protease is tolerant of DMSO at up to 10% (v/v) with only slight loss in activity. Higher levels of DMSO may be used, and may be compensated for by reducing the level of glycerol in the assay buffer to 10%.
6. Glycerol: Glycerol has been shown to increase the activity of HCMV protease severalfold. Glycerol concentrations in the range of 10–50% are useful, but samples become hard to pipet and mix at higher concentrations.
7. Enzyme behavior and assay temperature: At high concentrations, HCMV protease exists largely as a homodimer ***(10–12)***. On dilution it has been observed that the enzyme slowly reequilibrates to a mixture of monomer and dimer in a temperature- and concentration-dependent manner, reaching a steady-state rate after approx 15 min at 37°C, or 1 h at 25°C. This slow equilibration results in curved progress plots when the level of cleavage in the assays is measured against time. Although this will not significantly affect the identification of inhibitors in the assays described, the rate change must be considered in the use of these assays under real time measurement for kinetic analysis. For example, using the PNA

assay, kinetic parameters may be determined under both the initial and steady-state conditions. Similar dimerization behavior has also been observed with the HSV protease ***(13)*** suggesting that dimerization may be a general feature of herpesvirus proteases.

The dimerization behavior caused by changes in the assay temperature has two effects on the behavior of the protease. First, increased temperature increases the catalytic rate of the enzyme, resulting in increased initial rates in the assay, particularly when the enzyme is used directly from a concentrated stock. Second, increased temperature pushes the dimer:monomer equilibrium in the direction of monomer, an apparently less active species, decreasing the steady-state rate of the reaction. In the 60-min end point assay, these effects combine to give optimal enzyme activity at approx 25°C, but further temperature optimization may be useful if initial rates or longer incubation times are used.

8. Inhibitor kinetics: The IC_{50} determinations described herein provide a simple method of comparing protease inhibitors. However, it may be desirable to characterize the interactions of inhibitors with the enzyme in more detail. Both the chromogenic and fluorescence assays can be read in kinetics mode on the machines described to give real-time rate measurements for use in determining kinetic parameters.
9. Other herpes proteases: A major consideration in adapting these assays to identify inhibitors of other herpesvirus proteases is in the choice of an appropriate substrate. The herpesvirus proteases are highly conserved and have similar enzymatic properties, and several are able to share substrates. For example, EBV and MCMV protease can utilize the HCMV substrates described herein. HCMV and EBV proteases can also cleave peptides representing the HSV cleavage sites, including PNA derivatives (unpublished data). However, whereas HCMV protease is able to cleave HSV protein substrates, HSV protease cannot cleave HCMV protein substrates ***(14)***, and whereas EBV protease can cleave HCMV protein substrates, HCMV protease cannot cleave EBV protein substrates ***(15)***. For this reason, as a starting point, it is best to utilize peptide substrates that represent the natural maturation or release cleavage site of the protease of interest and, in addition, to ensure that sufficient sequence is provided on both the amino and carboxyl sides of the scissile bond ***(4,8,16)***. The PNA substrates require placement of the PNA group directly on the carboxyl side of the scissile bond, and therefore lack representation of the carboxyl amino acids. However, the authors have shown that at least the HCMV, EBV, and MCMV proteases are able to efficiently use these substrates, which suggests that they may be generally useful for herpesvirus proteases.

   Little additional modification to assay conditions should be required. Herpesvirus proteases are active at physiological pH, although the pH optima vary between pH 7.5 (HCMV) and pH 9.0 (EBV). Glycerol has been shown to generally improve enzyme activity.
10. From protease inhibitors to herpesvirus inhibitors: The ultimate goal of the identification of herpesvirus protease inhibitors is generally to identify antiherpes-

virus compounds, and hits should therefore be examined for potency against the virus of interest. Many inhibitors identified through biochemical screens will not work in antiviral assays owing to problems with stability, solubility, cell penetration, toxicity, and potency. However, biochemical screening programs have the potential to identify otherwise intractable leads that can be pursued, through synthesis and screening of related molecules, to finally develop useful antiviral compounds.

Acknowledgments

The authors would like to acknowledge the helpful contributions of their colleagues G. Hart, C. Roberts, S. Cary, C. Van Wely, V. Shield, E. Furfine, E. Littler, and R. Bethell in the preparation of this work.

References

1. Preston, V. G., Coates, J. A., and Rixon, F. J. (1983) Identification and characterisation of a herpes simplex virus gene product required for encapsidation of virus DNA. *J. Virol.* **45,** 1056–1064.
2. Gao, M., Matusick-Kumar, L., Hurlburt, W., DiTusa, S. F., Newcombe, W. W., Brown, J. C., McCann P. J., III, Deckman, I., and Colonno, R. J. (1994) The protease of herpes simplex virus type 1 is essential for functional capsid formation and viral growth. *J. Virol.* **68,** 3702–3712.
3. Welch, A. R., Woods, A. S., McNally, L. M., Cotter, R. J., and Gibson, W. (1991) A Herpesvirus maturational protease, *Assemblin:* identification of its gene, putative active site domain and cleavage site. *Proc. Natl. Acad. Sci. USA* **88,** 10,792–10,796.
4. Sardana, V. V., Wolfgang, J. A., Veloski, C. A., Long, W. J., LeGrow, K., Wolanski, B., Emini, E. A., and LaFemina, R. L. (1994) Peptide substrate cleavage specificity of human cytomegalovirus protease. *J. Biol. Chem.* **269,** 14,337–14,340.
5. Hall, D. L. and Darke, P. L. (1995) Activation of the herpes simplex virus type 1 protease. *J. Biol. Chem.* **270,** 22,697–22,700.
6. LaFemina, R. I., Bakshi, K. P., Long, W. J., Pramanik, B., Veloski, C. A., Wolanski, B. S., Marcy, A. I., and Hazuda, D. L. (1996) Characterization of a soluble stable human cytomegalovirus protease and inhibition by M-site peptide mimics. *J. Virol.* **70,** 4819–4824.
7. Baum, E. Z., Johnston, S. H., Bebernitz, G. A., and Gluzman, Y. (1996) Development of a scintillation proximity assay for human cytomegalovirus protease using ^{33}Phosphorous. *Anal. Biochem.* **237,** 129–134.
8. Handa B. K., Keech, E., Conway, E. A., Broadhurst, A., and Ritchie, A. (1995) Design and synthesis of a quenched fluorogenic peptide substrate for human cytomegalovirus proteinase. *Antiviral Chem. Chemother.* **6(4),** 255–261.
9. Holskin B. P., Bukhtiyarova, M., Dunn, B. M., Baur, P., de Chastonay, J., and Pennington, M. W. (1995) A continuous fluorescence-based assay of human cytomegalovirus protease using a peptide substrate. *Anal. Biochem.* **226,** 148–155.
10. Darke, P. L., Cole, J. L., Waxman, L., Hall, D. L., Sardana, M. K., and Kuo, L. C. (1996) Active human cytomegalovirus protease is a dimer. *J. Biol. Chem.* **271,** 7445–7449.

11. Cole, J. L. (1996) Characterization of human cytomegalovirus protease dimerisation by analytical centrifugation. *Biochemistry* **35,** 15,601–15,610.
12. Margosiak, S. A., Vanderpool, D. L., Sisson, W., Pinko, C., and Kan, C-C. (1996) Dimerisation of the human cytomegalovirus protease: kinetic and biochemical characterization of the catalytic homodimer. *Biochemistry* **35,** 5300–5307.
13. Schmidt, U. and Darke, P. L. (1997) Dimerisation and activation of the herpes simplex virus type 1 protease. *J. Biol. Chem.* **272,** 7732–7735.
14. Welch, A. R. and Villarreal, E. C. (1995) Cytomegalovirus protein substrates are not cleaved by herpes simplex virus type 1 proteinase. *J. Virol.* **69,** 341–347.
15. Donaghy, G. and Jupp, R. (1995) Characterization of the Epstein-Barr virus proteinase and comparison with the human cytomegalovirus proteinase. *J. Virol.* **69,** 1265–1270.
16. Mapelli, C., Dilanni, C. L., Tsao, J. F., Stevens, J. T., Weinheimer, S. P., O'Boyle, D. R., Drier, D. A., and Meyers, C. A. (1994) Substrate requirement of the HSV-1 and CMV proteases *in vitro* using peptides derived from their maturation and release sites in *"Peptides 1994"* (Maia, H. L. S., ed.), Proceedings of the 23rd European Peptide Symposium.

III

Human Immunodeficiency Virus

15

Testing Compounds for Antiviral Activity in Cell Cultures Infected with HIV

Donna Devine, Naomi Mathews, and Derek Kinchington

1. Introduction

This chapter describes the procedures that can be used to determine compounds that have antiviral activity against HIV. These include: maintenance of lymphoblastoid cell lines, preparation of peripheral blood mononuclear cells (PMMCs), and determination of the infectivity of the HIV stock-supernatant and antiviral assays. The assays described use both acutely and chronically infected cells. Toxicity of compounds is assessed by measuring ^{14}C uptake. These protocols are used for the evaluation of compounds that can be carried out by a single individual in a Category 3 containment laboratory. The number of compounds analyzed would be about 10, which is a convenient number to fill a single 96-well p24 enzyme-linked immunosorbent assay (ELISA) plate.

2. Materials

1. 96-well microtiter tissue culture plate (or sterile 6-mL tissue culture tubes; Falcon 2054).
2. Filter membranes (Helis Bio).
3. RPMI-1640 growth medium containing 10% fetal calf serum, 2 m*M* L-glutamine, 100 µg/mL penicillin, and 100 mg/mL streptomycin sulfate.
4. 2'3'-Dideoxycitidine (ddC) (Roche Products Ltd.).
5. Dimethyl sulfoxide (DMSO).
6. Ethanol.
7. Human immunodeficiency virus type 1 (HIV-1 IIIB).
8. HIV-1 p24 antigen kit (Coulter Electronics).
9. Ro 8959 Saquinavir (Roche Products UK, Ltd).
10. T-cell lines: C8166, H9, and HIV-1 chronically infected H9 cells (H9IIIB and H9RF).

From: *Methods in Molecular Medicine, vol. 24: Antiviral Methods and Protocols*
Edited by: D. Kinchington and R. F. Schinazi © Humana Press Inc., Totowa, NJ

11 0.1% Trypan blue.
12. Ficoll-Paque, research grade (Pharmacia).
13. 10% sodium hypochlorite.
14. 50 mL polypropylene centrifuge tubes.
15. Kova plastic disposable slides with grids (Hycor Biomedical Inc.).
16. Buffy coat from human blood donation.
17. ^{3}H-thymidine (Amersham UK, Ltd.).
18. ^{14}C protein hydrolysate (Amersham Life Sciences).
19. Cell harvester (*see* **Note 1**).
20. Scintillation counter.

3. Methods Using T-Lymphoblastoid Cells

HIV can be grown without any difficulty in transformed cell lines, such as C8166 and H9 T-lymphoblastoid cell lines. These are continuously growing cell lines and readily support HIV replication under controlled conditions. Experience has shown that these cell lines are useful in establishing structure–activity relationships when a large number of compounds are being investigated *(1–3)*.

3.1. Determination of Virus Infectivity in C8166 T-Lymphoblastoid Cells

Before beginning a program of testing, it is essential to prepare a volume of 100–200 mL seed stock of the virus with known infectivity. These supernatants should be frozen, in 0.5–1-mL aliquots, at –70°C (or in the vapor phase of liquid nitrogen). This volume will provide a standard virus stock for perhaps 12 mo when testing 10–20 compounds per week. The titration of seed stocks should to be carried out for each type of cell line used. The tissue culture infectious dose (TCID) is determined in replicate cultures of serial dilutions of the stock virus preparation (clarified culture supernatant). The titer of the virus stock is usually expressed as the 50% infective dose ($TCID_{50}$), which can be calculated more accurately than a negative end-point.

1. Split the target lymphoblastoid cells (e.g., C8166 or H9 cells) on d 0 into two or four parts depending on density and resuspend in 40 mL fresh medium (RPMI-1640 plus 10% bovine calf serum) in a 250-mL flask.
2. On d 1 mark up a 96-well flat-bottomed tissue culture plate so that the central 60 wells (10 horizontal and six vertical) are used **(Fig. 1)**. Pipet the cells, now in log phase growth, into two universals (20 mL each) and centrifuge at 1100 rpm for 5 min using a bench-top centrifuge. Resuspend the cells in 10–20 mL of fresh medium.
3. Making sure the cells are evenly dispersed, take 50 µL of these cells, mix with 50 µL of Trypan blue (10 mg/mL in phosphate-buffered saline [PBS]), and leave for 1 min. Carefully mix the solution and transfer 10 µL to a disposable plastic Kova counting chamber. Count the number of live (translucent) and dead (blue) cells in the sample (*see* **Note 2**).

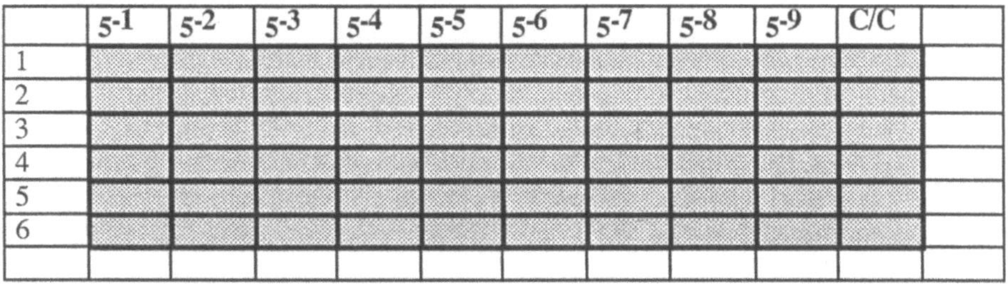

	5^{-1}	5^{-2}	5^{-3}	5^{-4}	5^{-5}	5^{-6}	5^{-7}	5^{-8}	5^{-9}	C/C	
1											
2											
3											
4											
5											
6											

Fig. 1. Typical 96-well layout for measuring the infectivity ($TCID_{50}$) of culture supernatant containing HIV-1.

4. To each marked well of the plate add 3×10^4 C8166 cells in 100 µL of culture medium.
5. Prepare a dilution series from 5^{-1} to 5^{-9} (i.e., 1 in 5 followed by serial 1 in 10 dilutions) of the original high-titer virus stock in 6-mL culture tubes. One milliliter of each dilution will suffice. Add 100 µL of the high-titer stock to the first column of wells and then add 100 µL of each virus dilution to subsequent columns. Each well will contain 200 µL. This will give a final dilution of 1/10 of the virus stock in the second column, 1/100 in the third, and so on. If the original virus stock has a very high titer then it may be necessary to extend the dilutions to 10^{-10} or below. Allow one column for cell control (c/c).
6. Add sterile PBS to the empty wells around the perimeter of the plate to reduce "edge effects" resulting from evaporation and incubate at 37°C in 5% CO_2.
7. Inspect the plate daily for cytopathic effect (CPE). The CPE caused by HIV-infected lymphoblastoid cells is clearly observed by the formation of syncytia, which are multinucleated giant cells. Syncytia may form in the first row within a few hours if the titer of virus is high **(Fig. 2) (Note 3)**.
8. Cellular respiration turns the color of the medium from pink to yellow as it becomes more acidic. With the C8166 cells CPE will be observed at about 72 h in some of the other wells. When no further CPE develops (usually d 4) the number of replicate wells showing CPE is recorded for each virus dilution (**Table 1**).
9. The $TCID_{50}$, i.e., the concentration when 50% of cultures become infected, is calculated using the method of Reed and Muench (Dulbecco, 1988)*(4)*. In this procedure the proportion of infected and uninfected cultures (wells) are pooled at all dilutions and the dilution giving 50% infected wells is estimated. The results of the titration in **Fig. 3** can be tabulated (**Table 2**). The 50% end-point, in this example, lies between the 7th and 8th dilutions. A simple interpolation is used to determine the 50% endpoint.

The $TCID_{50}$ of a the stock is determined by the following calculation. The figures are derived from the example in **Table 3**. The 50% end-point falls between 5^{-7} and 5^{-8} in **Table 2**.

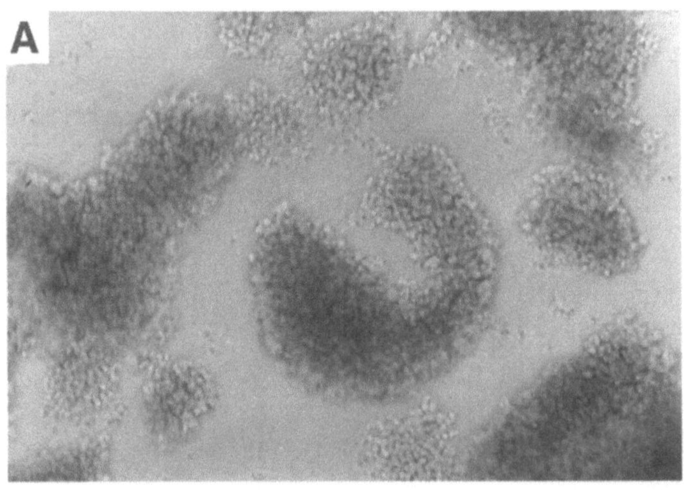

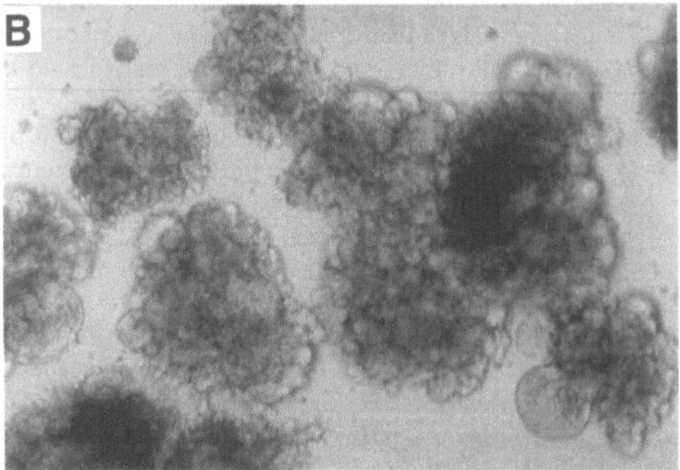

Fig. 2. **(A)** C8166 T-lymphoblastoid cells growing in culture. These grow characteristically in large clumps. Single cells can be seen at the edge of the clumps. **(B)** The same cells acutely infected with HIVIIIB. Large multinucleated cells are produced when sufficient viral proteins are expressed on the surface of the cells allowing fusion of cell membranes.

$$\frac{[(\%\ \text{infected wells at next dilution above } 50\%) - (50\%)]}{[(\%\ \text{infected wells at next dilution above } 50\%) - (\%\ \text{infected wells at next dilution below } 50\%)]} \quad (1)$$

$$(70 - 50)/(70 - 25) = 20/45 = 0.44 \quad (2)$$

The 50% endpoint is $5^{-7.44}$. To convert $5^{-7.44}$ to 10^x:

Table 1
Results Obtained in a Titration of HIV-1 in C8166 Cells

	Observed values		Accumulated values		
Virus dilution	Wells $^+$	Wells $^-$	Wells $^+$	Wells $^-$	% Infected
10^{-5}	6	0	18	0	100
10^{-6}	5	1	12	1	92.3
10^{-7}	4	2	7	3	70
10^{-8}	3	6	3	9	25
10^{-9}	0	6	0	15	0

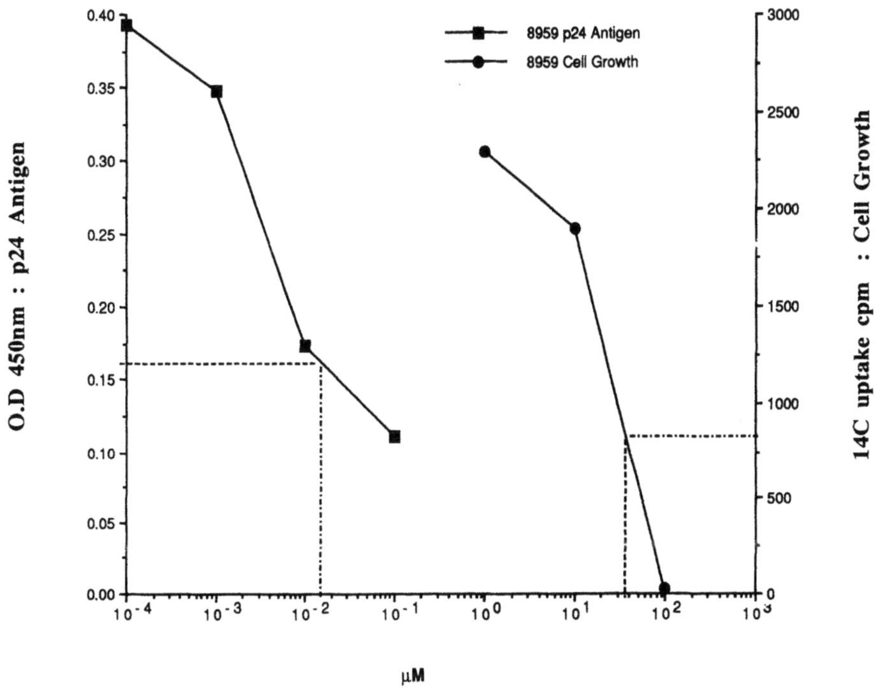

Fig. 3. Dose response for saquinavir in both the antiviral and the toxicity assay. The IC_{50} value in the p24 assay is given as 1.5×10^{-2} μ*M* (1.5 n*M*) and the CC_{50} value in the ^{14}C uptake assay is 36 μ*M*. The selectivity index (SI) for saquinavir is the ratio of the two ($36/1.5 \times 10^{-2}$) and is calculated as 2400.

$$(-7.44)(\log 5) = x \tag{3}$$

$$x = (-7.44)(0.699) = 5.2 \tag{4}$$

The 50% endpoint dilution is $10^{-5.2}$. The 50% titer is $10^{5.2}$. The $TCID_{50}$ is $10^{5.2}$/100 μL. To convert to per milliliter multiply by 10^1 (i.e., 100 μL × 10 = 1 mL)

$$10^1 \times 10^{5.2} = 10^{6.2} \quad (5)$$

The virus stock is $10^{6.2}$ $TCID_{50}$/mL or 1.59×10^6 $TCID_{50}$/mL. In the assay described in **Subheading 3.2.** the cells are infected with 10 $TCID_{50}$ / 2×10^5 cells. To calculate the volume of virus required using the above example for stock containing 1.59×10^6 $TCID_{50}$/mL.

$$1\ TCID_{50} = 1000\ \mu L/(1.59 \times 10^6) \quad (6)$$

$$10\ TCID_{50} = (1000\ \mu L \times 10)/(1.59 \times 10^6) \quad (7)$$

10 $TCID_{50}$ = 0.0063 µL/3×10^4 cells (i.e., cell concentration in original titration). For 100 samples the volume of virus stock required is $0.063 \times 100 = 6.3$ µL.

3.2. Testing Compounds for Antiviral Activity Using HIV-1 p24 Antigen as a Marker for Virus Growth in Acutely Infected C8166 Cells

The system described is for testing a small number of compounds simultaneously in 3×10^4 cells /200 µL grown in 96-well plates (*see* **Note 4**).

1. On d 0 split the target lymphoblastoid cells (e.g., C8166 or H9 cells) into two or four parts depending on density and resuspend the cells in 40 mL fresh medium (RPMI-1640 plus 10% bovine calf serum) in a 250-mL flask.
2. On d 1 weigh out the compounds under test and either dissolve them in 0.5–1 mL of water or solvent (DMSO) as a 10 m*M* stock or as 10 mg/mL stock if the molecular weight is not known. Prepare 1/10 dilutions giving a range of 10–0.01 m*M* or mg/mL. Each compound is tested in replicates of three.
   The stock solutions will be diluted 1/100 in the culture medium and will give a final concentration range of 100–0.0001 µ*M* or µg/mL. If an organic solvent is used, such as DMSO, then add 15 µL to the untreated controls. This gives a final concentration of the solvent of 1% (**Note 5**). The final concentrations of the controls in the culture medium will be: ddC (2, 0.2, 0.02, and 0.002 µ*M*), ZDV (0.1, 0.01, 0.001, and 0.0001 µ*M*), and saquinavir (0.1, 0.01, 0.001, and 0.0001 µ*M*).
3. Calculate the number of cells needed for the antigen assay: Each compound is tested at 4 concentrations in replicates of three; three untreated samples (for each solvent) are needed for the standard curve. Each sample contains 3×10^5 C8166 cells. Twenty percent extra cells are used to allow for pipeting and for monitoring growth in a flask. The number of samples is calculated as $12N+3S$.The total number of cells required is

   $$[(12N + 3S) \times 2 \times 10^5] \times 120/100 \quad (8)$$

   Where N= number of compounds and S = number of solvents used.
4. Spin down the total number of cells required for the antigen assay and resuspend in 1 mL of media in a plastic universal. Carry out **steps 5–13** in a Category 3 level containment laboratory.

5. Add a volume of the HIV-IIIB virus supernatant equivalent to 10 $TCID_{50}/3 \times 10^4$ cells and mix cells and virus supernatant by gently pipeting up and down.
6. Infect the cells in the universal for 1.5 h at 37°C in 5% CO_2.
7. Add 20 mL of culture medium to the infected cells in the universal and spin at 1100 rpm in a bench centrifuge for 5 min.
8. Wash the cells three more times by resuspending them in 20 mL of fresh culture medium and centrifuging at 1100 rpm. These washing steps remove the unabsorbed HIV particles.
9. Resuspend the infected cells in the total volume of culture media to give 3×10^4 cells/200 µL in a 75 cm^2 mL flask (i.e., the volume needed is the number of samples × 200 µL).
10. Pipet 2 µL of the stock dilution series for each compound and the reference antiviral agents into the empty tubes. (Use an 0.5–10-µL pipet for accuracy.)
11. Using a 1-mL disposable plastic pipet, pipet cells up and down frequently to distribute cells evenly throughout the column. Add 200 µL of the infected cells to each sample tube.
12. Leave the excess infected untreated cells in the flask and incubate with the sample tubes at 37°C, 5% CO_2 for 72 h.
13. On d 4 inspect the cells in the flask for syncytia formation using an inverted microscope. If there are fewer than 12 syncytia per field of view, 100 µL of the supernatant can be tested (care should be taken not to remove any cells); if there are 12–30 syncytia a 1 in 2 dilution is required; for >30 syncytia a 1 in 5 dilution is tested.

3.2.1. Carrying Out the p24-Antigen Assay

Set up a standard curve for the p24 antigen as follows:

1. Label four tubes 1, 0.5, 0.25, and 0.125 and pipet 100 µL media into those labeled 0.5, 0.25, and 0.125.
2. Add 100 µL supernatant from each of the three control tubes (the untreated cultures) into the tube labeled 1 and mix well.
3. Carry out a serial dilution, transferring 100 µL each time. Thoroughly mix at each transfer.
4. Add 100 µL of the four standard curve dilutions and 100 µL of each sample (or a dilution of each sample) to the appropriate wells of the ELISA plate. All samples are in replicates of three and each replicate should be allocated its own well in the ELISA plate. This is best noted on a 96-well plate—plan while adding the samples to the plate. Finally, add 100 µL of medium to each well to bring the final volume to 200 µL, which is the volume required for accurate p24 analysis.
5. Carry out the antigen assay according to the manufacturer's instructions.
6. Plot p24 against concentration to generate a dose response curve and determine the IC_{50} concentration **(Fig. 3)**.
7. Using the p24 antigen standard provided with the kit, the OD values for the samples can be converted to pg/mL of HIV-1 p24. This is done by incorporating a known concentration of the antigen provided with the kit.

3.3. Testing Compounds in Chronically Infected C8166 Cells for Antiviral Activity Using HIV-1 p24 Antigen as a Marker for Virus Growth

Compounds that are targeted against postintegration events in the replication cycle of HIV can be evaluated in chronically infected cells. The proteinase inhibitors block the late-stage maturation process. If the antiviral activity of this assay is compared with its activity in an acute assay then the site of action of an compound can be shown to be pre- or postintegration *(5)*.

1. On d 0 split the target chronically infected lymphoblastoid cells (e.g., H9IIIB or H9RF cells) into two or four parts depending on density and resuspended in 40 mL fresh medium (RPMI-1640 plus 10% bovine calf serum) in a 250-mL flask.
2. On d 1 spin down these cells in two universals at 1100 rpm for 5 min, pour off the supernatants, centrifuge, and resuspend in fresh culture medium. Repeat this procedure three more times to remove HIV particles from the supernatant.
3. After the final wash resuspend the cells in 20 mL RPMI and count the cells using the Kova plastic slides.
4. Calculate the number of cells needed for the antigen assay: Each compound is tested at four concentrations in replicates of three; three untreated samples (for each solvent) are needed for the standard curve. Each sample contains 3×10^4 H9IIIB cells. Twenty percent extra cells are taken to allow for pipeting and for monitoring growth in a flask (*see* **Subheading 3.2.**).
5. Add the cells to fresh culture medium in a 75-mL flask to give a final concentration of 3×10^4 cells/200 µL.
6. Pipet 2 µL of the compound dilutions and controls into 96-well plates. Controls should be those compounds that target postintegration events. A proteinase inhibitor, such as saquinavir, is appropriate. (*See* **Subheading 3.2.** for making up stock solutions for test and reference compounds.)
7. Add 200 mL of the H9IIIB cells to each tube.
8. Incubate the tubes at 37°C, 5% CO_2 for 72 h.
9. Test the supernatants by using a commercial ELISA. It may be necessary to dilute all supernatants by 1:2. (Ensure that the final volume in each well in the ELISA plate is 200 µL.)

3.4. Testing Compounds for Antiviral Activity Using a Back Titration Method

Some compounds may not actually reduce the amount of p24 released from the cell but cause the release of noninfectious virus particles. Such examples are the glycosidase inhibitors. In this assay, supernatants from the primary screen containing different concentrations of the drug are added to indicator cells and the extent of the CPE produced in the indicator cells gives a measure of the antiviral activity. C8166 and CEM cells form syncytia readily but MT2, MT4, and JM cells form syncytia that are more discrete and easier to count.

The infectivity in the original supernatant and hence the antiviral effect is assessed by the reduction in CPE.

1. Add 3×10^4 uninfected MT2 cells/100 µL fresh culture medium to the wells of a 96-well plate.
2. Titrate by serial dilution the supernatants (100 µL) from each tube of the primary cultures containing different concentrations of compounds onto the indicator cells. Ensure that the final volume in the wells containing the indicator cells is 200 µL.
3. Inspect the plate each day and score the formation of syncytia, either on a semiquantitative basis (+++++/+++/+/–) or by counting individual syncytia (*see* **Note 6**).

3.5. Mixed Cell Assays That Measure the Effect of Compounds Blocking Cell Surface Molecules

This method is used to test the effect of such compounds as soluble CD4 that bind to gp120 expressed on the surface of infected cells. Similarly, this system could be used to investigate the antibodies or small molecules that may bind to the family of coreceptors (CXR4 and CCR5, and so forth) required for the entry of HIV into cells. Compounds that selectively kill HIV-infected cells may also be investigated with this technique *(6)*. If CPE or cell viability (vital staining) is used as an end-point then plates should be treated as described in **Note 6.**

The experiment can be carried out in using four different combinations to investigate differential effects. Cells are mixed 10 uninfected:1 infected: untreated infected cells with untreated uninfected cells, treated infected cells with untreated uninfected cells, untreated infected cells with treated uninfected cells, or treated infected cells with treated uninfected cells.

1. Split the target lymphoblastoid cells (e.g., C8166 or MT2 and H9IIIB cells) on d 0 into two or four parts depending on density and resuspended in 40 mL fresh medium (RPMI-1640 plus 10% bovine calf serum) in a 75-cm^2 flask.
2. On d 1 count the required number of chronically infected cells and uninfected cells for the four different combinations listed.
3. Incubate each treated culture overnight in a 50-mL flask. Three concentrations of the compounds can be used. Place the untreated cells in similar flasks.
4. On d 2 cells should be mixed (10:1, uninfected:infected) as shown above, giving final concentrations of 2×10^4 plus 2×10^5/mL in 200 µL.
5. Plates should be inspected on a daily basis, over a 4-d period either on a semiquantitative basis (+++++/+++/+/–) or by counting individual syncytia.

If the end-point is to be p24 then all cultures should washed and resuspended three times following overnight preincubation with the compounds to remove HIV in the supernatants from the chronically infected cells.

3.6. Time-Course Experiments

Adding compounds at increasing times postinfection (1.5–48 h) will also discriminate between compounds that act either early or late in the replication cycle of HIV. Reverse-transcriptase inhibitors will lose activity after about 6 h postinfection, whereas proteinase inhibitors will still retain significant activity at 48 h postinfection (references). The methodology is the same as that described in **Subheadings 3.2.** and **3.2.1.** These experiments are typically only carried out with a single compound of interest together with an appropriate reference compound. A number of replicate assays are set up and dilutions of the compound added at 2, 4, 6, 12, 24, and 48 h. Dose responses are drawn for each time-point or responses are shown for each concentration at all time-points *(7)*.

3.7. Testing for Compound Toxicity

3.7.1. With Uninfected T-Lymphoblastoid Cells

The preliminary evaluation of new drugs often starts with screening for toxicity in the culture system to be used. This ensures that the drugs will eventually be tested in the appropriate concentration range when tested against the virus. A crude measure of toxicity can be obtained simply by including a series of dilutions of the drug in maintenance medium added to cell cultures in cluster plates and observing the cells for evidence of obvious toxicity. Staining of the cells with a vital stain after exposure to the drug can be used and is most suitable for assessing toxicity in cultures of nonadherent cells. Repeated passage of the cells in the presence of the compound, accompanied by total and viable cell counts, provides a more discriminating method of detecting cytotoxicity. However, to cope with 10–20 compounds at a time using nonautomated methods the use of radioisotopes is a satisfactory compromise.

A sensitive method to measure toxic effects of drugs is to monitor cellular metabolism by incorporation of ^{3}H-thymidine or ^{14}C-protein hydrolysate. ^{14}C-protein is used in preference to ^{3}H-thymidine when it is necessary to avoid competition in uptake between the labeled thymidine and an unlabeled nucleoside reverse-transcriptase inhibitor. These methods are used mainly to monitor sublethal toxicity after initial screening or when comparing structure–activity relationships. The assays described here are carried out using 6-mL culture tubes (**Note 1**). These assays are carried out in parallel with the antiviral assay.

1. Split the target lymphoblastoid cells (e.g., C8166 or H9 cells) on d 0 into two or four parts depending on density and resuspend in 40 mL fresh medium (RPMI-1640 plus 10% bovine calf serum) in a 250-mL flask.
2. Calculate the number of cells needed for the toxicity assay: Each compound is tested in replicates of three. Three untreated samples (for each solvent) are needed as the standard. Each sample contains 3×10^4 C8166 cells (*see* **Subheading 3.3.**).

3. Pipet 2 µL of the same concentration range of each compound as used in the antiviral assay. Add 200 µL of the uninfected cells. If an organic solvent, such as DMSO, is used then add 2 µL to the untreated controls. This gives a final concentration of the solvent of 1%.
4. Incubate aliquots of uninfected cells in the presence of the compounds at the appropriate concentrations for 72 h in 5% CO_2. *See* **Subheading 3.** for making up stock solutions. To find the maximum concentration tolerated by the uninfected cell cultures it may be necessary to increase the concentration of the original stock solutions by 10- or 100-fold.
5. The T-cells form a pellet at the bottom of the tube. The appearance of this pellet and the color of the culture medium are reliable indicators of toxicity. A dispersed pellet and/or pink color indicate poor growth. Pour off the supernatant into chloros and allow to drain.
6. On d 3, add 0.5 µCi/well of the ^{14}C label in 5 µL of medium to each well. On d 4 harvest the cells on a filter mat at the same time as supernatants from infected cells are tested for p24.
7. Measure incorporated or ^{14}C-protein hydrolysate in a b-scintillation counter. Plot the concentration against the ^{14}C- uptake values and calculate the 50% cytotoxicity value (CC_{50}) (**Table 1**).

3.7.2. With Infected T-Lymphoblastoid Cells

If a cell harvester is available in the Category 3 laboratory and usually installed in a Class 3 cabinet then the preceding protocol may be followed as described. If this equipment is not available then for most purposes comparison of growth of the uninfected cells, in this case H9, can be made compared with the effect of the compound on HIV-1 antigen production (*see* **Table 1**).

3.8. Assays Using Peripheral Blood Mononuclear Cells

The use of PBMCs is usually reserved for those few compounds that show good activity in the primary screen. PBMCs are more difficult to infect than lymphoblastoid cells and more virus is used: 100 $TCID_{50}$. The release of sufficient p24 for measurement usually takes at least 5 d. If only a few compounds are to be evaluated at one time it is possible to increase the number of replicates at each concentration (5–10) since more variation is observed between wells. PBMCs are prepared from human blood donations either from a transfusion center or from a donor panel of healthy volunteers. Transfusion centers can provide a "buffy coat," which is a leukocyte concentrate of one unit of blood containing red blood cells (RBCs) and platelets. It is usually necessary to obtain ethical permission to work with PBMCs from donors because their blood will be tested for p24. The method describes the separation of PBMCs from a buffy coat or a heparinized whole-blood donation from a healthy volunteer.

3.8.1. Preparation of PBMCs

1. On d 0 leave Ficoll-Paque to warm to room temperature if stored at +4°C.
2. PBMCs should be prepared in a Class 2 cabinet and latex gloves should be worn. Cut the top left hand tubing on the buffy coat bag. Use round-ended scissors wiped with 70%. Carefully pour 25-mL aliquots of the contents of the bag into 50-mL centrifuge tubes.
3. Add 25 mL RPMI wash medium to each tube, thus diluting the buffy coat 1:2. Depending on the volume of the buffy coat 4–6 tubes will be needed. Pipet up and down several times to mix.
4. Invert the Ficoll-Paque and check that it has reached room temperature and add 15 mL to four sterile centrifuge tubes. If the buffy coat has a large volume (>80 mL), then **steps 5–13** can be repeated if the maximum number of PBMCs present are required.
5. Using a 10 mL plastic pipet, carefully layer 25 mL of the buffy coat-RPMI mixture on top of the Ficoll-Paque. This is achieved by allowing the buffy coat to run slowly down the inside of the centrifuge tube. The centrifuge tube should contain no more than 40 mL at this stage.
6. Centrifuge the 50-mL tubes in a bench centrifuge at 1800 rpm at room temperature for 40 min.
7. Transfer the buckets to the cabinet and carefully remove the centrifuge tubes. The RBCs should form the bottom layer leaving the lymphocytes in a band above the Ficoll layer.
8. Remove the "opaque ring of lymphocytes" by either placing a 10-mL pipet directly into the lymphocyte layer and aspirating or by first removing the plasma layer above the lymphocytes and then the lymphocytes. Take care to aliquot the maximum volume of lymphocytes while obtaining the minimum volume of Ficoll-Pacque and avoiding the RBCx.
9. Dispense 20-mL aliquots of lymphocytes into sterile 50-mL centrifuge tubes. Add an equal volume of RPMI-wash medium and centrifuge at 1500–1700 rpm for 10 min.
10. The lymphocytes will form a pellet at the bottom of the tubes. There may also be some residual red cells present. Pour off the supernatant into 10% hypochlorite and "flick" the tubes to dislodge the pellets. Add a few milliliters of RPMI-wash to each centrifuge tube. Pool these preparàtions into one tube and add more RPMI-wash to give a total volume of 20 mL. Gently pipet up and down mix and break up clumps of cells.
11. Count the cells using a plastic disposable counting chamber and seed cells at 2×10^6 cells/mL in warmed RPMI growth medium in a 75-cm^2 tissue culture flask.
12. Place the flask vertically in a 37°C CO_2 incubator, leaving the cap slightly loosened unless the cap has a "built in" filter. (N.B.: If the flask is placed horizontally the macrophages may strongly adhere to the surface of the flask.
13. Resuspend cells in fresh medium the next day.

3.8.2. Activation of PBMC

1. On d 1 take the required number of PBMCs as for both the p24 and toxicity assay (*see* **Subheading 3.3.**) and resuspend in fresh medium containing phytohemagglutinin (10 mg/mL).

3.8.3. Infection of PBMCs with HIV

1. On d 4 centrifuge at 1000 rpm for 5 min. Resuspend the cells in 20 mL of medium.
2. Mix the PBMCs gently and remove a volume containing the required number of cells for the antigen assay. With PBMCs the concentration of cells needed is 2×10^5/200 µL growth medium. Spin down and resuspend the PMBC in 1 of medium and incubate with 100 $TCID_{50}$ HIVIIIB for 1.5 h at 37°C (*see* **Note 7**).
3. Thoroughly wash three times and resuspend in the total volume required for the assay.
4. Add stock IL-2 (1000 U/mL) to this culture to give a final IL-2 concentration of 10 U/mL (i.e., 1/100 dilution).
5. Transfer cell aliquots (2×10^5/200 µL) to 6-mL culture tubes containing dilutions of the drugs (2 µL) under investigation, reference compounds, and controls for plotting the standard curve.
6. Incubate for 5 d.
7. On d 9 test the supernatants for p24 using the commercial ELISA.

3.8.4. Testing for Compound Toxicity in PBMCs

1. On d 4 take the second aliquot of PBMCs and resuspend in the total volume of medium required for this assay.
2. Add stock IL-2 (1000 U/mL) to this culture to give a final IL-2 concentration of 10 U/mL (i.e., 1/100 dilution).
3. Transfer cell aliquots (2×10^5 /200 µL) to 6-mL culture tubes containing dilutions of the drugs (2 µL) under investigation, reference compounds, and controls for plotting the standard curve (*see* **Subheading 3.7.**).
4. Incubate for 5 d.
5. On d 9, add 0.5 µCi/well of the ^{14}C label in 5 µL of medium to each well. On d 4 harvest the cells on a filter mat at the same time as supernatants from infected cells are tested for p24 (*see* **Subheading 3.7.** and **Note 1**).

4. Notes

1. The toxicity method described in **Subheading 3.7.** is carried out in 96-well plates and the cells are harvested using a standard 96-well cell harvester (e.g., Skatron). If 6-mL tubes are used, cells are harvested using an Ilicon harvester adapted to aspirate 12 6-mL tubes simultaneously. This allows cells to be grown under the same conditions as those for p24 analysis (*see* **Note 4**). However, experience has shown that similar end-points for toxicity are obtained using either 96-well plates or 6-mL culture tubes.

2. Cultures in which dead cells make up more than 10% of the sample should be discarded. In well-maintained lymphoblastoid cell lines the dead cells usually make up about 3% of the population following log phase growth for 18 h.
3. Fusion from without occurs when syncytia form quickly with high-titer virus. Fusion from within occurs when low-titer HIV requires several rounds or replication to occur, in a culture, before sufficient virus particles are present to cause the fusion of cell membranes.
4. When a small number of compounds is being tested the use of 6-mL culture tubes containing 2×10^5 cells/ 1.5 mL culture medium has several advantages over 96-well plates containing 3×10^4 cells/200 μL : Edge effects do not pose a problem and it is easy to sample 200 mL supernatant required for the antigen assay without contaminating the sample with cells, since the carryover of infected cells into the ELISA well would significantly change the p24 value. Further, more 200-μL aliquots may be taken for analysis if repeat measurements are required.
5. It is important to include control tubes for each solvent used because p24 antigen levels can be affected by such solvents as DMSO, resulting in a changed standard curve when compared to water.
6. These experiments are more satisfactorily carried out in 24- or 96-well plates because end-points are calculated by qualitative evaluation or by counting CPE. Plates can be placed in a shallow plastic sandwich box and placed on the stage of a binocular microscope. It may be necessary to wipe the moisture off the underside of the plate lid (in the Class 3 hood) before viewing.
7. If wild-type and resistance clinical isolates of HIV are to be evaluated then seed stock of these strains need to be prepared (ref) and their infectivity determined as described in **Subheading 2.**

References

1. Roberts, N. A., Martin, J. A., Kinchington, D., Broadhurst, A. V., Craig, J. C., Duncan, I. B., Galpin, S. A., Handa, B. K., Kay, J., Krohn, A., Lambert, R. W., Merrett, J. H., Mills, J. S., Parks, K. E. B., Redshaw, S., Ritchie, A. J., Taylor, D. L., Thomas, G. J., and Machin, P. (1990) Rational design of peptide-based HIV proteinase inhibitors. *Science* **248,** 358–361.
2. Holmes, H. C., Mahmoud, N., Karpas, A., Petric, J., Kinchington, D., O' Connor, T., Jeffries, D. J., De Clercq, E., Pauwels, R., Desmyter, J., and Hay, A. (1991) Screening of compounds for activity against HIV: a collaborative study. *Antiviral Chem. Chemother.* **2,** 287–293.
3. Pauwels, R., Balzarini, J., Baba, M., Snoeck, R., Schols, D., Herdewijn, P., Desmyter J., and De Clercq, E. (1988) Rapid and automated tetrazolium-basd colorimetric assay for the detection of anti-HIV compounds. *J. Virol. Methods* **20,** 309–321.
4. Dulbecco, R. (1994) Endpoint method—measurement of the infectious titer of a viral sample, in *Virology,* 2nd ed., Lippincott, Philadelphia, pp. 22–25.
5. Galpin, S., Roberts, N. A., O' Connor, T., Jeffries, D. J., and Kinchington, D. (1993) Antiviral properties of the HIV proteinase inhibitor RO 31-8959. *Antiviral Chem. Chemother.* **5,** 43–45.

6. Kinchington, D., Randall, S., Winther, M., and Horrobin, D. (1993) Lithium gamma-linolenate-induced cytotoxicity against cells chronically infected with HIV-1. *FEBS Letts.* **330,** 219–221.
7. Pauwels, R., Andries, K., Debyser, Z., Kukla, M., Schols, D., Desmyter, J., De Clercq, E., and Janssen, P. A. (1992) TIBO derivatives: a new class of highly potent and specific inhibitors of HIV-1 replication. *Biochem. Soc. Trans.* **20(2),** 509–512.

16

Evaluation of Compounds That Prevent Reactivation of HIV-1 in OM-10.1 Cells

Salvatore T. Butera

1. Introduction

It is critically important that new therapeutic compounds and targets for therapeutic intervention be identified in the battle against the human immunodeficieny virus type 1(HIV-1). Many of the currently existing therapeutic approaches target virus-specific factors involved in steps along the HIV-1 life cycle prior to proviral integration. These preintegrative or afferent therapeutic approaches initially appeared quite promising (like reverse transcriptase [RT] inhibitors and soluble CD4) but have shown disappointing clinical benefit. With the recent appreciation of suppression of HIV-1 fusion by selected chemokines, more development of afferent inhibitors is certainly on the horizon.

The postintegrative or efferent phase of the HIV-1 life cycle also provides several attractive therapeutic targets if viral-specific factors can be identified. The recent excitement over the clinical benefit from HIV-1 protease inhibitors, which disrupt viral protein processing during the efferent phase, demonstrate the potential for intervention targeting these steps. Other attractive efferent components include viral transcription, assembly, and release. Furthermore, many cellular factors are involved in completing these steps of the viral life cycle and are potential targets of intervention if selectivity can be achieved.

To test and evaluate novel therapeutic compounds inhibiting steps along the efferent portion of the HIV-1 life cycle, several chronically infected, cloned cell models have been developed *(1)*. Because of several unique features, one cell model, OM-10.1, has proven particularly convenient and informative in the evaluation of efferent HIV-1 inhibitors. OM-10.1 cells were cloned following an acute HIV-1_{LAI} infection of HL-60 promyelocytes *(2)*. In a clonal fashion, these cells harbor a single HIV-1 provirus, constitutively express little

From: *Methods in Molecular Medicine, vol. 24: Antiviral Methods and Protocols*
Edited by: D. Kinchington and R. F. Schinazi © Humana Press Inc., Totowa, NJ

viral protein, and remain CD4 positive. On exposure to tumor necrosis factor-alpha (TNF-α), OM-10.1 cells activate HIV-1 transcription, down-modulate cell surface CD4 secondary to viral envelope protein expression within 24 h, and express large amounts of HIV-1 into the culture supernatant within 48 h *(2)*. Therefore, the OM-10.1 culture system can be used to rapidly and conveniently screen novel therapeutic compounds for an ability to inhibit HIV-1 transcription, translation, or particle maturation and release ***(3–5)***.

2. Materials

1. Complete growth medium: RPMI-1640 growth medium containing 10% heat-inactivated fetal bovine serum, 2 m*M* L-glutamine, 1% Pen-Strep (Gibco, Grand Island, NY).
2. Recombinant human TNF-α (Genzyme, Cambridge, MA) at 200,000 U/mL.
3. Trypan blue 0.1% (Gibco).
4. 48- (or 24-) and 96-well plates (sterile).
5. Phycoerythrin-conjugated, anti-human CD4 monoclonal antibody (Leu-3a, Becton Dickinson, San Jose, CA).
6. RT assay cocktail: filtered, distilled water containing 0.05% NP-40, 50 m*M* Tris, pH 7.8, 75 m*M* KCl, 2 m*M* dithiothreitol (DTT), 5 m*M* $MgCl_2$, 1 mg/mL poly-A template (Pharmacia, Piscataway, NJ) and 31.25 mU (absorption at A_{260})/mL oligo dT_{12-18} primer (Pharmacia).
7. Flow cytometry wash buffer: standard phosphate-buffered saline (PBS, pH 7.4) containing 0.2% sodium azide, 0.1 % bovine serum albumin, and 2% human AB^+ serum. Filter by suction through a 0.45-μ*M* filter.
8. 1% paraformaldehyde prepared in PBS.
9. Radioactive material from standard commercial sources: ^{3}H-thymidine (1 mCi/mL) and [α-^{32}P]-TTP (10 mC/mL).
10. Test compounds or vehicle (DMSO, water, ethanol, and so on).
11. 1.5X SSC: distilled water containing 225 m*M* sodium chloride and 22.5 m*M* sodium citrate.
12. Diethylamino ethyl (DEAE) cellulose paper (DE81, Whatman, Maidstone, UK).

3. Methods

3.1. Drug Treatment and HIV-1 Activation in OM-10.1 Cultures

1. Split OM-10.1 culture the day before the assay to $< 5 \times 10^5$ cells/mL to insure log phase growth.
2. Count OM-10.1 cells using trypan blue and a hemocytometer and collect by centrifugation sufficient cells to perform the assay (7.5×10^5 cells needed for each test well).
3. Resuspend the cell pellet in complete growth medium to 5×10^5 cells/mL and seed 1.5 mL/test into a well of a 24- or 48-well plate.
4. Pretreat (4 h is generally aufficient, *see* **Note 2**) the culture with the appropriate drug concentrations (ideally, a titration of each unknown test compound should be performed) or vehicle.

5. Treat the culture with TNF-α at 20 U/mL (prepare a 1:100 dilution of the 200,000 U/mL TNF-α stock in complete growth medium and then add 15 μL to the 1.5 mL culture [final dilution = 1:10,000 of stock]).
6. Resuspend the cells by pipeting and, for associated toxicity evaluation, transfer 100 μL aliquots into five individual wells of a 96-well plate.
7. Culture both the 24- or 48-well and the 96-well plates at 37°C in a humidified atmosphere of 7% CO_2 and 93% air.

3.2. Determination of HIV-1 Activation

Insight into the mechanisms of drug inhibition can be obtained by evaluating multiple determinants of HIV-1 activation in OM-10.1 cultures. Because CD4 downmodulation is dependent only on HIV-1 transcription and translation, inhibitors of virion maturation or release will reduce RT activity of culture supernatant whereas the loss of surface CD4 appears unaffected. A flowchart of analysis is presented in **Fig. 1**.

3.2.1. Determination of Cell Surface CD4 Expression by Flow Cytometry

1. After 24 h of culture, resuspend the OM-10.1 cells in the 24- or 48-well plate culture by pipeting, and transfer 0.5 mL of cell suspension into a small tube appropriate for the flow cytometer to be used. Return the plate to the incubator for the determination of supernatant RT activity after an additional 24 h.
2. Add 3 mL of flow cytometry wash buffer and pellet the cells by centrifugation.
3. Decant the supernatant into 10% bleach solution, allowing the last 100–200 μL to return to the bottom of the tube.
4. Add 10 μL of Leu-3a into the remaining buffer and gently vortex to resuspend the cell pellet.
5. Incubate in the dark (at room temperature or 4°C) for 30 min.
6. Add 4 mL of PBS to wash out unbound antibody and pellet the cells by centrifugation.
7. Decant as much of the supernatant as possible and add 0.5 mL of 1% paraformaldehyde, vortex to resuspend the cells, and incubate at 4°C in the dark for a minimum of 20 min to fix and inactivate HIV-1.
8. Read samples for CD4 surface levels by standard flow cytometry using a medium-maintained OM-10. 1 culture as a positive for surface expression (>90% $CD4^+$) and a TNF-α-treated OM-10.1 culture as a negative for surface expression (<15% $CD4^+$ by 24 h).

3.2.2. Determination of RT Activity in OM-10.1 Culture Supernatants

1. After 48 h of culture and being careful not to disturb the cells at the bottom of the well, transfer 100–150 μL of cell-free culture supernatant from the individual cultures in the 24- or 48-well plate into a storage plate (a new 96-well plate is ideal). This storage plate can be kept at –70°C until the RT assay is performed.
2. Prepare radioactive reverse transcriptase assay solution by adding [α-^{32}P]-TTP to a final concentration of 20 μCi/mL of RT cocktail. Mix well and distribute 25 μL of this mixture/well into a U- or V-bottomed 96-well plate.

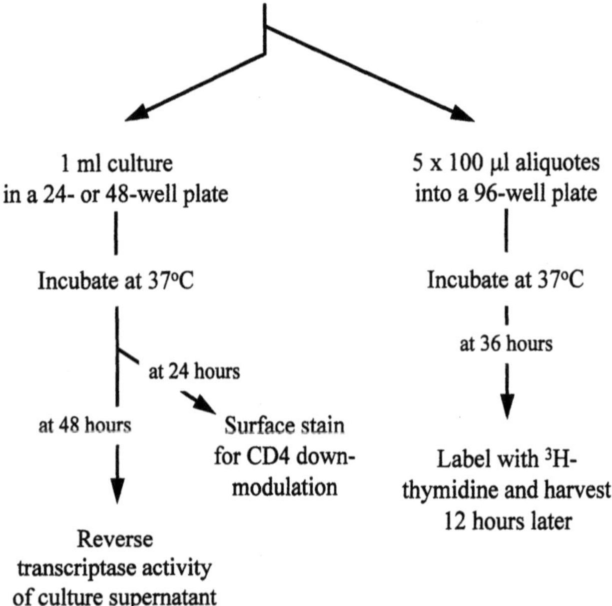

Fig. 1. Schematic flowchart of OM-10.1 culture standard setup for evaluating drug inhibition of HIV-1 reactivation.

3. Add 5 µL of the culture supernatants into the individuals wells containing the radioactive RT assay solution. Duplicate reaction wells for each supernatant are recommended. If the culture supernatants are stored in a 96-well plate, a small-volume multichannel pipeter can be conveniently used for this addition.
4. Incubate the RT reaction plate at 37°C for 1.5 h.
5. Design a 96-well template and stencil it, using pencil or permanent ink, onto DEAE paper. A handheld stamp designed to mimic the wells of a 96-well plate is convenient and can be custom-produced at some local office supply companies.
6. After the incubation period, spot 6 µL of the RT reaction onto the DEAE template. Again, if the template is designed to mimic the spacing of a 96-well plate, a small-volume multichannel pipeter can be conveniently used. Allow the spotted paper to dry for 5–10 min.
7. Wash the paper five times in approx 250 mL of 1.5X SSC. Discard the first three washes as liquid radioactive waste.
8. Wash the paper twice more in approx 250 mL of 95°C ethanol and allow to dry after the final wash.

9. Quantitate the radioactivity, as a measure of RT activity in 1 μL of the culture supernatant, either by liquid scintillation counting (cut out the spots and place them directly into scintillation fluid), by phosphorimage analysis and quantitation of relative pixel units, or by autoradiography and laser densitometry.

3.3. Determination of Relative Drug Toxicity on OM-10.1 Cultures

1. After 36 h of culture, add 1 μCi of ^{3}H-thymidine in a small volume of complete growth medium to each replicate in the 96-well plate.
2. Culture for an additional 12 h to allow DNA incorporation of label.
3. Harvest cultures onto filter paper using an automated cell harvester, as directed by the manufacturer.
4. Determine thymidine uptake by liquid scintillation counting as a measure of drug-induced cytostatic or toxicity.

4. Notes

1. Because OM-10.1 cells remain CD4+, the possibility of superinfection exists *(6)*. Superinfection of OM-10.1 cells results in a higher level of constitutive HIV-1 expression by the culture. This can be prevented or reduced by periodic treatment of OM-10.1 cultures with 10 μg/mL AZT for 72 h *(2,6)*. Remove AZT by washing and allow the culture to expand for 24 h before using the cells for any further experiments. After AZT treatment, the constitutive level of $CD4^-/HIV^+$ cells should be approx 5%.
2. Extending the period of exposure to the drug before TNF-α induction beyond 4 h is necessary in some instances to observe the full inhibitory effect of certain compounds.
3. Phorbol esters (such as PMA) also activate HIV-1 expression from OM-10.1 cells *(2)* and can be used to study drug inhibition of viral activation mediated by pathways somewhat divergent from those involved in TNF-α signal transduction *(3,4)*. However, because phorbol ester treatment results in CD4 downmodulation independent of HIV-1 expression, changes in cell surface CD4 expression cannot be used as an indirect indicator of HIV-1 transcription and translation.
4. Because OM-10.1 cells are derived from HL-60 promyelocytes, these cells differentiate toward more mature cellular phenotypes when exposed to established agents (including phorbol esters, vitamin D3, retinoic acid, sodium butyrate, and DMSO). Therefore, cellular differentiation in the presence of test compounds can indicate selectivity of drug inhibition for HIV-1 activation *(4)*.
5. Supernatant RT levels can be lowered owing to a cytostatic effect of drug treatment, giving the false impression of HIV-1 inhibition In these instances, CD4 downmodulation, which is independent of culture expansion, can still be used as a reliable indicator of HIV-1 inhibitory effects.
6. OM-10.1 cells express passagable virus *(2)*, although viral titers do not recover on serial passage indicating some viral defect. Therefore, increased end point HIV-1 titers after TNF-α induction can be used to evaluate drug effects in place of or in addition to supernatant RT activity. Furthermore, appropriate biosafety level containment should always be observed when working with OM-10.1 cultures or products.

References

1. Butera, S. T. and Folks, T. M. (1992) Application of latent HIV-1 infected cellular models to therapeutic intervention. *AIDS Res. Human Retroviruses* **8,** 991–995.
2. Butera, S. T., Perez, V. L., Wu, B.-Y., Nabel, G. J., and Folks, T. M. (1991) Oscillation of the human immunodeficiency virus surface receptor is regulated by the state of viral activation in a CD4+ cell model of chronic infection. *J. Virol.* **65,** 4645–4653.
3. Critchfield, J. W., Butera, S. T., and Folks, T. M. (1996) Inhibition of HIV activation in latently infected cells by flavonoid compounds. *AIDS Res. Human Retroviruses* **12,** 39–46.
4. Butera, S. T., Roberts, B. D., Critchfield, J. W., Fang, G., McQuade, T., Gracheck, S. J., and Folks, T. M. (1995) Compounds that target novel cellular components involved in HIV- 1 transcription. *Mol. Med.* **1,** 758–767.
5. Feorino, P. M., Butera, S. T., Folks, T. M., and Schinazi, R. F. (1993) Prevention of activation of HIV-1 by antiviral agents in OM-10.1 cells. *Antiviral Chem. Chemother.* **4,** 55–63.
6. Besansky, N. J., Butera, S. T., Sinha, S., and Folks, T. M. (1991) Unintegrated human immunodeficiency virus type 1 DNA in chronically infected cell lines is not correlated with surface CD4 expression. *J. Virol.* **65,** 2695–2698.

17

Assessment of Activity of Topical Virucidal Agents

Timothy O'Connor

1. Introduction

There is currently considerable interest in the possibility of developing a potent, nontoxic anti-HIV agent that could be used intravaginally to reduce the risks of transmission of HIV. Worldwide up to 80% of HIV infections have been acquired heterosexually. Projections suggest that by the year 2000 approx 25 million individuals worldwide will have been infected by heterosexual transmission. This spread of infection is particularly rapid in parts of Africa, Asia, and Latin America. In the absence of a prophylactic vaccine, there is an urgent need to develop safe, effective, female-controlled, topical virucidal preparations to prevent sexual transmission of HIV and other sexually transmitted diseases (STDs). Many assays directed against the virus have had problems with removal of the presumptive agents, which in many cases are toxic to the cell culture system. Methods have includes dilution, centrifugation, and erythrocyte ghost preparations, but these have problems with virus dilution and an inability to examine the kinetics of inactivation.

A number of substances have been identified that have either a specific virucidal effect on HIV or prevent infection of cells in vitro. The virucidal activity of potential topical agents can be assessed against cell-free and cell-associated virus using these assay systems. They allow the measurement of precise contact times between the HIV and virucides, enable the protective effect of preparations to be examined, and allow removal of the virucide from the system prior to assessment of cell viability.

2. Assay for Determining Virucidal Activity Using Cell-Free Viruses

2.1. Materials

1. Commercial HIV P24 antigen assay (Coulter UK)
2. HIV 111B strain (MRC AIDS Reagent Project #ADP 101).

From: *Methods in Molecular Medicine, vol. 24: Antiviral Methods and Protocols*
Edited by: D. Kinchington and R. F. Schinazi © Humana Press Inc., Totowa, NJ

3. Human T-lymphoblastoid cell line C8166 (MRC AIDS Reagent Project #ADP 013).
4. Hydrochloric acid (Sigma # H7020).
5. Isopropanol (Sigma # I 9516).
6. MTT (Sigma # M 2003).
7. Phosphate-buffered saline (Dulbecco A) (PBS).
8. Plate reader (wavelengths 450 + 570 nm).
9. Plate reader (wavelengths 540 + 690 nm).
10. Poly-L-lysine hydrobromide (Sigma # P1399).
11. RPMI 1640 growth medium (Labtech) containing 10% fetal calf serum, 2 m*M* L-glutamine, 100 µg/mL penicillin, and 100 mL/mL streptomycin.
12. Tissue culture plates (Nunclon, 96-well flat bottom, sterile).
13. Trypan blue (Sigma # T8154).

2.2. Method (see Fig. 1)

1. 50 µL of 50 µg/mL poly-L-lysine is added to a sterile flat-bottomed 96-well tissue culture plate (Nunc) and incubated at room temperature for 1 h.
2. Using a multichannel pipeter, the coated plate is gently washed (twice) with sterile PBS.
3. 25 µL of RPMI 1640 medium, containing HIV IIIB (50 $TCID_{50}$) is then added to each well and incubated for 1 h at room temperature.
4. At this stage plates can be frozen at –70°C for later use.
5. The plate is gently hand washed (twice) with sterile PBS.
6. 30 µL of the dilution series of the presumptive virucide are added to each well (Use four wells per dilution). Contact time can be varied (1–120 min in our assays), allowing the kinetics of inactivation to be studied.
7. After the required exposure, the wells are washed twice with sterile PBS to remove the virucide.
8. 300 µL of growth medium (RPMI 1640) containing 4×10^4 of the target cells (C8166s) are added to each well. The outer ring of wells were left uncoated and are filled with 250 µL of sterile water to counter the effects of evaporation.
9. After 72 or 96 h the plates are examined and scored for cytopathic effect (CPE). Carefully remove 200 µL from each well or 50 µL from each replicate of four for testing to evaluate levels of HIV p24 antigen production in the wells. Testing in this laboratory was with the Coulter UK P24 antigen assay.
10. CPE and HIV P24 antigen levels are expressed as a percentage of reduction (if any occurs) of control well levels. The concentration that causes 50 or a 90% reduction (IC_{50}, IC_{90}) in HIV P24 antigen can be plotted from this data.

3. Method

A virucide must operate quickly and effectively in preventing infection of vulnerable target cells. The previous assay looked at the effect of the virucide on free virus, and was removed prior to challenge of the target cells. This assay looks at the protective effects of virucides on the target cells prior to challenge with virus. We have found that certain substances can mediate the efficacy of

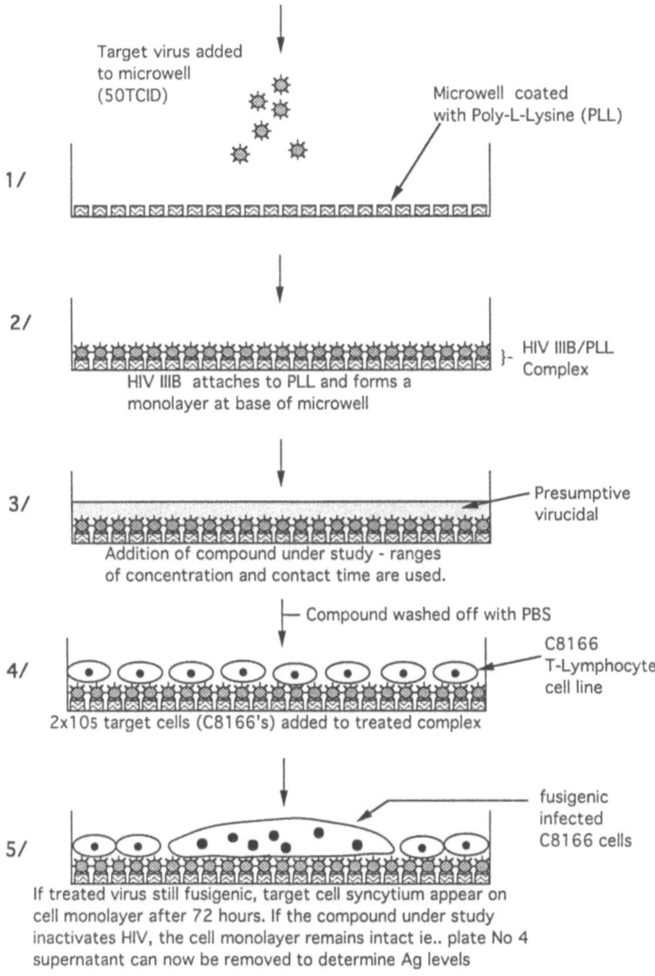

Fig. 1. Viral adhesion microassay.

agents, i.e., certain topical virucides that rely on binding to cellular sites and locking out the virus have been shown to be sensitive to presence or absence of semen. Thus, target cells can be treated with virucide/protein/genital secretion combinations prior to challenge.

3.1. Assay to Determine Protection of Target Cells from Virucide

1. 50 µL of 50 µg/mL poly-L-lysine is added to a sterile flat-bottomed 96-well tissue culture plate (Nunc) and incubated at room temperature for 1 h.
2. Using a multichannel pipeter, the coated plate is gently washed (twice) with sterile PBS.

3. 200 μL of growth medium (RPMI 1640) containing 4×10^4 of the target cells (C8166s) are added to each well. The outer ring of wells were left uncoated and are filled with 250 μL of sterile water to counter the effects of evaporation. This step can be performed on the day of the assay, leaving the cells for a minimum of 1 h, or for maximum adhesion the cells can be left overnight in a 37°C/5% CO_2 incubator.
4. Using a multichannel pipeter the growth medium is gently removed from the cells.
5. A minimum of 50 μL of the virucide under test is added to appropriately labeled wells. This step needs to be carried out immediately after **step 4** to prevent the cells from drying out. The virucide must be diluted in a suitable diluent, i.e., growth medium or PBS. If only soluble in toxic agents, i.e., DMSO or alcohol, the concentration can be adjusted to give 100× the required amount and diluted into growth medium or PBS in the well. Cells can survive 1% concentrations of DMSO or alcohol for 72 h (or higher for short periods, i.e., 4% DMSO for 60 min). Control wells are treated with PBS
6. The compound is left to absorb for a suitable period, i.e., 60 min.
7. At this stage the treated cells are challenged with 50 TCID HIV IIIB. The virus may be added in the presence/absence of the virucide by washing/not washing the wells with PBS after **step 6**. Other cofactors, such as semen, can be mixed with the virus challenge to simulate the in vivo state.
8. The wells are incubated at 37°C/5% CO_2 for 90 min.
9. Using a multichannel pipetter, the treated wells are gently washed (twice) with sterile PBS to remove the challenge mixture.
10. 300 μL of growth medium (RPMI 1640) is added to each well. The outer ring of wells are left uncoated and are filled with 250 μL sterile water to counter the effects of evaporation.
11. After 72 or 96 h the plates are examined and scored for cytopathic effect (CPE). Carefully remove 200 μL from each well or 50 μL from each replicate of four for testing to evaluate levels of HIV p24 antigen production in the wells. Testing in this laboratory was with the Coulter UK P24 antigen assay.
12. CPE and HIV P24 antigen levels are expressed as a percentage of reduction (if any occurs) of control well levels. The concentration that causes 50% reduction (IC_{50}) in HIV P24 antigen can be plotted from this data

3.2. Toxicity Assessment

When considering the cytotoxic effect of topical virucides the parameters are somewhat wider than those applied to systemic agents. Compounds, such as nonoxynol 9, have a selective index of <2 (selectivity = CC_{50} value divided by the IC_{50} value). This nonionic surfactant would never have passed the first round of toxicity testing if it were to be used systemically. Thus, agents that have an equally destructive effect on cells as well as the virus are not to be discarded from a test program. In some situations this dual activity could be advantageous, such as activity against cells and virus in HIV-positive semen.

The toxicity assays employed to look at topical agents are not used to exclude but to alert researchers to any potential problems that may arise if these compounds are used in vivo at high concentrations.

3.3. Trypan Blue Exclusion

Steps 1–6 are the same as the previous assay (the period of contact between the cells and the virucide should be the same as that selected for the antiviral assays).

7. Add 50 μL stock trypan blue solution (10 mg/mL in PBS) to each well and leave for 1 min.
8. Count the number of live cells (translucent: trypan blue is excluded) and the number of dead cells (blue: trypan blue is not excluded) using a hemocytometer. Calculate the percentage of live cells in the well

$$\% \text{ of viable cells} = (\text{no. of live cells})/(\text{total no. of cells}) \times 100 \quad (1)$$

Compare these values for a dilution series of a compound with that obtained for the control to determine the CC_{50} (50% cytotoxic concentration) if any.

3.4. Colorimetric MTT (Formazan) Method

This assay was developed and used in anti-HIV screening programs (Pauwels et al. 1988). The tetrazolium salt MTT [3-(4,5-dimethyl thiazol-2-yl)-2,5-diphenyltetrazolium bromide] is converted to dark blue formazan by living cells but not by dead cells or culture medium. These assays are carried out in 96-well plates.

1. To a 96-well culture plate add 3×10^4 cells in 150 μL of fresh growth medium (RPMI 1640) to each well.
2. Add 100 μL medium with and without drug to be tested at the appropriate dilutions and incubate cells at 37°C in 5% CO_2 for 3–5 d in a humidified environment. Compounds should be tested in triplicate wells at each concentration.
3. Using a multichannel pipet, carefully remove 150 μL growth medium.
4. Add 10 μL of 5 mg/mL MTT to the remaining 100 μL of culture fluid containing the cells and incubate the plates in 5% CO_2 for a further 4 h.
5. Remove supernatants and add 150 μL acid-isopropyl alcohol (0.04 *N* HCl in isopropanol) to all wells.
6. Mix thoroughly to dissolve the dark blue crystals of formazan that are formed.
7. Incubate for 5–10 min to ensure all the crystals are dissolved.
8. Read the plates on a plate reader at 540 nm and with a reference wavelength of 690 nm. The absorbance measured at 690 nm is subtracted from the absorbance at 540 nm; this eliminates the effects of nonspecific absorbance. The 50% cytotoxic dose (CD_{50}) is given as the concentration of compound that reduces the absorbance (OD540) of the uninfected cell samples by 50% when compared to the control wells.

4. Notes

1. Contact times in these assays should reflect the in vivo condition as much as possible, i.e., preparations in a pessary or applicator may only remain in the genital lumen a matter of hours. Preparations introduced via a slow release method, i.e., sponge or ring, may be in contact with the cells for days.
2. Binding of cells or virus seems to vary depending on the tissue culture plate used. When non-Nunc plates were used, variations in binding quality were noticed.
3. Although the coating of cells onto poly-L-lysine can be carried out in 1 h, the monolayer is delicate, and care must be taken at all washing steps. The overnight incubation gives a much more robust coat.

18

Assays That Measure Selective Killing of Virus-Infected Cells

Sharon Randall

1. Introduction

When evaluating potential antiviral compounds, determining the effect of the drug on virus replication is usually the prime concern. However, since virus replication is dependent on the host cell, in circumstances where virus infection is not rapidly lytic to cells, the effect of these compounds on cell growth and viability merits consideration. Differential host cell metabolism has been reported for cells infected with viruses, e.g., HIV, measles, and HSV, and therefore it is possible that cells infected with viruses have different susceptibilities to antiviral drugs, depending on the their mode of action. Experience with HIV and a potential anti-HIV drug, EF13, showed that HIV-chronically infected cells were markedly more susceptible to EF13 than their parent uninfected cells *(1)*; however, acutely HIV-infected cells showed a similar susceptibility as uninfected cells to EF13 *(2)*. In addition, cells containing actively replicating HIV-1 were more susceptible to EF13 than either uninfected cells or cells infected with but not producing HIV-1 *(3)*.

Methods used to determine selective killing of virus-infected cells over uninfected cells can be very simple; for example, the Trypan blue exclusion test, which merely distinguishes between live and dead cells on the basis of whether the cell membrane is intact (for live cells) or perforated (for dead cells). Trypan blue will potentially stain all dead cells by staining the cell cytoplasm. Slightly more sophisticated dyes, for example, acridine orange and ethidium bromide, can distinguish between live and dead cells by differential staining of cell nuclei and hence are useful for viability determinations when anucleated cells in cultures can be ignored, e.g., red blood cells in PBMC cultures. Still more sophisticated techniques, such as flow cytometry, can indicate specifi-

From: *Methods in Molecular Medicine, vol. 24: Antiviral Methods and Protocols*
Edited by: D. Kinchington and R. F. Schinazi © Humana Press Inc., Totowa, NJ

cally which cells are both infected and dead or vice versa. The methods outlined in this chapter will be described with reference to HIV; however, they can be applied to any virus-infected cells providing the necessary reagents are available.

2. Materials

1. Trypan blue stain (0.2% w/v stock solution in phosphate-buffered saline [PBS]).
2. Acridine orange:ethidium bromide stain; 20 mg acridine orange and 10 mg ethidium bromide dissolved in 10 mL PBS. Dilute 1:100 in PBS before use.
3. Cell cultures to be tested.
4. Light microscope.
5. Epifluorescent light microscope.
6. Cell counting chamber (Hemocytometer or disposable Kova* slides).
7. Liquid handling equipment.
8. Ethidium monoazide bromide (EMA; stock solution 50 μg/mL in PBS).
9. FITC-conjugated monoclonal antibody (MAb) against an intracellular viral antigen. In the case of HIV-1 a specific anti-p24 MAb, KC57, is available from Coulter Electronics Ltd. (UK).
10. FITC-conjugated murine immunoglobulin (if using a mouse monoclonal) of the same class as the virus-specific MAb to be used.
11. Fluorescent light source, 40 W.
12. Bench-top centrifuge.
13. Permeabilizing agent, e.g., Permeafix (Ortho Diagnostics, UK), saponin.
14. FACS-wash A (PBS containing 0.5% BSA [bovine serum albumin]).
15. FACS-wash B (PBS containing 3% BSA, 10% calf serum, and 0.0055% EDTA.
16. FACS-fix (flow cytometer sheath fluid containing 1.0% formaldehyde).
17. Flow cytometer (e.g., Becton Dickinson FACScan).

3. Methods

3.1. Trypan Blue Exclusion Test for Cell Viability

1. Culture uninfected cells and virus-infected cells, under optimal conditions for the particular cell type to be tested, in the presence and absence of increasing concentrations of the potential antiviral compound. Harvest cell samples daily and perform viability staining.
2. Resuspend the cells thoroughly to avoid clumping of cells because this will cause inaccuracies in cell counting. For adherent cells, monolayers will require prior trypsinization. Remove the growth medium from the cell monolayer and rinse the monolayer twice with PBS to remove any traces of calf serum. Add sufficient trypsin solution (0.25%) to cover the monolayer. Leave the trypsin solution in

---

*Kova slides are plastic disposable counting slides useful for counting cells in Category 3 laboratories where use of glass is inadvisable. Kova slides are available from Bio-Stat Diagnostics (Stockport, UK) or Hycor Biomedical Inc. (California).

contact with the cells for 1 min, then pour off the excess and incubate the culture flask, in a horizontal position, monolayer on the base, at 37°C for 5–10 min. Test that the cells have become detached by holding the culture flask in a vertical position and tapping. If the cells begin to slide off the surface of the flask they are ready for resuspension. Add medium containing calf serum to the flask and resuspend the cells by gentle repeated pipeting.

3. Aim to count a suspension of cells at approx 6×10^5–6×10^6 cells/mL. With practice, the approximate order of the cell count can be estimated by the turbidity of the suspension. If necessary, dilute the cell suspension 1:10, 1:100, and so forth, in cell medium prior to counting.
4. Take 20 µL of cell suspension and mix well with 20 µL of 0.2% Trypan blue solution.
5. Fix a coverslip to the counting chamber and apply the stained cell suspension to each side of the chamber. If using disposable Kova slides, these are provided complete with coverslips and require calibration for accuracy.
6. Observe under the light microscope for blue-stained (dead) and unstained (live) cells. With Trypan blue staining, cells should be observed between 2 and 5 min after staining for consistent results. **Figure 1** shows the appearence of the center square of the counting grid of a hemocytometer. The center square is edged by triple lines and divided into 16 smaller squares. Count all cells within the center square, aiming to count between 30 and 300 cells (counting outside of these limits can be inaccurate). Only count cells that lie within the square; exclude any cells that fall in the triple line edge. The formula for converting the cell count to a count per mL of culture medium is

$$\text{cells/mL} = \text{cell count} \times \text{dilution factor in Trypan blue} \times 10^4 \quad (1)$$

The dilution factor in this instance is 2 (equal volumes of cells and stain were mixed) but may be any dilution you choose. The 10^4 accounts for the volume of cells counted and the surface area under the grid.

Space between the coverslip and the top of the slide = 0.1 mm
Each square encloses = 1.0 mm^2
Therefore volume of culture counted ($1 \times 1 \times 0.1$ mm) = 0.1 mm^3 = 0.1 µL
Therefore number of cells/mL = count $\times 10^4$

For detecting selective toxicity, express the count as % dead cells.

$$\%\ \text{dead cells} = (\text{number of blue cells})/(\text{total number of cells}) \quad (2)$$

7. For statistical analysis, the greater the number of counts per culture the more accurate will be the statistics. The absolute minimum is triplicate values. **Figure 2** shows the selective toxicity of EF13 for HIV-chronically infected cells over uninfected cells established using the Trypan blue exclusion test.

3.2. Acridine Orange and Ethidium Bromide Staining for Cell Viability

Follow the protocol given for Trypan blue staining, substituting the acridine orange/ethidium bromide stain for the Trypan blue. Observe the stained cells

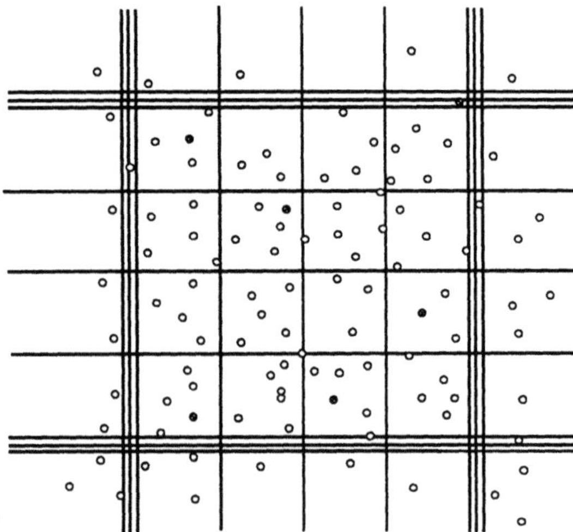

Fig. 1. Hemocytometer counting grid. The center square of the hemocytometer is divided into 16 smaller squares and is edged by triple lines. Count all cells within the triple lined square, but exclude any cells that fall on the triple lines. For accurate counts, aim to count between 30 and 300 cells in each square.

under epifluorescent light provided by a halogen lamp. It is not necessary to have a darkened room to observe the fluorescence, but placing the microscope away from sunlight is necessary. A small amount of light is helpful for focusing on the counting grid. Dead nucleated cells will fluoresce orange and live nucleated cells will fluoresce green. Again, express the count as % dead cells.

3.3. Cell Viability and Infectivity by Flow Cytometry

1. Culture uninfected cells and virus-infected cells, under optimal conditions for the particular cell type to be tested, in the presence and absence of predetermined concentrations of the potential antiviral compound. Harvest cell samples at predetermined intervals and perform viability/infectivity staining.
2. Resuspend the cells thoroughly to avoid clumping of cells as this will cause inaccuracies in cell counting.
3. Dispense 2×10^5 cells into 6 mL plastic, round-bottomed FACS tubes (Falcon, UK). For each culture, four tubes will be required per sampling; one for control staining, one for EMA only, one for virus-specific FITC-conjugated MAb only, and one for dual EMA and virus-specific FITC-conjugated MAb staining. Wash the cells with FACS-wash A and centrifuge the tubes at 1100 rpm for 5 min to pellet the cells. Discard the supernatant by inversion and resuspend the cells in the residual fluid (~100 μL).
4. Add EMA to two of the four tubes per sample to a final concentration of 1–5 μg/mL. (Each batch of EMA should be titrated to find the optimum concentration, which should be between 1 and 5 μg/mL.) Add an identical volume of FACS-

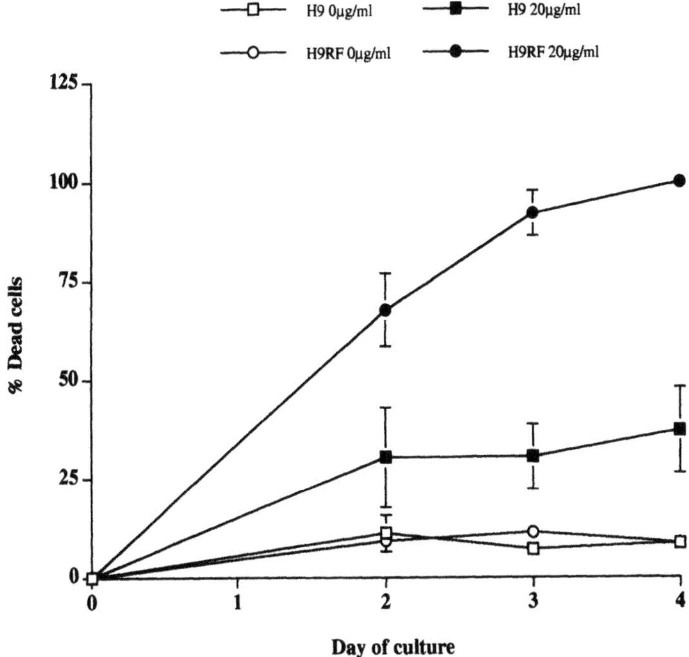

Fig. 2. Selective toxicity of EF13 for C8166 cells chronically infected with HIV-1. Uninfected (H9) and chronically HIV-infected (H9RF) cells were cultured for 4 d in the presence of EF13, a potential anti-HIV compound. Cell samples were taken daily and counted in the presence of Trypan blue to determine the proportion of cells that were live and dead. The data points represent the mean of 5 counts plus error bars of one standard deviation.

wash A to the remaining two tubes. Vortex all of the tubes gently to mix and incubate for 15 min on ice under fluorescent light at a distance of 18 cm from the source.

5. Pellet the cells and wash twice with 1 mL FACS-wash A, vortexing gently and centrifuging the cells at 1100 rpm with each wash, then fix and permeabilize the cells in Permeafix (1 mL) for 40 min at room temperature (*see* **Subheading 3.3.1.** for saponin permeabilization).
6. Pellet the cells by centrifugation at 1800 rpm and wash once in FACS-wash B, recentrifuging the cells at 1800 rpm for 5 min.
7. Add 100 μL of a 1:300 dilution* of KC57-FITC (anti-p24), diluted in FACS-wash B minus the EDTA, to one EMA-stained tube and one unstained tube per sample and add 100 μL of a 1:300 dilution of mouse-immunoglobulin-FITC-conjugate to the remaining tubes. Incubate at room temperature for 40 min.

*Antibody dilutions require prior determination.

8. Wash the cells three times with FACS-wash B, centrifuging the cells at 1800 rpm, then resuspend the cells in 500 µL FACS-fix. Finally, gently vortex and store away from light at 4°C until analysis.

3.3.1. Saponin Permeabilization

Follow **steps 1–4** in **Subheading 3.3.**

5. Pellet the cells and wash twice with 1 mL FACS-wash A, vortexing gently and centrifuging the cells at 1100 rpm with each wash. After discarding the final wash, add 100 µL of 1:300 KC57-FITC (anti-p24) diluted in FACS-wash A containing 0.3% saponin to each of two tubes, one containing EMA-stained cells and the other containing unstained cells. To the remaining two tubes of cells add 100 µL of mouse immunoglobulin FITC-conjugate diluted 1:300 in FACS-wash A containing 0.3% saponin. Incubate at room temperature for 20 min.
6. Wash the cells three times with 0.1% saponin-containing FACS-wash A, gently vortexing and centrifuging at 1500 rpm with each wash. Finally, fix the cells in 500 µL FACS-fix and store away from light at 4°C until analysis.

Note: The above methods employ FITC-conjugated antibodies because FITC has a different emission wavelength to EMA on the flow cytometer. When using different fluorolabels be sure their emission wavelengths can be distinguished from that of EMA. If conjugated primary antibodies are not available, unlabeled antibodies can be used followed by three washes and incubation with a secondary conjugated antispecies antibody.

3.3.2. Flow Cytometric Analysis

The flow cytometer is used to determine the percentage of cells stained with the different fluorophores and also their relative fluorescent intensity. The following brief description is based on the Becton Dickinson FACScan and Lysis II acquisition software but is applicable to other instruments. If you are not used to the flow cytometer much time will be saved by obtaining instruction from a regular instrument user. Initially, forward and right-angle (side) light scatter measurements are used to identify cell populations, differentiate among morphologically different cells (important when using primary cells, such as PBMC, when the differential staining of the cell types is required), and eliminate as much debris as possible from the following analysis. Even the best prepared samples contain debris. Gating is used to isolate the cell population(s) that will be analyzed by the computer. In essence, a polygon, box, or elipse is drawn around the cells of interest; however, specific gating techniques vary from instrument to instrument. Also, when using more than one stain, compensation among the emission channels is required to overcome any spectral overlap for the fluorochromes.

3.3.2.1. Helpful Notes for the Becton Dickinson FACScan

1. When starting up the FACScan, ensure that all the channels you wish to use are switched on. You may be given the option to choose which channels you wish to open during the set-up procedure; otherwise you will have to check the protocol window to see which channels are on and which are off. For the above protocol, channels 1 and 2 are required.
2. With the instrument in "set-up" mode, apply the control unstained cell tube to the FACScan probe. While in "set-up" mode, parameters can be adjusted and data is not recorded. When ready to collect data the instrument must be switched to "normal" mode. In "set-up" mode, alter the forward light scatter (FSC) and side light scatter (SSC) parameters to visualize the cell populations in a dot-plot window of FSC-height against SSC-height. This dot-plot will display all cells and debris dependent on size and granularity of the cells. Fluorescence is not taken into account at this stage. Debris will usually appear in the bottom left-hand corner of the dot-plot but may disperse, and live and dead cells may appear as separate populations depending on the changes in granularity and size of cells as they die. A threshold, below which data is not recorded, can be set on either axis to eliminate as much of the debris as possible, leading to more accurate analyses. Gates can be drawn prior to acquisition of data, in which case the option to acquire data only from within those gates is available; however, there are advantages to acquiring all data and applying gates at the analysis stage, in which case setting of a threshold prior to acquisition avoids debris being counted as events as accumulative data are collected.
3. For determination of viability, a large gate is required that will encompass as many of the cells as possible. Using the region tool in the dot-plot window menu, draw a large gate around the cells to be analyzed. Attempt to exclude any debris if possible.
4. Display the data from within the gate in a second dot-plot of channel 2 height (FL2-H) against channel 1 height (FL1-H). FL2-H will show EMA staining and FL1-H will show FITC staining. Since these control cells are not stained with EMA or specific viral MAb, the cell population will appear in the lower left-hand corner of the dot plot (**Fig. 3A**).
5. Change the unstained cell sample for the EMA-only cell sample. This time the gated population displayed on an FL2-H against FL1-H dot plot will display two cell populations (**Fig. 3B**). Dead cells stained with EMA will be in an elevated position on the FL2-H axis and live unstained cells will appear lower on the FL2-H axis. If compensation between the FL1 and FL2 channels has not been set, the cells will curve away from the FL2 axis to the right and instead of forming a discreet population of cells may form a diagonal line (*see* **Subheading 3.3.2.2.**). The live (unstained) cells may not appear in the same location on the FL2-H axis because the previously unstained control cells, i.e., they may move slightly upward. This is caused by background staining and is quite distinct from positive staining.
6. Replace the EMA-only tube with a positive anti-p24-FITC-only tube (i.e., known infected cells). On the FL2-H against FL1-H dot plot there should be a movement

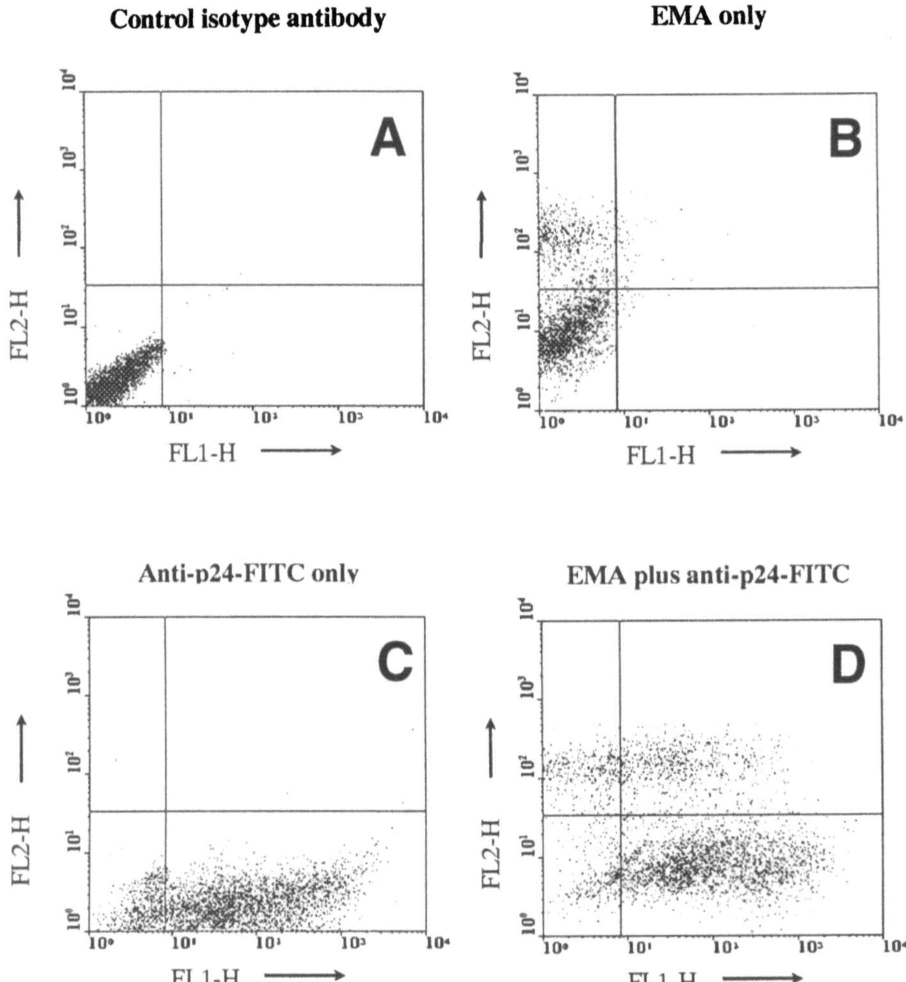

Fig. 3. FACScan analysis of C8166 cells. C8166 cells infected with HIV-1, 4 d postinfection, were stained with **(A)** control FITC-conjugated isotype antibody, **(B)** ethidium monoazide bromide (EMA), **(C)** HIV-specific anti-p24 FITC-conjugated MAb, and **(D)** dual stained with EMA and anti-p24-FITC. Dual staining allows determination of the proportion of cells that are either live or dead or infected or uninfected and hence the proportion of cells that are both dead and infected, dead and uninfected, live and infected, or live and uninfected. Comparison of the proportion of cells that are dead/live/infected/uninfected with potential antiviral drug-treated and untreated cells will give an indication of whether the drug is selectively toxic for virus-infected cells or cytotoxic regardless of infection. Data were acquired on a Becton Dickinson FACScan and analyzed using WinMDI software.

of cells to the right, along the FL1-H axis, if the cells are positive for intracellular p24 (**Fig. 3C**). This time, there may be a continuous band of cells instead of discreet positive and negative cell populations. In acutely infected cultures there will be both infected and uninfected cells and as cells become increasingly positive for intracellular p24 the they will appear further to the right. Again, if the compensation has not been set the cells will form a diagonal streak across the dot-plot and compensation should be checked.

7. Replace the FITC-only cells with cells that are dual stained with anti-p24-FITC and EMA. For infected cells, populations will appear in each of four quadrants of the FL2-H against FL1-H dot-plot (**Fig. 3D**). In the lower left-hand quadrant there will be live uninfected cells, in the lower right-hand quadrant there will be live infected cells, in the upper left-hand quadrant there will be dead uninfected cells, and in the upper right-hand quadrant there will be dead infected cells.
8. Once all parameters are satisfactorily set, switch the instrument to "normal" mode and acquire data. Always include uninfected cells to control for nonspecific staining of the virus-specific intracellular MAb in addition to the EMA staining for viability.
9. Instruments are supplied with software for data analysis. These programs may also be purchased for use on personal computers, which is advantageous if time on the flow cytometer is in great demand. Alternatively, free analysis software is available on the internet for research purposes only *(4)*.

3.3.2.2. Setting Compensation Between Channels

Compensation between instrument channels is required where the emission spectra of the fluorochromes overlap. Compensation is necessary between channels 1 and 2 and between channels 2 and 3 but is not required between channels 1 and 3 because these spectra should not overlap. To set compensation use the compensation parameter menu and cell samples of known positivity for the fluorochromes that are being used, in this case known dead cells and known infected cells, and also negative controls.

1. Apply the negative control sample to the FACScan probe. Create a FSC-H against SSC-H dot-plot visualizing the cells by altering the FSC-H and SSC-H parameters. Gate the desired cell population. Create an FL2-H against FL1-H dot-plot for the gated cells. The unstained cells should fall in the lower left-hand corner of the dot-plot.
2. Apply the EMA only known dead cells to the FACScan probe. The cells will probably form a thin diagonal line across the dot-plot. Access the compensation tools and increase the FL2-FL1 parameter until the cells form a discreet population in the upper region of the FL2-H axis. Over compensation will result in the cells disappearing off the left-hand edge of the dot-plot.
3. Now apply the FITC-anti-p24-only stained known positive cells to the FACScan probe. This time increase the FL1-FL2 parameter until the infected cell population falls to the right of the FL1-H axis in the lower half the dot-plot.
4. Applying a dual stained cell population should now give four cell populations (three if there are no uninfected live cells present) placed in four distinct quad-

rants of the dot-plot. Now stats bars can be applied between the cell populations on the dot-plot to divide the quadrants and the computer can determine the proportion of cells in each quadrant.

5. Once the compensation has been set, the sample data can be acquired by the flow cytometer. Identify each sample as the data is acquired and indicate the number of events (cells) to be counted; the computer will do the calculations.

4. Notes

1. Significant internal p24 staining was not detectable until after 36 h of infection in the flow cytometric assay using C8166 cells infected with a HIV-1 clinical isolate at a multiplicity of infection of 1:500. Experimental conditions will require optimization according to the virus/cell model used.
2. It is important to test virus-specific antibodies in uninfected cells as well as infected cells to determine the level of nonspecific staining for that antibody. Several MAbs may have to be tried before finding one with acceptable levels of nonspecific staining.
3. Stained cells can be analysed immediately or fixed and stored at 4°C. If storing at 4°C, storage should be for >6 h. During this window of 6 h results may be inconsistent if comparing with cells analyzed immediately after staining.
4. The flow cytometric method may not be suitable for potential antiviral compounds that significantly alter the host cell membranes because this may alter the appearance (size or granularity) or permeability and hence the staining of the cells.

References

Additional reading for those interested in the technical details and further applications of flow cytometry can be found in *Flow Cytometry: A Practical Approach* edited by M. G. Ormerod and published by IRL Press. Chapter 1 of this publication, Introduction to the principles of flow cytometry, N. P. Carter and E. W. Meyer, also contains diagrams of dual stained cells before and after spectral overlap compensation.

1. Kinchington, D., et al. (1993) Lithium γ-linolenate-induced cytotoxicity against cells chronically infected with HIV-1. *FEBS Lett.* **330(2),** 219–221.
2. Randall, S., et al. (1997) Inhibition of HIV infection and down modulation of CD4 and CXCR4 surface molecules by lithium γ-linolenic acid. *AIDS*, submitted.
3. Mpanju, O., et al. (1997) Selective toxicity of lithium γ-linolenic acid in human T-cells chronically and productively infected with HIV. *Antiviral Ther.* **2(1),** 17–23.
4. For more information about WinMDI software contact trotter@scripps.edu.

19

Evaluating Clinical Isolates for Their Phenotypic and Genotypic Resistance Against Anti-HIV Drugs

**Anne-Mieke Vandamme, Myriam Witvrouw,
Christophe Pannecouque, Jan Balzarini, Kristel Van Laethem,
Jean-Claude Schmit, Jan Desmyter, and Erik De Clercq**

1. Introduction

The high replication rate of HIV, together with the low fidelity of its reverse transcriptase, provides the virus with an unprecedented genomic flexibility. This allows a fast adaptation to selective pressure, including antiviral drugs, resulting in the development of drug-resistant strains. The present improvements in the treatment of AIDS patients are at least partly owing to antiviral therapy. To assess the implications of HIV drug resistance on patient management, drug resistance assays for clinical HIV isolates are widely being used. Ideally, monitoring drug resistance should help clinicians in their treatment decisions. If patients would really benefit clinically from this strategy, then the gain from clinical improvement and from omitting drugs to which the virus is already resistant would outweigh the cost of drug resistance testing. In the next few years, researchers should consolidate the clinical benefit of antiviral drug resistance testing, and for this they need fast, reliable and cheap assays. All present assays are in vitro assays, which can only partly mimic the in vivo situation with confounding factors, such as cellular resistance *(1)*. Efforts are presently made to establish in vivo assays (*2*; *see also* Chapter 10).

Both genotypic and phenotypic drug resistance assays are valuable tools in this respect. Where genotypic tests are fast and relatively cheap to monitor the presence of known resistance-related mutations, they suffer from known and unknown synergistic and antagonizing effects of combinations of mutations. Only phenotypic assays can measure the actual inhibitory effects of the antiviral drugs on the clinical HIV-1 isolate. Specific reverse transcriptase (RT) and

From: *Methods in Molecular Medicine, vol. 24: Antiviral Methods and Protocols*
Edited by: D. Kinchington and R. F. Schinazi

protease enzyme tests should be able to provide fast answers on resistance toward RT and protease inhibitors, respectively. The present tests, however, lack sensitivity and reproducibility or even fail to detect resistance against particular drugs (e.g., AZT; *3*), and replication-based tests are still the most widely used phenotypic assays.

One of the first standardized phenotypic tests was the HeLa CD4$^+$ plaque reduction assay *(4)*. Although this assay is easy to perform, inexpensive and has a high reproducibility, it is rather labor-intensive and is only suitable for syncytium-inducing (SI) strains. Most patient isolates contain nonsyncytium-inducing (NSI) strains or a mixture of SI and NSI strains. The necessary in vitro cultivation of patient isolates to obtain a high-titer standardized SI-inoculum selects for a subpopulation of SI variants.

In most labs that perform sensitivity tests on clinical HIV isolates, the HeLa CD4$^+$ plaque reduction assay has been replaced by the more generally useful peripheral blood mononuclear cell (PBMC)-based culture system. More than 80% of clinical isolates can be grown in PBMCs, but selection of variant strains cannot be excluded. Japour et al. *(5)* developed a widely used standardized protocol for drug susceptibility testing in PBMCs. This protocol can be considered the present standard and is called ACTG-DoD protocol (AIDS Clinical Trials Group, Department of Defense). It is described in **Subheading 2.**

The ACTG-DoD protocol is time-consuming, less reproducible than the HeLa CD4$^+$ plaque reduction assay, and very expensive, because it uses the expensive p24 antigen enzyme-linked immunosorbent assay (ELISA) to measure virus replication. This is because almost all clinical trials do not produce a clear cytopathogenic effect that can be scored visually or in a cell-killing color test. To circumvent this problem, an elegant assay was devised by Kellam and Larder *(6)* and later adapted by Boucher et al. *(7)*. This recombinant virus assay (RVA) allows the generation of viable virus by homologous recombination of a polymerase chain reaction (PCR)-pool of patient-derived RT gene into an RT-deleted laboratory HIV-1 strain. This recombinant virus retains the sensitivity toward RT drugs of the clinical isolate, whereas replication can now be measured by fast, easy, and cheap tests, designed for lab strains. The first RVA was developed for evaluation of susceptibility toward RT drugs. The second RVA, described by Maschera et al. *(8)* allows recombination of clinical HIV-1 protease genes with laboratory strains. The assay protocol is almost identical to the RT-RVA, except that the PCR is designed to amplify the patient-derived protease gene, and that a different clone is used—a protease deleted proviral clone. The biggest disadvantage of this protease-RVA is that the recently reported mutations in the protease cleavage sites *(9)* are not recombined and thus cannot be evaluated. To what extent selection can bias the results has not been evaluated for the RVA. Selection can occur at the level of the PCR reaction (primer-related sequence selection), with the recombination event and the virus culture depending on the cell line used. In **Subheading 3.** the RVAs will be described and in **Subheading 4.** several replication assays for lab strains that can be used in association with the RVA will be described.

In **Subheading 5.** a few genotypic tests will be described. Using phenotypic assays, clinical isolates that display various levels of resistance to particular drugs have been identified. Often the researcher wants to know what mutations are responsible for this phenotypic resistance, in an attempt to understand and possibly to anticipate the development of the resistance. Because present-day clinical anti-HIV drugs are RT or protease inhibitors, sequencing protocols for clinical HIV-1 RT and protease genes will be described. Once researchers have established a stable relationship between resistance and particular mutations, tests that identify specific mutations may be very valuable and much faster than any other method. In this respect, the protocol for two amplification refractory mutation systems (ARMS) will be described, which use mutation-specific PCRs. Other useful assays are the point mutation assay ***(10)*** and LiPA (*see also* Chapter 10).

2. Assays in PBMCs: ACTG-DoD Protocol

2.1. Experiment Outline

The purpose of these experiments is to determine the dose effect relationship of drugs inhibiting HIV replication in clinical isolates of patients under antiretroviral therapy. By comparison of the obtained IC_{50} values of the different drugs for the patient virus with the values obtained for the wild-type virus, the extent of resistance can be measured.

PBMCs are an interesting research tool because they are the primary target of HIV in humans. The disadvantage of an assay using PBMC in comparison with other cells, e.g., the MT-4 cells, is that it is more labor-intensive and the final evaluation with a p24 sandwich ELISA is expensive.

In general, isolating good-quality PBMCs is the most delicate process in this protocol, and usually requires some experience.

When growing a patient's HIV on donor PBMC in vitro, success is dependent on the viral load and thus on the clinical condition of the patient, e.g., it is more difficult with samples obtained from asymptomatic patients or patients under antiretroviral therapy.

The different steps in the assay are as follows:

1. Isolation and culture of PBMCs of a healthy donor.
2. The growth of a virus stock from the patient's isolates.
3. Determination of the titer of the obtained virus stock.
4. IC_{50} determination for drugs used in anti-HIV therapy.

2.2. Materials

1. Buffy coat of a healthy blood donor.
2. Fetal calf serum (FCS), heat-inactivated for 30 min at 56°C.
3. Gentamycin stock solution (50 mg/mL).
4. L-glutamine stock solution (200 m*M*).
5. Interleukin-2 (IL-2). Used as solution of 200 U/mL in RPMI medium supplemented with 15% heat-inactivated FCS, 2 m*M* L-glutamine, 0.1% sodium bicarbonate, and 20 µg/mL gentamycin. This solution is stored at –20°C.
6. Lymphoprep™ (Nycomed Pharma As, Oslo, Norway).
7. Phytohemagglutinin (PHA-P). Used as a solution of 160 µg/mL in RPMI medium supplemented with 15% heat-inactivated FCS, 2 m*M* L-glutamine, 0.1% sodium bicarbonate, and 20 µg/mL gentamycin. This solution is stored at –20°C.
8. RPMI-1640 medium with 20 m*M* HEPES buffer (Life Technologies, Merelbeke, Belgium), supplemented with 15% (v/v) heat-inactivated FCS, 2 m*M* L-glutamine, 0.1% sodium bicarbonate, and 20 µg/mL gentamycin (equals complete medium for PBMCs).
9. Phosphate-buffered saline (PBS).
10. Trypan blue.
11. p24 antigen ELISA.

2.3. Isolation of the PBMCs from a Buffy Coat

1. Use freshly prepared buffy coat (within 12 h after blood collection), which is available from blood transfusion centres or blood banks.
2. Dilute the buffy coat 1/2 with PBS.
3. Pipet 15 mL of Lymphoprep in a 50-mL conical tube.
4. Hold the tube at a slant and carefully pipet 20 mL of the diluted buffy coat on the Lymphoprep layer. Do this very carefully to avoid any mixing of the layers.
5. Centrifuge at 1450 rpm (±430*g*) for 30 min (the acceleration and deceleration should be kept low).
6. During this 30 min, thaw the IL-2 solution (200 U/mL) that was stored at –20°C.
7. Carefully remove the clear solution at the top of the tube with a pipet and discard.
8. Collect the white intermediate layer operating a slow and smooth circular movement and transfer it to another 50-mL conical tube. (If treating more tubes, bring the intermediate layer from three tubes in one).
9. Add PBS up to 50 mL.
10. Centrifuge at 1200 rpm (±300*g*) for 10 min at 25°C.
11. Remove the supernatant by pouring and keep the pellet.
12. Add 45 mL of PBS and mix carefully.
13. Centrifuge again at 1200 rpm (±300*g*) for 10 min.
14. Remove the supernatant by pouring.
15. Add 10 mL of peripheral blood lymphocytes (PBL) medium to each tube (this volume should be correctly measured as cells will be counted).
16. Join the content of the different tubes in one tube and make homogeneous.

17. Take a sample of 100 μL and add 900 μL of medium or PBS. (This dilution step is necessary to facilitate the cell count).
18. Count the lymphocytes using the Trypan blue exclusion method.
19. Make cell cultures at ± 1,750,000 PBMC/mL in complete medium for PBMCs. Add 2 mg/mL of PHA-P and 5 U/mL IL-2.
20. Incubate for 3 d in a vertical position, after 3 d clusters are visible.

2.4. Making a Virus Stock on PBMCs

2.4.1. Growing a Patient's HIV

An aliquot, usually 1 mL of a patients plasma sample is added to a pellet of 10×10^6 3-d stimulated PBMCs (1200 rpm [±300*g*], 10 min, 25°C) and is incubated for 1–2 h in a humidified CO_2 (4.5%) incubator at 37°C. These (infected) PBMCs are cultured at 10×10^6 cells in 10 mL of complete medium for PBMCs with 10 U/mL IL-2.

Every 7 d an aliquot of cell culture is evaluated for p24 antigen production. When p24 is beyond 50,000 pg/mL, the new stock can be aliquoted. If the level of 50,000 pg/mL is not reached, the culture is made homogeneous by gentle mixing with a pipet and half of it is discarded, and 10×10^6 cells 3-d stimulated PBMCs in 5 mL complete medium for PBMCs with 20 U/mL IL-2 are added. This is done for 4–5 wk. Then, if the p24 then still has not reached the desired level, the whole procedure should be repeated.

2.4.2. Storage of a Patient's HIV

The infected cell culture is brought into 50-mL tubes and the cells are pelleted, and the supernatant is carefully distributed in aliquots of 1 mL in cryotubes. The cryotubes are labeled with a virus stock number. The number and the content are indexed on the list of virus stocks and the tubes are stored at –80°C. For delicate strains, the freezing procedure might damage the virus. Therefore, the titration of the virus stock should be done on a similar frozen aliquot as for the susceptibility testing. In rare cases, freezing abolishes infectivity, and virus has to be left at room temperature for a few days until the susceptibility test can be initiated.

2.5. Titration of a Virus Stock in PBMCs

1. Count 3-d stimulated PBMC cells. For each testing plate, 4.2 million cells are required. Calculate the volume of cell culture necessary to perform the titration experiment.
2. Pipet the calculated volume of homogeneous suspension of PBMCs in a 50-mL tube. Sediment at approx 1000 rpm (±200*g*) for 10 min at 20°C. Discard the supernatant by pouring.
3. Adjust the PBMC pellet to obtain a concentration of 4 million PBMCs/mL in complete medium for PBMCs supplemented with 20 U/mL IL-2. Keep this suspension in the incubator until **step 9**.

Table 1
Microtiter Plate Formatting for the Titration of a Virus Stock in PBMCs

	1	2	3	4	5	6	7	8	9	10	11	12
A[a]	PBS	PBS	PBS	PBS	PBS	PBS	PBS	PBS	PBS	PBS	PBS	PBS
B	PBS	PBS	PBS	PBS	PBS	PBS	PBS	PBS	PBS	PBS	PBS	PBS
C	PBS	PBS	4^{-2}	4^{-3}	4^{-4}	4^{-5}	4^{-6}	4^{-7}	4^{-8}	PBS	PBS	PBS
D	PBS	PBS	4^{-2}	4^{-3}	4^{-4}	4^{-5}	4^{-6}	4^{-7}	4^{-8}	PBS	PBS	PBS
E	PBS	PBS	4^{-2}	4^{-3}	4^{-4}	4^{-5}	4^{-6}	4^{-7}	4^{-8}	PBS	PBS	PBS
F	PBS	PBS	PBS	PBS	PBS	PBS	PBS	PBS	PBS	PBS	PBS	PBS
G	PBS	PBS	PBS	PBS	PBS	PBS	PBS	PBS	PBS	PBS	PBS	PBS
H	PBS	PBS	PBS	PBS	PBS	PBS	PBS	PBS	PBS	PBS	PBS	PBS

[a]A1–H12 represent microtiter plate wells.

4. Bring 200 µL of PBS in rows A, B, F, G, and H in **Table 1** and in the wells of columns 1, 2, and 10–12 of rows C–E (75 wells × 200 µL = 15 mL).
5. Bring 150 µL of culture medium in each well of columns 4–9 of rows C–E (18 wells × 150 µL = 2.7 mL).
6. Rapidly thaw the virus stock in a water bath at 37°C or in an incubator at 37°C until only a small crystal of ice remains. Dilute the stock 1/12 in complete medium for PBMCs (100 µL stock + 1.100 mL of medium).
7. Bring 200 µL of the 1/12 diluted virus stock in the wells C, D, and F of column 3.
8. Transfer 50 µL of wells C, D, and F of column 3 to the respective wells in column 4 using a multichannel. Mix the content, and blow out the tips. Take new tips and continue the transfer. The 50 µL removed from column 9 have to be discarded.
9. Dispense 50 µL of the PBMC suspension of **step 3** to the wells of rows C–E of columns 3–9, moving from the right to the left (from less concentrated virus to more concentrated).
10. Cover the plate and incubate at 37°C and 4.5% CO_2 in a humidified incubator.
11. On d 4, resuspend the cells with a multichannel, moving from the right to the left (from less concentrated virus to more concentrated) by mixing, removing, and discarding 125 µL of the cell suspension. Add 150 µL of complete medium for PBMCs supplemented with 10 U/mL IL-2 to each well of rows C–E, moving from the left to the right.
12. On d 7, carefully remove 100 µL of the supernatant of the wells and store it at –80°C until the HIV-1 p24 Core Profile ELISA is performed. A dilution of 1/10 of the sample is used for p24 antigen quantification.
13. A well is scored positive if the HIV-1 p24 antigen is >50 pg/mL ***(12)***.
    a. Calculation of the TCID50/mL is done using Spearman-Karber calculations for plates as currently formatted.
    b. The 50% titer = $4^{[8 + (0.5–1/3 \times \#neg.)]}$, where #neg. is the total number of negative scores (p24 < 50 pg/mL) observed in the test plate as currently formatted.
    c. The $TCID_{50}$/mL of the virus stock is given by the formula (*see also* **Note 1**).
    d. $TCID_{50}/mL = 5 \times 4^{[8 + (0.5–1/3 \times \#neg.)]}$.

2.6. Virus Susceptibility for Anti-HIV Drugs

1. Count 3-d stimulated PBMCs. For each well, 200,000 cells should be used and an excess of ± 10% should be taken.
2. Pipet the calculated volume of homogeneous suspension of PBMCs in a 50-mL conical tube. Sediment at 1000 rpm (±200*g*) for 10 min at 20°C. Discard the supernatant by pouring.
3. Adjust the volume to obtain 4×10^6 PBMCs/mL in complete medium for PBMCs.
4. Take one-fourth of the volume and add the same volume of complete medium for PBMCs. Keep this in a humidified CO_2 (4.5%) incubator.
5. The remaining three-fourths of the original volume are centrifuged at 1000 rpm (±200*g*) for 10 min at 20°C.
6. The supernatant is discarded by pouring.
7. The virus is added to the pellet. The amount of virus stock required is calculated as follows : #mL of virus stock required = #cells to infect/(1000 × $TCID_{50}$/mL). The infected pellet is kept in a humidified CO_2 (4.5%) incubator for 1–2 h.
8. A serial dilution of the anti-HIV drugs is prepared in complete medium for PBMCs supplemented with 10 U/mL IL-2, usually between five and eight dilution steps. The solutions are made in a concentration that is twice as high as the concentrations that are to be evaluated.
9. Add 100 µL of the dilutions to the adequate wells, start at the lowest concentration and move up to the highest concentrations.
10. Resuspend the cells from **step 4** and dispense 100 µL in the row for toxicity evaluation. Move from the lowest concentration to the highest concentration.
11. Resuspend the infected cells from **step 7** and dispense 100 µL in the wells for activity determination moving from the lowest to the highest concentration (*see* **Table 2**).
12. Incubate the plates in a humidified CO_2 (4.5%) incubator for 4 d.
13. On d 4, microscopically evaluate the PBMCs. Resuspend the cells in the wells and remove 125 µL from each well, using a multichannel pipet. Move from the lowest concentration to the highest concentration.
14. Dilute the solutions of the tested compounds from **step 8** mentioned above one-half with complete medium for PBMCs supplemented with 10 U/mL IL-2.
15. Add 150 µL of the solution to the adequate wells, always paying attention not to contaminate the "toxicity" wells with virus.
16. Incubate in a humidified CO_2 (4.5%) incubator for three more days.
17. On d 7, aliquots of 100 µL supernatant are carefully taken using a multichannel pipet. These samples are stored at –80°C until p24 antigen ELISA is performed.
18. The median value of the triplicate is used for the calculation of the IC_{50} value. The percent protection is calculated for each concentration of the compound as follows:
    a. Percent protection = [1– (p24 value of test concentration/p24 value of untreated control)] × 100% (*see* **Note 2**).
    b. log IC_{50} = log conc. HPP – [(HPP – 50)/(HPP – LPP) × log d] (*see* **Note 3**), where HPP = highest percent protection (PP), the PP closest to 50% but higher than 50%; LPP = lowest percent protection, the PP closest to 50% but lower than 50%; conc. HPP = drug concentration where the HPP was

Table 2
Microtiter Plate Formatting for the Determination of Virus Susceptibility for Anti-HIV Drugs in PBMCs

	1	2	3	4	5	6	7	8	9	10	11	12
A[a]	PBS	PBS	PBS	PBS	PBS	PBS	PBS	PBS	PBS	PBS	PBS	PBS
B	PBS	PBS	PBS	PBS	PBS	PBS	PBS	PBS	PBS	PBS	PBS	PBS
C	PBS	PBS	Activity	Activity	Activity	Activity	Activity	Activity	Activity	Activity	PBS	PBS
D	PBS	PBS	Activity	Activity	Activity	Activity	Activity	Activity	Activity	Activity	PBS	PBS
E	PBS	PBS	Activity	Activity	Activity	Activity	Activity	Activity	Activity	Activity	PBS	PBS
F	PBS	PBS	Toxicity	Toxicity	Toxicity	Toxicity	Toxicity	Toxicity	Toxicity	Toxicity	PBS	PBS
G	PBS	PBS	PBS	PBS	PBS	PBS	PBS	PBS	PBS	PBS	PBS	PBS
H	PBS	PBS	PBS	PBS	PBS	PBS	PBS	PBS	PBS	PBS	PBS	PBS

[a]A1–H12 represent microtiter plate wells.

Table 3
Scoring for HIV p24 Positivity and Calculating $TCID_{50}$/mL

	1	2	3	4	5	6	7	8	9	10	11	12
A[a]	PBS	PBS	PBS	PBS	PBS	PBS	PBS	PBS	PBS	PBS	PBS	PBS
B	PBS	PBS	PBS	PBS	PBS	PBS	PBS	PBS	PBS	PBS	PBS	PBS
C	PBS	PBS	+	+	+	–	–	–	–	PBS	PBS	PBS
D	PBS	PBS	+	+	+	–	–	–	–	PBS	PBS	PBS
E	PBS	PBS	+	+	+	–	–	–	–	PBS	PBS	PBS
F	PBS	PBS	PBS	PBS	PBS	PBS	PBS	PBS	PBS	PBS	PBS	PBS
G	PBS	PBS	PBS	PBS	PBS	PBS	PBS	PBS	PBS	PBS	PBS	PBS
H	PBS	PBS	PBS	PBS	PBS	PBS	PBS	PBS	PBS	PBS	PBS	PBS

[a]A1–H12 represent microtiter plate wells.

observed; conc. LPP = drug concentration where the LPP was observed; and d = dilution factor.

19. The toxicity is evaluated by trypan blue exclusion method. The percent toxicity is calculated for each concentration of the compound as follows:
    a. Percent toxicity = [1– (# cells conc. x/# cells conc. 0)] × 100%
    b. The log CC_{50} = log conc. {HPT – [(HPT – 50)/(HPT – LPT) × log d}; where HPT = highest percent toxicity, the value closest to 50% but higher than 50%; LPT = lowest percent toxicity, the value closest to 50% but lower than 50%, conc. HPT = concentration of drug where the HPT was observed, conc. LPT = concentration of drug where the LPT was observed.

2.7. Notes

1. Spearman-Karber formula for calculating $TCID_{50}$/mL in test plate format as described under **Subheading 2.5.**
   a. An example of scoring the plate for HIV p24 antigen positivity (>50 pg/mL) as shown in **Table 3**:
   b. Calculating $TCID_{50}$/mL; xk = dose of highest dilution; r = number of "–" responses; d = spacing between dilutions; n = wells per dilution; and $\sum r$ = sum of r.
   c. Spearman-Karber formula:
   $$\begin{aligned} M &= xk + d[0.5 - (1/n)(\Sigma r)] \\ &= 8 + 1[0.5 - (1/3)(12)] \\ &= 8 + 1[0.5 - 4.0] \\ &= 4.5 \end{aligned}$$
   d. The 50% end point is $4^{-4.5}$, converting to 10^x: $x = 4.5 \cdot \log_4 = 4.5 \cdot 0.602 = 2.7$;the 50% titre is $10^{2.7}$. To calculate the $TCID_{50}$/mL of virus stock, the original dilution must be corrected by multiplying by 5 (200 µL of 1 mL).
   e. $TCID_{50}/\text{mL} = 5 \cdot 10^{2.7}$
   $$5 \times 4^{[8 + (0.5 - 1/3 \times \#\text{neg.})]}$$
2. Formula to calculate % protection (or PP) for a given compound concentration: PP = [1 – (p24 value of test concentration/p24 value of untreated control)] × 100%. Example = [1 – (6.176/18.763)]·100% = 67%.

3. Formula to calculate IC_{50} for a given compound:
   a. HPP = highest PP, the PP closest to 50% but higher than 50%; LPP = lowest PP, the PP closest to 50% but lower than 50%; conc. HPP = drug concentration where the HPP was observed; conc. LPP = drug concentration where the LPP was observed; and *d* = dilution factor
   b. $\log IC_{50} = \log \text{conc. HPP} - [(HPP - 50)/(HPP - LPP) \times \log d]$. Example for an experiment in which 10 μ*M* gives 67% protection and 2 μ*M* gives 34% protection:
   $= \log 10 - [(67 - 50)/(67 - 34) \times \log_5]$
   $= 1 - (17/33 \times 0.699)$
   c. $\log IC_{50} = 1 - 0.36 = 0.64$.
   d. $IC_{50} = 4.37$ μ*M*.

3. Recombinant Virus Assays

3.1. Experiment Outline

The RVA aims at putting a patient-derived RT or protease (PRO) gene in a lab-strain genetic environment with the purpose to perform fast, cheap, and reproducible phenotypic drug assays that are developed for lab strains. The lab strain genetic environment is generated through a proviral RT or PRO deleted clone, propagated in a plasmid (*see* **Fig. 1**). The clinical HIV-1 RT or PRO gene is generated by PCR. The viable virus is obtained through homologous recombination of the RT or PRO deleted provirus with the RT or PRO-PCR product from the clinical isolate. Several research groups are working on a combined RT and PRO deleted clone, which will probably become available soon. RT-PRO-PCR product can easily be obtained. This double-deleted clone will only require a single recombinant virus stock that can be used to measure susceptibility of the clinical isolate to both RT and PRO inhibitors.

The experiments in this section describe the procedures to obtain a high-titer recombinant virus stock either through recombination of RT-PCR product with RT-deleted proviral DNA or PRO-PCR product with PRO deleted proviral DNA. The susceptibility testing is outlined in **Subheading 4.** The following steps are described (**Fig. 1**):

1. Plasmid preparation to obtain linearized proviral HIV-1 DNA in which the entire RT or PRO is deleted.
2. Amplification (PCR) of patient-derived HIV-1 RT or PRO gene.
3. Recombination of the proviral clone and the clinical HIV-1 RT or PRO gene; virus propagation.

3.2. Materials

1. TE-buffer: 10 m*M* Tris-HCl, pH 8.0, 1 m*M* EDTA.
2. Electrocompetent JM109 *Eschericha coli* cells (Life Technologies, Merelbeke, Belgium).
3. Glycerol.

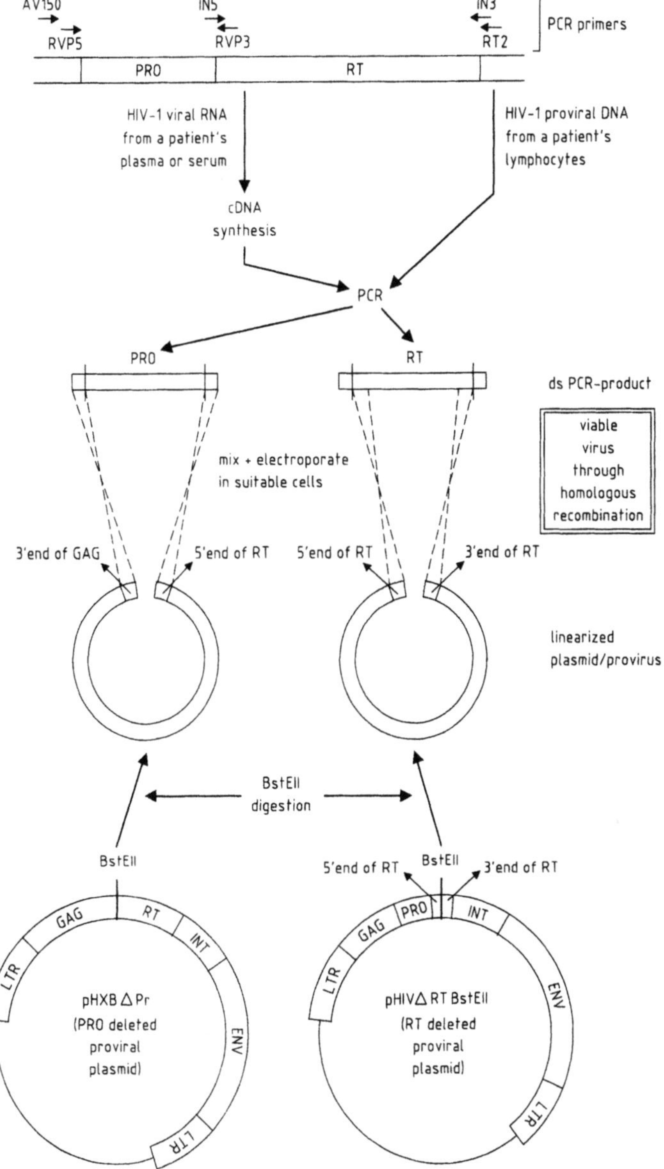

Fig. 1. Schematic representations of the recombinant virus procedure.

4. LB agar (LB medium + 15 g/L bacto agar, mix and autoclave to dissolve), and plates filled with LB agar containing 50 µg/mL ampicillin. Ampicillin is added before plating but after cooling to 40°C.
5. Ampicillin (stock solution: 50 mg/mL ampicillin in water/ethanol [1/1], working concentration: 50 µg/mL ampicillin), it is added to the medium immediately before use.

6. LB medium (for 1 L):10 g bacto-tryptane, 5 g bacto yeast extract, 10 g NaCl in water, adjust to pH 7.0 with 5 *M* NaOH.
7. JETSTAR Plasmid Lit (Genomed, ImTec, Antwerpen, Belgium).
8. Isopropanol.
9. Ethanol.
10. Restriction enzymes *Bst*EII, *Xba*I, *Bal*I, and enzyme digestion buffers (Life Technologies).
11. Phenol, chloroform, isoamylalcohol (25/24/1).
12. 4 *M* NaAc.
13. Seakem LE agarose (Sanver-Tech, Boechout, Belgium.
14. 50X TAE (for 1 L): 242 g Trisbase, 57.1 mL acetic acid, 37.2 g Na_2EDTA in water.
15. Molecular weight marker.
16. 10X loading buffer: 50 m*M* Tris-borate, 1 m*M* EDTA, 0.1% xylene cyanol, 0.1% bromophenol blue, in 100% formamide.
17. Ethidium bromide (stock solution: 20 mg/mL in water, working solution : 2.5 µg/mL in 1X TAE).
18. TRIZOL LS reagent (Life Technologies).
19. Water treated with diethylpyrocarbonate (DEPC) as RNase-free water.
20. Carrier RNA (10 mg/mL tRNA).
21. 10X PCR buffer II: 100 m*M* Tris-HCl, pH 8.3, 500 m*M* KCl; Perkin Elmer, Brussels, Belgium.
22. 25 m*M* $MgCl_2$.
23. dNTPs. The nucleotides can be ordered from several companies. They are mixed in equal concentrations and stored, e.g. when provided as 10 m*M* dATP, 10 m*M* dCTP, 10 m*M* dGTP, 10 m*M* dTTP, a mix of equal volumes of all four nucleotides will result in a stock solution of 2.5 m*M* of each dNTP.
24. cDNA and PCR primers. The primers can be ordered from various companies that synthesize user designed primers. A stock solution of 20 µ*M* in desionized (MilliQ) water is prepared. The primers used are listed in **Table 7**.
25. GeneAmp RNA-PCR kit (Perkin-Elmer) including the following solutions (RNase-free): 20 U/µL RNase inhibitor, 50 U/µL MuLV-RT, 5 U/µL Ampli*Taq* DNA polymerase, 10X PCR buffer II (100 m*M* Tris-HCl, pH 8.3, 500 m*M* KCl), 25 m*M* $MgCl_2$, 10 m*M* dATP, 10 m*M* dCTP, 10 m*M* dGTP, 10 m*M* dTTP, and RNase-free water
26. QIAamp Blood Kit (DNA extraction kit from QIAgen, Westburg, Leusden, The Netherlands).
27. 5 U/µL Ampli*Taq* DNA polymerase (Perkin-Elmer).
28. 40% Acrylamide/bisacrylamide in water (29/1) stock solution from Bio-Rad.
29. 10X TBE (for 1 L: 108 g Trisbase, 55 g boric acid, 9.3 g Na_2EDTA in water).
30. Ammonium persulphate (1.6% = 16 g/L).
31. Tetramethylethyleendiamine (TEMED).
32. Microcon Microconcentrators (Amicon, Millipore, Brussels, Belgium).
33. Phosphate-buffered saline (PBS): 8 g NaCl, 0.2 g KCl, 1.44 g Na_2PO_4, 0.24 g KH_2PO_4, pH 7.4, in 1 L water, sterilize by autoclaving.

34. MT-4 cells can be obtained from the Medical Research Council (MRC) or from the National Institutes of Health (NIH).
35. RPMI-1640 medium with 20 m*M* HEPES buffer (Life Technologies), supplemented with 10% (v/v) heat-inactivated FCS, 2 m*M* L-glutamine, 0.1% sodium bicarbonate and 20 μg/mL gentamicin (equals complete medium).
36. Equipment: Petri dishes, culture tubes, and flasks, shaking incubator, UV/Vis spectrophotometer, water bath, centrifuge, horizontal (Bio-Rad, Nazareth, Belgium), and vertical (SE250 Mighty Small II, Hoefer) gel electrophoresis system, power supply, UV transilluminator and photographing instrument (ImageMaster Amersham Pharmacia Biotech, Roosendaal, The Netherlands), microwave oven, vortex, thermal cycler, electroporator, and cuvets.

3.3. Plasmid

3.3.1. Transformation and Storage of Transformed Bacteria

Aliquots of the plasmids pHIVΔRT*Bst*EII for the RT-RVA and pHXBΔPr for the PRO-RVA can be obtained from the respective designers ***(6,8)*** or from the MRC. To produce large amounts of plasmid, an *E. coli* lab strain (e.g., DH5α) has to be transformed and can then be stored for a long time as a glycerol stock at –80°C. The selective medium to maintain the plasmid contains ampicillin. Always start from single colonies to make a glycerol stock. This is done on an LB-agar ampicillin-containing plate. Work on a sterile bench or in a sterile laminar air cabinet reserved for bacterial culture.

1. Chill the electroporation cuvets on ice before beginning the electroporation.
2. Thaw electrocompetent cells on ice. Add to 40 μL cells 10–100 ng plasmid in 1–5 μL TE buffer, mix gently and incubate for a few minutes on ice.
3. Electroporate using the following conditions: 12.5 kV/cm and a time constant of approx 5 ms.
4. Immediately transfer sterile 960 μL LB medium to the cuvet. Then transfer the mixture to a sterile culture tube and incubate the suspension at 37°C for 1 h with shaking.
5. Fill four sterile tubes with 1 mL LB medium and prepare four successive 1/10 dilutions starting from the electroporated cells. Spread 50-μL aliquots of each dilution onto a plate, using a triangular-shaped, sterile glass rod. Incubate the plates at 37°C overnight.
6. To make a small, freshly saturated culture, remove the cap from a sterile culture tube and work quickly to minimize contact of the tube with possibly contaminated air. Use a sterile pipet to transfer 5 mL of LB medium, with ampicillin, into the tube.
7. Inoculate the liquid with a single bacterial colony by touching the colony with a sterile inoculating needle, making certain that some of the cells have been transferred to the needle. Take at least two different colonies and grow them each in a different tube.
8. Dip the needle into the medium and shake it a bit.

9. Close the tube and incubate it at 37°C in a shaking incubator (300 rpm) for at least 6 h.
10. Perform a plasmid miniprep on 2 mL of bacterial culture mainly as described in **Subheading 3.3.3.** using the JETSTAR Plasmid Kit (GENOMED, ImTec) with the following differences: in point 1 use 2 mL of E4, in 2 use 2 mL of cells, in 3 use 0.4 mL of E1, in 4 use 0.4 mL of E2, in 5 use 0.4 mL of E3, in 8 use 2 times 2.5 mL of E5, in 9 use 0.9 mL of E6, in 12 wash with 1 mL 70% EtOH.
11. Perform a restriction digest on one-fifth of the obtained plasmid DNA without spectrophotometrically determining the plasmid yield as described in **Subheading 3.3.4.** Use *Xba*I, *Bal*I, and *Bst*EII, each separately.
12. Put the restriction digest mix on an agarose gel as described in **Subheading 3.3.5.** pHIVΔRT*Bst*EII will produce 1 band of ± 3000 bp and 1 band of ± 11,300 bp when using *Xba*I, ± 1670 bp and ± 13,800 bp with *Bal*I, and one band of ± 14,300 bp with *Bst*EII. pHXBΔPr will produce 1 band of ± 3000 bp and 1 band of ± 12, 450 bp when using *Xba*I, ± 520 bp and ± 13,800 bp with *Bal*I, and one band of ± 15,450 bp with *Bst*EII.
13. Add 150 µL sterile glycerol to 850 µL bacterial culture of the correct colony. Vortex the culture to ensure that the glycerol is evenly dispersed. Freeze the culture in ethanol-dry ice and then transfer the tube to –70°C for long-term storage.

3.3.2. Starting a Culture from a Frozen Glycerol Stock

1. Scrape the frozen surface of the glycerol culture with a sterile inoculating needle and streak the bacteria across one side of an LB agar plate containing ampicillin.
2. Sterilize the needle in a flame and pass once through the first streak across a fresh part of the plate. Repeat this process at least once more.
3. Incubate the plate overnight at 37°C.
4. Return the frozen glycerol culture to storage at –70°C.
5. To make a small, freshly saturated culture, proceed as described in **Subheading 3.3.1, steps 6–9.**
6. Inoculate a 500-mL culture with 5 mL of the small culture. Use a flask with a volume at least five times the volume of the culture.
7. Grow the culture overnight at 37°C with vigorous shaking (300 rpm) to ensure proper aeration.

3.3.3. Plasmid Isolation

JETSTAR Plasmid Kit (GENOMED):plasmid isolation kit, based alkaline lysis of the bacterial cell. Chromosomal DNA sticks to the cell wall and coprecipitates with the cell debris, whereas plasmid DNA remains solubilized. An anion exchange resin, provided in columns, binds the plasmid DNA under high salt conditions, the DNA is washed and eluted in low salt conditions. The solutions are provided in the kit: E1 (cell resuspension buffer: 50 m*M* Tris-HCl, pH 8.0, 10 m*M* EDTA), E2 (cell lysis solution: 200 m*M* NaOH, 1% SDS), E3 (neutralization buffer: 3.2 *M* KOAc/HOAc, pH 5.5), E4 (column equilibration buffer: 100 m*M* NaOAc/HOAc, pH 5.0, 600 m*M* NaCl, 0.15% Triton X-100), E5 (column wash buffer: 100 m*M* NaOAc/HOAc, pH 5.0, 800 m*M* NaCl), E6 (DNA elution buffer: 100 m*M* Tris/HCl, pH 8.5, 1250 m*M* NaCl).

1. For a midiprep, equilibrate a column by applying 10 mL solution E4, containing 100 µg RNase/mL. Allow the column to empty by gravity flow. Do not force out remaining solution.
2. Pellet 100 mL cells by centrifugation at 4500 rpm (±4000*g*) for 20 min. Remove all traces of medium carefully.
3. Add 4 mL solution E1 to the pellet and resuspend the cells until the suspension is homogeneous. Transfer the suspension to another tube.
4. Add 4 mL solution E2 and mix gently by inverting the tube five times to lyse the cells. Do not vortex! Incubate at room temperature for 5 min.
5. Add 4 mL solution E3 and mix immediately, but gently, by inverting the tube five times to neutralize. Do not vortex!
6. Centrifuge the mixture at 20°C and 14,000 rpm (±20,000*g*) for 10 min. Transfer the supernatant to a new tube and repeat the centrifugation to remove all cell debris.
7. Apply the supernatant promptly to the equilibrated column. Allow the lysate to run by gravity flow.
8. Wash the column with 10 mL solution E5 twice. Each time allow the column to empty by gravity flow.
9. Elute the DNA with 5 mL E6 solution. Do not force out remaining solution.
10. Precipitate the DNA by adding 0.7 vol isopropanol, previously equilibrated to room temperature, and mix by vortexing.
11. Pellet the DNA by centrifugation at 14,000 rpm (±20,000*g*) for 30 min at 4°C.
12. Discard the supernatant carefully and wash the pellet by adding 5 mL 70% ethanol and centrifuging at 11,000 rpm (±16,000*g*) for 10 min. Wash the pellet again with 1 mL 70% ethanol in a 1.5-mL microtube and recentrifuge for 10 min at 14,000 rpm (±20,000*g*).
13. Air-dry the pellet for 10 min, and redissolve the DNA in a suitable volume of water.
14. Determine the plasmid yield spectrophotometrically. Dilute an aliquot of the DNA in water and measure the optical density (OD) at 260 nm, which allows the calculation of the concentration of nucleic acid in the sample. An OD of 1 at 260 nm corresponds to approx 50 µg/mL for double-stranded DNA. The ratio between the readings at 260 and 280 nm (OD_{260}/OD_{280}) provides an estimate of the purity of the nucleic acid. Pure preparations of DNA have ratios of 1.8. If there is contamination with protein, the OD_{260}/OD_{280} will be significantly less than 1.8, and accurate quantification of the amount of DNA will not be possible.

3.3.4. Linearization of the Plasmid

1. Add 50 µL of the proper restriction enzyme digestion buffer (buffer 2 if the enzyme and the buffer is supplied by Life Technologies) and 20 µL restriction enzyme *Bst*EII (6 U/µL) to 100 µg of either pHIVΔRT*Bst*EII for the RT-RVA or pHXBΔPr for the PRO-RVA. Mix with sufficient water to give a volume of 500 µL.

2. Incubate the mixture for 1.5 h at 60°C.
3. Evaluate the digestion by applying 0.5 µg of the DNA on an agarose gel.
4. As the enzyme *Bst*EII is completely resistant to heat inactivation, purify the rest of the DNA from the reaction mixture by extraction with phenol and precipitation in ethanol.

3.3.5. Agarose Gel Electrophoresis

To monitor the restriction enzyme digest, the linearized plasmid is evaluated by agarose gel electrophoresis. Completely linearized pHIVΔRT*Bst*EII and pHXBΔPr should give one clear band at approx 14.3 and 15.3 kb, respectively. No supercoiled (moving faster) or nicked (moving slower) plasmid should be visible.

1. Add the desired amount of Seakem LE powder to a volume of 1X TAE sufficient for constructing a 0.5% agarose gel.
2. Melt the agarose in a microwave and swirl to ensure even mixing. Let the melted agarose cool without gelling before pouring onto the gel-casting tray.
3. Pour the melted agarose in the casting tray and insert the gel comb, making sure that no bubbles are trapped underneath the comb and that all bubbles on the surface of the agarose are removed before the gel sets.
4. After the gel has solidified, withdraw the gel comb, taking care not to tear the sample wells. Place the gel-casting tray containing the gel in the electrophoresis tank. Add 1X TAE to cover the gel completely.
5. Add 10X loading buffer to the samples. Load the samples and a molecular weight marker each in separate wells.
6. Run the gel at 110 V until the light blue dye has migrated for at least 4 cm.
7. Remove and carefully stain the gel for 5 min in ethidium bromide, then rinse in water. Place the gel onto an ultraviolet (UV) transilluminator and photograph with a red filter (Kodak 22A wratten).

3.3.6. Extraction with Phenol/Chloroform/Isoamyl Alcohol and Ethanol Precipitation

1. Add an equal volume of phenol/chloroform/isoamyl alcohol to the nucleic acid and vortex the mixture until an emulsion is formed.
2. Centrifuge at 14,000 rpm (±15,000*g*) for 5 min. Carefully transfer the aqueous phase containing the DNA to a fresh tube. Discard the interface and organic phase.
3. Add an equal volume of chloroform and repeat the centrifugation and the transferring of the aqueous phase.
4. Add 1/10 vol 4 *M* NaAc and 22/10 vol 100% EtOH. Mix by vortexing and place in crushed dry ice for at least 5 min.
5. Centrifuge at 14,000 rpm (±15,000*g*) for 20 min and remove the supernatant.
6. Add 1 mL 70% ethanol and invert the tube several times.
7. Centrifuge at 14,000 rpm (±15,000*g*) for 5 min. Remove the supernatant and dry the pellet.

8. Dissolve the dry pellet in an appropriate volume of water to obtain a concentration of 1 μg DNA/μL.

3.4. PCR

3.4.1. Viral RNA Extraction and cDNA Synthesis

1. Add 750 μL TRIZOL LS Reagent (Gibco-BRL, Life Technologies) to 250 μL sample (plasma, serum) and shake vigorously. Incubate the homogenized samples for 5 min at room temperature to permit the complete dissociation of nucleoprotein complexes.
2. Add 200 μL of chloroform and 1 μL of carrier RNA (10 mg/mL, e.g., tRNA) per 750 μL of TRIZOL LS Reagent. Shake tubes vigorously by hand for 15 s and incubate them at room temperature for 2–15 min.
3. Centrifuge the samples at 14,000 rpm (±15,000*g*) for 15 min at 4°C. Following centrifugation, the mixture separates into a lower red, phenol-chloroform phase, an interphase, and a colorless upper aqueous phase. RNA remains exclusively in the aqueous phase. The volume of the aqueous phase is about 70% of the volume of TRIZOL LS Reagent used for the homogenization. Transfer the aqueous phase to a clean tube.
4. Precipitate the RNA from the aqueous phase by mixing with isopropyl alcohol. Use 500 μL of isopropyl alcohol per 750 μL TRIZOL LS Reagent used for the initial homogenization. Incubate samples at room temperature for 10 min.
5. Centrifuge at 14,000 rpm (±15,000*g*) for 10 min. The RNA precipitate, often invisible before centrifugation, forms a gel-like pellet on the side and bottom of the tube. Remove the supernatant.
6. Wash the RNA pellet once with 75% ethanol, adding at least 1 mL of 75% ethanol per 750 μL of TRIZOL LS Reagent used for the initial homogenization. Mix the sample by vortexing.
7. Centrifuge at 14,000 rpm (±15,000*g*) for 5 min at 4°C. Discard the supernatant.
8. Briefly dry the RNA pellet. Do not dry the RNA pellet by centrifugation under vacuum. It is important not to let the RNA pellet dry completely as this will greatly decrease its solubility.
9. Dissolve RNA in 25 μL RNase-free water by vortexing and incubating for 10 min at 55–60°C.
10. Perform the cDNA synthesis in a 20-μL reaction volume (e.g., with the GeneAmp RNA-PCR kit from Perkin-Elmer) containing 10 m*M* Tris-HCl, pH 8.3, 50 m*M* KCl, 5 m*M* $MgCl_2$, 1 m*M* dNTPs, 1 U/μL RNase inhibitor, 1 μ*M* RT2 (reverse PCR outer primer), and 2.5 U/μL MuLVRT, using 10.2 μL of RNA. Before adding the RNA to the reaction mixture, denature the secondary structures by incubating the RNA samples at 70°C for 2 min. Incubate the mixtures for 1 h at 42°C to perform the cDNA synthesis. Stop the reaction by incubating the mixtures for 5 min at 70°C.

3.4.2. DNA Extraction

QIAamp Blood Kit (QIAgen): total DNA isolation kit, based on protease digestion of the cellular structures. A silica-based membrane, provided in columns, binds the DNA under specific salt and pH conditions, the DNA is washed and eluted in low-salt conditions. The solutions are provided in the kit, including Buffer AL (cell lysis buffer), and Buffer AW (column wash buffer).

1. Add 25 µL QIAGEN Protease stock solution and 200 µL Buffer AL to 10^7 lymphocytes in 200 µL PBS. Mix immediately by vortexing for 15 s. In order to ensure efficient lysis, it is essential that the sample and Buffer AL are mixed immediately and thoroughly to yield a homogeneous solution. Do not add QIAGEN Protease directly to Buffer AL. Incubate at 70°C for 10 min.
2. Add 210 µL of 96–100% ethanol to the sample and mix again by vortexing. Place a QIAamp spin column in a 2-mL collection tube. Carefully apply the mixture to the QIAamp spin column, taking care that the liquid settles on the membrane and not on the rim, without damaging the membrane. Close each spin column in order to avoid aerosol formation during centrifugation and centrifuge at 14,000 rpm (±15,000*g*) for 1 min.
3. Remove the QIAamp spin column and place it in a clean 2-mL collection tube. Discard the tube containing the filtrate. Carefully open the QIAamp spin column and add 500 µL of Buffer AW.
4. Centrifuge at 14,000 rpm (±15,000*g*) for 1 min. Remove the QIAamp spin column, place it in a clean 2-mL collection tube, and discard the collection tube containing the filrate. Carefully open the QIAamp spin column and add another 500 µL of Buffer AW.
5. Centrige at 14,000 rpm (±15,000*g*) for 1 min. Discard the filtrate and replace the QIAamp spin column in the same collection tube.
6. Centrifuge at full speed for a further 2 min. The additional full-speed spin removes all traces of Buffer AW from the QIAamp spin column before elution.
7. Place the QIAamp spin column in a clean 1.5-mL microfuge tube and discard the collection tube containing the filtrate. Carefully open the QIAamp spin column and elute the DNA by applying 200 µL of distilled water preheated to 70°C. Incubate at room temperature for 1 min.
8. Centrifuge at 14,000 rpm (±15,000*g*) for 1 min. The eluate now contains the extracted DNA.

3.4.3. Polymerase Chain Reaction

1. Amplify 10 µL of cDNA or proviral DNA in a 50 µL outer PCR containing 10 m*M* Tris-HCl, pH 8.3, 50 m*M* KCl, 2 m*M* $MgCl_2$, 200 µ*M* dNTPs, 0.2 µ*M* outer primers (AV150 and RT2), and 0.025 U/µL Ampli*Taq* DNA polymerase. The outer cycling conditions are 45 s 95°C, 30 s 55°C, 1 min 72°C for 40 cycles on a PE9600 thermal cycler. The same outer PCR product is used for both the RT and PRO inner PCR. When using AmpliTaq from Perkin-Elmer, the buffer reagents are provided including the following stock solutions: 10X PCR buffer II and 25 m*M* $MgCl_2$.
2. For the RT inner PCR, amplify 2 µL outer PCR product in a 100 µL inner PCR containing 10 m*M* Tris-HCl, pH 8.3, 50 m*M* KCl, 4 m*M* $MgCl_2$, 200 µ*M* dNTs, 0.5 µ*M* inner primers (IN5 and IN3), and 0.025 U/µL Ampli*Taq* DNA poly-

merase. The inner cycling conditions are 30 s 94°C, 30 s 55°C, 1 min 72°C for 30 cycles on a PE9600 thermal cycler.

3. For the PRO inner PCR, amplify 2 µL outer PCR product in a 100 µL inner PCR containing 10 m*M* Tris-HCl, pH 8.3, 50 m*M* KCl, 3 m*M* $MgCl_2$, 200 µ*M* dNTPs, 0.5 µ*M* inner primers (RVP5 and RVP3), and 0.025 U/µL Ampli*Taq* DNA polymerase. The inner cycling conditions are 45 s 95°C, 30 s 60°C, 1 min 72°C for 30 cycles on a PE9600 thermal cycler.

3.4.4. Detection of the PCR Products

For small PCR products, acrylamide gels give a better resolution than agarose gels.

1. Assemble clean glass plates, aluminum oxide plates, and spacers for casting the gel.
2. Prepare the gel solution. For 10 minigels (SE250 Mighty Small II, Amersham Pharmacia Biotech) 150 mL is adequate. For a 6% acrylamide gel, mix the following: 22.5 mL 40% acrylamide/bisacrylamide, 15 mL 10X TBE, 6 mL 1.6% ammonium persulfate, 106.5 mL water, and 150 µL TEMED.
3. Pour the acrylamide gel mix between the plates and insert the appropriate comb. Allow to polymerize at room temperature for at least 45 min.
4. After polymerization of the gel, remove the comb and rinse the sample wells with water. Place the gel into the electrophoresis apparatus. Fill upper and lower buffer chamber with 1X TBE so that the wells are submerged.
5. Add 10X loading buffer (mix 1/10) to the DNA samples. Load the samples and a molecular weight marker on the gel. Run the gel at 200 V until the dark blue dye has reached the bottom of the gel.
6. Detach the gel plates from the electrophoresis apparatus and remove the gel from the plates.
7. Stain the gel for 5 min in ethidium bromide and rinse with water.
8. Place the gel onto a UV transilluminator and photograph.

3.4.5. Desalting and Concentrating PCR Product

The Microcon Microconcentrator (Microcon -50, with a cutoff of 50 kDa) consists of a membrane immobilized in a column. The pore size of the membrane is chosen so that the PCR product is retained on the membrane. Buffer, salt, nucleotides, and primers are smaller and will cross the membrane.

1. Place a Microcon (Amicon) into a vial and add 200 µL PCR product onto the membrane of the Microcon. Dilute the PCR product with water up to the rim of the column.
2. Centrifuge for 10 min at 13,000 rpm (±15,000*g*) to concentrate and desalt the sample. Try to avoid centrifuging the Microcon completely dry; if this does happen, add 10 µL water and shake to redissolve the PCR product that has dried onto the membrane.
3. Recover the DNA by inverting the Microcon in a new vial and centrifuging for 5 min at 5000 rpm (±2000*g*).

3.5. Recombination

Although this is the most crucial step in the recombinant virus assay, the procedure is easy and simple. In general, 10 µg of proviral plasmid and 2 µg of PCR are used for recombination. In most cases, less PCR product will also perform well, but it may take somewhat longer before the virus breaks through. In difficult cases, more PCR product can be used, but one should be aware that, in these cases, the recombinant virus might not be representative for the virus population in the patient. The virus obtained can be directly used for stock titration as described in the protocol for the MT-4/MTT assay in **Subheading 4.1.3.1.**

1. Split the MT-4 cells 1:2 in complete medium approx 24 h before electroporation to obtain actively deviding cells. Incubate the cells in a humidified CO_2 (5%) incubator.
2. Pellet the cells (10 min 1200 rpm [±300*g*] at 4°C) and resuspend them in ice-cold PBS at 3.125×10^6 cells/mL.
3. Mix 0.8 mL resuspended cells with 10 µg of the pHIVΔRT*Bst*EII clone and 2 µg of RT PCR product, or with 10 µg of the pHIVΔPRO*Bst*EII clone and 2 µg of PRO PCR product, in an electroporation cuvet and electroporate using an EASYJECT (Eurogentec, Seraing, Belgium). The electroporation conditions are 300 V and 300 µF. Chill the cells shortly on ice to dissipate excess heat produced during the electroshock.
4. Place the cuvets in a 20°C water bath for 30 min to improve the uptake of DNA by the cells.
5. Add the electroporated cells to 5 mL complete medium and incubate at 37°C.
6. After 48 h, add 5 mL fresh complete medium. Incubate the cells at 37°C with changes of medium as required.
7. Harvest the recombinant virus when full cytopathogenic effect (CPE) is observed in the culture by centrifuging the cell culture for 10 min at 2000 rpm (±800*g*). In general, CPE is already visible after 3–4 d; full CPE takes approx 6 d.
8. Aliquot and store the virus supernatant at –80°C.

4. Replication Assays for Recombinant Strains

4.1. MT-4/MTT Assay

4.1.1. Experiment Outline

The purpose of these experiments is to determine the inhibitory effect (IC_{50}) of drugs on the HIV-induced CPE in human T4 lymphocyte MT-4 cell cultures. MT-4 cells are highly susceptible to the CPE of HIV.

4.1.2. Materials

1. MT-4 cells can be obtained from the MRC or from the NIH.
2. RPMI-1640 medium with 20 m*M* HEPES buffer (Life Technologies), supplemented with 10% (v/v) heat-inactivated FCS, 2 m*M* L-glutamine, 0.1% sodium bicarbonate, and 20 µg/mL gentamicin (equals complete medium).
3. Stocks of recombinant virus, minimal 4.5 log U/mL.

4. Titertek[R] Multidrop dispenser (ICN Biomedicals, Asse-Relegem, Belgium).
5. Biomek 2000 robot (Beckman, Fullerton, CA).
6. 7.5 mg/mL 3-(4,5-dimethylthiazol-2-yl)-2,5-diphenyltetrazolium bromide (MTT) (Sigma, St. Louis, MO) in PBS. Filtrate, aliquot, and store the solution at –20°C.
7. 10% (v/v) Triton X-100 in acidified isopropanol (2 mL concentrated HCl per 500 mL solvent).
8. Eight-channel computer-controlled Titertek Microplate Reader and Stacker (Multiskan, MCC, ICN).
9. Light microscope.

4.1.3. Methods

4.1.3.1. Virus Stock Titration

1. Maintain MT-4 cells at 37°C in a humidified atmosphere of 5% CO_2 in air. Every 3–4 d and always 2 d before starting the experiment, seed cells at 3×10^5 cells/mL; count the cells under the microscope, pellet them (5 min at 1000 rpm [±200*g*] at 20°C), and resuspend them in the appropriate volume of complete medium.
2. Fill flat-bottomed, 96-well microtiter trays with 100 µL of complete medium.
3. Add virus stock in 25 µL vol to the six middle cups (sixfold titration) of the second column of the microtiter tray (2B up to 2G). Present volume in these wells is 125 µL. Be aware that freezing can influence the virus titer: use identical aliquots for virus titration and for antiviral testing.
4. Make nine serial, fivefold dilutions of the virus directly in the microtiter trays using the Biomek 2000 robot or a multichannel pipet: take 25 µL out of column 2 and add it to column 3, mix, change tips, and again take 25 µL out of column 3 and repeat the dilution up to column 10. Leave row 11 without virus, as control (*see* **Table 4**).
5. Centrifuge exponentially growing MT-4 cells 5 min at 900 rpm (±140*g*) and discard the supernatants.
6. Resuspend the MT-4 cells at 3×10^5 cells/mL complete medium in a flask that is connected with an autoclavable dispensing cassette of a Titertek Multidrop dispenser (or use a multichannel pipet).
7. Transfer under light magnetic stirring 100 µL cell suspension to the microtiter tray wells, except to the outer row wells (columns 1 and 12, row A and H). As a consequence, final virus dilutions are 1/10, 1/50, and so on.
8. Fill the outer row wells with an additional 100 µL of medium (or PBS).
9. Incubate the plates at 37°C in a humidified atmosphere of 5% CO_2 in air.
10. Five days after infection, examine the cell cultures under the light microscope for HIV-induced CPE. A well is scored positive if CPE is observed. Calculation of the $CCID_{50}$ using Reed and Muench calculations as currently formatted are described in **Note 1**.

4.1.3.2. Anti-HIV Assay

1. Prepare MT-4 cells as described in **Subheading 4.1.3.1.**
2. Fill flat-bottomed, 96-well microtiter trays with 100 µL of complete medium (*see* **Table 5**).

Table 4
Microtiter Plate Formatting for the Titration of a Virus Stock in MT-4 Cells

	1	2	3	4	5	6	7	8	9	10	11	12
A[a]	Medium	Medium	Medium	Medium	Medium	Medium	Medium	Medium	Medium	Medium	Medium	Medium
B	Medium	Virus 1/5	Virus 1/25	Virus 1/125	Virus 1/625	Virus 1/3125	Virus 1/15625	Virus 1/78125	Virus 1/390625	Virus 1/1953125	No virus	Medium
C	Medium	Virus 1/5	Virus 1/25	Virus 1/125	Virus 1/625	Virus 1/3125	Virus 1/15625	Virus 1/78125	Virus 1/390625	Virus 1/1953125	No virus	Medium
D	Medium	Virus 1/5	Virus 1/25	Virus 1/125	Virus 1/625	Virus 1/3125	Virus 1/15625	Virus 1/78125	Virus 1/390625	Virus 1/1953125	No virus	Medium
E	Medium	Virus 1/5	Virus 1/25	Virus 1/125	Virus 1/625	Virus 1/3125	Virus 1/15625	Virus 1/78125	Virus 1/390625	Virus 1/1953125	No virus	Medium
F	Medium	Virus 1/5	Virus 1/25	Virus 1/125	Virus 1/625	Virus 1/3125	Virus 1/15625	Virus 1/78125	Virus 1/390625	Virus 1/1953125	No virus	Medium
G	Medium	Virus 1/5	Virus 1/25	Virus 1/125	Virus 1/625	Virus 1/3125	Virus 1/15625	Virus 1/78125	Virus 5 1/390625	Virus 1/1953125	No virus	Medium
H	Medium	Medium	Medium	Medium	Medium	Medium	Medium	Medium	Medium	Medium	Medium	Medium

[a]A1–H12 represent microtiter plate wells.

Table 5
Microtiter Plate Formatting for the Determination of Virus Susceptibility for Anti-HIV Drugs in MT-4 Cells

	1	2	3	4	5	6	7	8	9	10	11	12
HIV-infected rows												
A[a]	Medium	Medium	Medium	Medium	Medium	Medium	Medium	Medium	Medium	Medium	Medium	Medium
B	Medium	Drug 1/5	Drug 1/25	Drug 1/125	Drug 1/625	Drug 1/3125	Drug 1/15625	Drug 1/78125	Drug 1/390625	Drug 1/1953125	No drug	Medium
C	Medium	Drug 1/5	Drug 1/25	Drug 1/125	Drug 1/625	Drug 1/3125	Drug 1/15625	Drug 1/78125	Drug 1/390625	Drug 1/1953125	No drug	Medium
D	Medium	Drug 1/5	Drug 1/25	Drug 1/125	Drug 1/625	Drug 1/3125	Drug 1/15625	Drug 1/78125	Drug 1/390625	Drug 1/1953125	No drug	Medium
Mock-infected												
E	Medium	Drug 1/5	Drug 1/25	Drug 1/125	Drug 1/625	Drug 1/3125	Drug 1/15625	Drug 1/78125	Drug 1/390625	Drug 1/1953125	No drug	Medium
F	Medium	Drug 1/5	Drug 1/25	Drug 1/125	Drug 1/625	Drug 1/3125	Drug 1/15625	Drug 1/78125	Drug 1/390625	Drug 1/1953125	No drug	Medium
G	Medium	Drug 1/5	Drug 1/25	Drug 1/125	Drug 1/625	Drug 1/3125	Drug 1/15625	Drug 1/78125	Drug 1/390625	Drug 1/1953125	No drug	Medium
H	Medium	Medium	Medium	Medium	Medium	Medium	Medium	Medium	Medium	Medium	Medium	Medium

[a]A1–H12 represent microtiter plate wells.

3. Add stock solutions (10X final test concentration) of compounds in 25 µL volumes to the six middle cups of the second column of the microtiter tray (2B up to 2G). Present volume in these wells is 125 µL.
4. Make nine serial, fivefold dilutions of the compound directly in the microtiter trays using the Biomek 2000 robot or a multichannel pipet: take 25 µL out of column 2 and add it to column 3, mix, and again take 25 µL out of column 3 and repeat the dilution up to column 10. Leave row 11 without drug, as control.
5. Add 50 µL of HIV at 100–300 CCID50 medium, respectively, to the upper (rows B–D) and lower part (rows E–G) of the microtiter tray.
6. Centrifuge exponentially growing MT-4 cells 5 min at 900 rpm (±140*g*) and discard the supernatants.
7. Resuspend the MT-4 cells at 6×10^5 cells/mL complete medium in a flask that is connected with an autoclavable dispensing cassette of a Titertek Multidrop dispenser (or use a multichannel pipet).
8. Transfer under light magnetic stirring 50 µL cell suspension to the microtiter tray wells, except to the outer row wells (columna 1 and 12, rows A and H).
9. Fill the outer row wells with an additional 100 µL of medium (or PBS).
10. Incubate the plates at 37°C in a humidified atmosphere of 5% CO_2 in air.
11. Five days after infection, examine spectrophotometrically the viability of HIV (upper part)- and mock (lower part)-infected cells by the MTT method as described in **Subheading 4.1.3.1.** *(11)*.

4.1.3.3. MTT Assay

The MTT assay is based on the reduction of the yellow-colored MTT by mitochondrial dehydrogenase of metabolically active cells to a blue formazan that can be measured spectrophotometrically.

1. Add to each well (except the outer row) of the microtiter trays 20 µL of MTT (7.5 mg/mL) using the Titertek Multidrop (or a multichannel pipet).
2. Incubate the trays at 37°C in a CO_2 incubator for 1 h.
3. Remove a constant volume of medium (e.g., 150 µL) from each cup using the Biomek 2000 robot (or a multichannel pipet) without disturbing the MT-4 cell clusters containing the formazan crystals.
4. Lyse the cells and solubilize the formazan crystals by adding 100 µL of the Triton X-100 isopropanol mix to each cup using the Biomek 2000 robot (or a multichannel pipet).
5. Complete dissolution of the formazan crystals will be obtained after placing the trays on a plate shaker for 10 min.
6. Finally, the absorbances should be read in a an eight-channel computer-controlled Titertek Microplate Reader and Stacker at two wavelengths (540 and 690 nm). Subtract the absorbance measured at 690 nm from the absorbance at 540 nm, to eliminate the effects of cell debris scattering. Use the first column wells for background subtraction because they contain all reagents except MT-4 cells, virus, and compounds.

7. 50% cytotoxic concentration (CC_{50}) and 50% inhibitory concentration (IC_{50}): the CC_{50} is the concentration of compound that reduced the absorbance (OD_{540}) of the mock-infected control sample by 50%. Calculate the PP achieved by the compounds in HIV-infected cells by the following formula: $[(OD_T)_{HIV} - (OD_C)_{HIV}]/[(OD_C)_{mock} - (OD_C)_{HIV}] \times 100$, where $(OD_T)_{HIV}$ is the OD measured with a given concentration of the test compound in the HIV-infected cells; $(OD_C)_{HIV}$ is the OD measured for the control untreated HIV-infected cells (column 11), which stands for 100% infection-related CPE; and $(OD_C)_{mock}$ is the OD measured for the control untreated mock-infected cells (column 11), which stands for 0% infection-related CPE. The concentration achieving 50% protection according to the above formula is defined as the IC_{50}.

4.1.4. Notes

1. Reed and Muench *(14)* formula for calculating $CCID_{50}$ in test plate format as described under **Subheading 4.1.3.1.**
   a. An example of scoring the plate for HIV-induced CPE is shown in **Table 6**.
   b. Calculating $CCID_{50}$: Reed and Muench *(14)* formula:
      y_1 = percent of positive-scored wells closest to 50% but higher than 50% at a certain dilution.
      y_2 = percent of positive-scored wells closest to 50% but lower than 50% at a certain dilution.
      x_1 = log(dilution of virus where y_1 was observed).
      x_2 = log(dilution of virus where y_2 was observed).
      M = dilution of virus stock for 1 $CCID_{50}$.
      $M = \text{inv log}\{x1 + [(x2 - x1)\cdot(50 - y1)/(y1 - y2)]\}$
      $= \text{inv log}\{3.097 + [(3.796 - 3.097)\cdot(50 - 66.6)/(66.6 - 33.3)]\}$
      $= \text{inv log}[3.097 + (0.699\cdot 0.5)]$
      $= \text{inv log}3.447 = 2799$
2. The OD ratio of $(OD_C)_{mock}$ and $(OD_C)_{HIV}$ should be at least 5.
3. Always include reference compounds (e.g., AZT, nevirapine, ritonavir, and so on) with known antiviral activity.

4.2. CEM, Molt-4 (Clone 8), C8166 Syncytium Assay

4.2.1. Experimental Outline

This assay is based on the HIV-induced giant cell (syncytium) formation in human T-4 lymphocyte CEM, Molt-4 (clone 8), or C8166 cell cultures and is aimed at evaluating drugs for their inhibitory activity against a primary HIV-1 or HIV-2 infection (replication) in established laboratory cell lines. The chosen cell lines are highly susceptible to the HIV-induced cytopathicity. Giant cell formation can be easily recorded under the light microscope.

4.2.2. Materials

1. CEM, Molt-4, and C8166 can be obtained from the American Tissue Culture Collection (Rockville, MD).

Table 6
Scoring HIV-Induced CPE and Calculating $CCID_{50}/m^2$

	1	2	3	4	5	6	7	8	9	10	11	12
A[a]	Medium	Medium	Medium	Medium	Medium	Medium	Medium	Medium	Medium	Medium	Medium	Medium
B	Medium	+	+	+	+	–	–	–	–	–	–	Medium
C	Medium	+	+	+	+	–	–	–	–	–	–	Medium
D	Medium	+	+	+	–	+	–	–	–	–	–	Medium
E	Medium	+	+	+	+	+	–	–	–	–	–	Medium
F	Medium	+	+	+	–	–	–	–	–	–	–	Medium
G	Medium	+	+	+	+	–	–	–	–	–	–	Medium
H	Medium	Medium	Medium	Medium	Medium	Medium	Medium	Medium	Medium	Medium	Medium	Medium

[a]A1–H12 represent microtiter plate wells.

2. RPMI-1640 medium is supplemented with 10% (v/v) heat-inactivated (30 min at 56°C) FCS, 2 m*M* L-glutamine (Gibco), and 0.075% sodium bicarbonate (Life Technologies).
3. Stocks of HIV-1 or HIV-2 are at least >1000 $CCID_{50}$/mL (titrated on CEM cell cultures) or >100,000 $CCID_{50}$ (titrated on MT-4 cell cultures).
4. Flat-bottomed, 96-well microtiter plates.
5. Humidified CO_2-controlled incubator at 37°C.
6. Light microscope.

4.2.3. Assay Methods

4.2.3.1. Virus Stock Titration

HIV-1 or HIV-2 stocks are obtained from the supernatants of HIV-infected MT-4 cell cultures. Cells and cell debris were removed from the supernatants of HIV-infected cell cultures by centrifugation at 3000*g* for 10 min at a time at which cytopathicity of HIV reaches completion in the infected MT-4 cell cultures. Virus-containing supernatants are aliquoted in 1.5 mL-cryotubes (~0.5–1.0 mL of supernatant) and frozen at –70°C or (preferably) in liquid nitrogen before use.

4.2.3.2. Anti-HIV Assays

1. Fill flat-bottomed, 96-well microtiter plates with 100 µL of serial drug dilutions (twofold, threefold, fivefold, or 10-fold; advisable for compounds that have never been tested before: fivefold dilutions, starting at 1000 or 200 µ*M* as the highest drug concentration, followed by 6–10 serial drug dilutions). Drug dilutions have to be made in culture medium. Be sure to have at least four wells in each microtiter plate that contain culture medium without drug.
2. Use CEM, Molt 4/clone 8, or C8166 cells grown in cell cultures that were subcultured or supplied with fresh culture medium (±10 mL fresh medium added to a 15–20 mL cell culture) 1 d before initiation of the experiment. Pellet the cells (10 min at 1200 rpm (±300*g*), room temperature), resuspend in a few milliliters of culture medium, count the cell number by an automated Coulter counter (Analis, Gent, Belgium), and adjust the cell number by adding an appropriate volume of culture medium in order to obtain a cell density of ±500,000 cells/mL.
3. Add a virus inoculum to the cell suspension in order to obtain ±200 $CCID_{50}$/mL. One $CCID_{50}$ is defined as the minimal amount of virus that is able to infect 50% of a series of identical cell cultures (should not be confused with the amount of virus that is able to infect 50% of one cell culture).
4. Add carefully 100 µL of the HIV-infected cell suspension to each microtiter plate well. Each time use a new tip when going from high to low drug concentrations. (One tip can be used for each drug when going from low to high drug concentrations.) Make sure that the cell suspension is properly mixed from time to time in order to add a homogenous cell suspension to the microplate wells.
5. Incubate the plates at 37°C in a humidified, CO_2-controlled incubator.

6. Four to 5 d after infection, the cell cultures can be examined under the light microscope. The number of giant cells should be estimated and quantified as the percentage of the cell cultures (~10% [±], 25% [+], 50% [++], 90% [+++], or 100% [++++]) converted to giant cells. The amount of giant cells in the control cultures are set at 100% (++++). Usually, one microscopic field of an HIV-infected control cell culture (magnification ×200) contains approx 100 giant cells.
7. The 50% effective concentration (EC_{50}) is defined as the compound concentration required to inhibit HIV-induced giant cell formation by 50%.

4.2.4. Notes

1. Drugs can be insoluble or poorly soluble in cell culture medium. Therefore, stock solutions of the drugs can be made in 100% dimethylsulfoxide (DMSO) at 50 m*M*. The highest testable drug concentration should preferably not contain DMSO concentrations higher than 1% to avoid toxicity of DMSO to the cell cultures.
2. The cell number of exponentially growing control CEM, Molt, or C8166 cell cultures should increase by 5- to maximum 10-fold within the time period of the incubation.
3. There exist clones of CEM and Molt cells that are not or are poorly susceptible to HIV-1- or HIV-2-induced cytopathicity. Be sure to work with the right sensitive cell clone.
4. At least one or two reference compounds with known antiviral activity should be included to make sure that the assay has been properly performed.
5. The 96-well microplates containing the virus-infected cell cultures should always be closed with their lid on transfer to the incubator. They should also preferably be placed in a plastic box of which the lid has been left opened slightly to allow a free exchange of humidified air and CO_2, to ensure a constant temperature during incubation (in case the doors of the incubator are frequently opened and closed during the day), and to avoid direct HIV-containing medium spills in the incubator.

5. Genotypic Assays

5.1. Sequencing Protocols

5.1.1. Experiment Outline

The protocols described in this section include the preparation of patient-derived HIV viral RNA or proviral DNA, as also described in **Subheading 3.** The RT and PRO genes are amplified and directly sequenced (without cloning) using a cycle sequencing protocol adapted for the ABI sequencer. The direct sequencing approach has the advantage that the average sequence of the clinical isolate is seen. Thus, sequence information of the predominant variant is gathered in a single run. This is much faster than cloning the PCR product and sequencing several clones, which has the disadvantage that PCR artifacts cannot be discriminated from patient-derived variants. However if one needs to know the sequence of minor variants, cloning is the only alternative.

5.1.2. Materials

1. Isopropanol.
2. Ethanol (95% and a dilution in water of 75%).
3. Phenol, chloroform, isoamylalcohol (25/24/1).
4. 3 *M* NaAc, pH 5.2.
5. Seakem (Sanver-Tech) LE agarose.
6. 50X TAE: for 1 L: 242 g Trisbase, 57.1 mL acetic acid, 37.2 g Na_2EDTA in water.
7. Molecular weight marker.
8. 10X loading buffer: 50 m*M* Tris-borate, 1 m*M* EDTA, 0.1% xylene cyanol, 0.1% bromophenol blue, in 100% formamide.
9. Ethidium bromide: stock solution: 10 mg/mL in water, working solution: 2.5 µg/mL in water.
10. TRIZOL LS reagent (Life Technologies).
11. Water treated with DEPC as RNase-free water.
12. Carrier RNA (10 mg/mL tRNA); however, when random priming is performed then use glycogen as carrier (20 mg/mL stock solution).
13. 10X PCR buffer II: 100 m*M* Tris-HCl, pH 8.3, 500 m*M* KCl; Perkin Elmer.
14. 25 m*M* $MgCl_2$.
15. dNTPs. The nucleotides can be ordered from several companies. They are mixed in equal concentrations and stored, e.g., when provided as 10 m*M* dATP, 10 m*M* dCTP, 10 m*M* dGTP, 10 m*M* dTTP; a mix of equal volumes of all four nucleotides will result in a stock solution of 2.5 m*M* of each dNTP.
16. cDNA and PCR primers. The primers can be ordered from various companies that synthesize user-designed primers. A stock solution of 20 µ*M* in desionized (MilliQ) water is prepared. For details on the primers *see* **Table 7**.
17. GeneAmp RNA-PCR kit (Perkin-Elmer) including the following solutions (RNAse-free): 20 U/µL RNase inhibitor, 50 U/µL M-MLV-RT, 5 U/µL Ampli*Taq* DNA polymerase, 10X PCR buffer II (100 m*M* Tris-HCl, pH 8.3, 500 m*M* KCl), 25 m*M* $MgCl_2$, 10 m*M* dATP, 10 m*M* dCTP, 10 m*M* dGTP, 10 m*M* dTTP, 50 µ*M* random hexamers, and RNase-free water
18. QIAamp Blood Kit (DNA extraction kit from QIAgen).
19. QIAquick Gel Extraction Kit (DNA extraction kit from QIAgen).
20. 5 U/µL Ampli*Taq* DNA polymerase (Perkin-Elmer).
21. 5 U/µL Ampli*Taq* Gold DNA polymerase (Perkin-Elmer).
22. 40% Acrylamide/bisacrylamide in water (29/1) stocksolution from Bio-Rad.
23. 10X TBE (for 1 L: 108 g Trisbase, 55 g boric acid, 9.3 g Na_2EDTA in water).
24. Ammonium persulfate (16 g/L).
25. TEMED.
26. Microcon Microconcentrators (–50) (Amicon, Millipore).
27. ABI PRISM Dye Terminator Sequencing Core Kit (Perkin Elmer).
28. TSR buffer (Perkin-Elmer).
29. Equipment: tips and filtertips, waterbath, heating block, microcentrifuge and tubes, horizontal (Bio-Rad) and vertical electrophoresis system (SE250 Mighty Small II, Amersham Pharmacia Biotech), power supply, UV transilluminator and

Table 7
Details on the Primers for PCR (Including RVA and ARMS) and Sequencing

A

Primers (reference)	Gene fragment	Technique	Sequence 5'-3'
A35 (17)	RT	ARMS	5'-TTGGTTGCACTTTAAATTTTCCCATTAGTCCTATT-3'
NE(1)35 (17)	RT	ARMS	5'-CTTACTAACTTCTGTATGTCATTGACAGTCCAGCT-3'
B (17)	RT	ARMS	5'-GGATGGAAAGGATCACC-3'
215WT (17)	RT	ARMS	5'-ATGTTTTTTGTCTGGTGTGGT-3'
215MT (17)	RT	ARMS	5'-ATGTTTTTTGTCTGGTGTGAA-3'
AV3 (18)	RT	ARMS, PCR, sequencing	5'-TACTGGATGTGGGTGATGCATA-3'
151WT	RT	ARMS	5'-CTGGTGATCCTTTCCATCCCTG-3'
151MT	RT	ARMS	5'-CTGGTGATCCTTTCCATCCCAT-3'
RT1 (19)	RT	PCR	5'-GTAGAATTCTGTTGACTCAGATTGG-3'
RT2 (19)	RT	PCR, RVA	5'-GATAAGCTTGGGCCTTATCTATTCCAT-3'
AV150	PRO	PCR, RVA	5'-GTGGAAAGGAAGGACACCAAATGAAAG-3'
M13USPA35 (16)	RT	PCR	5'-GTAAAACGACGGCCAGTTTGGTTGCACTTTAAATTTTCCCATTAGTCCTATT-3'
M13RSPNE(1)35 (16)	RT	PCR	5'-CAGGAAACAGCTATGACCTTACTAACTTCTGTATGTCATTGACAGTCCAGCT-3'
M13USP	RT	sequencing	5'-TGTAAAACGACGGCCAGT-3'
M13RSP	RT	sequencing	5'-CAGGAAACAGCTATGAC-3'
AV36 (16)	RT	sequencing	5'-CAGTACTGGATGTGGGTGATG-3'
AV44 (16)	RT	sequencing	5'-TACTAGGTATGGTAAATGCAGT-3'
IN5 (6)	RT	RVA, sequencing	5'-AATTTTCCCATTAGTCCTATTGAAACTGTACCAG-3'
IN3 (6)	RT	RVA, sequencing	5'-TCTATTCCATC(CT)AAAAATAGTACTTTCCTGATTCC-3'
RVP5 (8)	PRO	RVA, sequencing	5'-GGGAAGATCTGGCCTTCCTACAAGGG-3'
RVP3 (8)	PRO	RVA, sequencing	5'-GGCAAATACTGGAGTATTGTATGG-3'
AV15 (20)	RT	PCR	5'-GATAGGGGGAATTGGAGGTTTTATCAAAGT-3'
AV2 (18)	RT	PCR	5-'AGTGCTTTGGTTCCCCTAAGGAGTTTACA-3'
HP2080N (3)	RT	PCR, sequencing	5'-TTGCACTTTGAATTCTCCCATTAG-3'
AV4 (20)	RT	PCR, sequencing	5'-CATACAAATCATCCATGTATTG-3'

B

Primers (reference)	Gene fragment	Technique	Sequence 5'-3'
AV1 (17)	RT	PCR	5'-TTGGGCCTGAAAATCCATACAATACTCC-3'
AV7 (17)	RT	PCR	5'-CCCAAGCTTCTTCTTGGGCCTTATCTAT-3'
HP3797C (10)	RT	PCR, sequencing	5'-CTTATCTATTCCATCTAGAAATAGT-3'

photographing instrument (ImageMaster), microwave oven, vortex, thermal cycler, ABI PRISM 310 Automated Sequencer (Perkin Elmer).

5.1.3. Methods

5.1.3.1. Viral RNA Extraction and cDNA Synthesis, Proviral DNA Extraction

See **Subheadings 3.4.1.** and **3.4.2.**, but cDNA synthesis is with the reverse primer RT2, AV7, or AV150, depending on the PCR used for sequencing.

5.1.3.2. PCR and Detection of PCR Products

See **Subheadings 3.4.3.** and **3.4.4.** The PCRs used for sequencing and the corresponding details of the primers and the protocols are given in **Tables 7** and **8**, respectively.

5.1.3.3. Purification of PCR Product

The PCR product is purified on a Seakem LE agarose gel electrophoresis (*see* **Subheading 3.3.5.**). The concentration of the gel is 1% instead of 0.5%. The desired PCR fragment is excised from the gel and extracted using the QIAquick Gel Extraction Kit (Westburg):

Table 8
Cycling Conditions for PCR and Cycle Sequencing

Primers	Specifications	Primerconcentration	$MgCl_2$ concentration	Cycling conditions	Preheat step, cycle number and final step	PCR machine
A35 - NE(1)35	outer ARMS	0.2 µM	2.5 mM	15 sec 94°C 15 sec 55°C 60 sec 72°C	40 cycles + 10 min 72°C	GeneAmp PCR System 9600
B - 215WT / 215MT	inner 215 ARMS	0.4 µM	1.5 mM	30 sec 94°C 30 sec 45°C 45 sec 72°C	+ 10 min 94°C 25 cycles + 10 min 72°C	Biometra TRIO-Thermoblock
AV3 - 151WT / 151MT	inner 151 ARMS	0.4 µM	1.5 mM	15 sec 94°C 15 sec 45°C 30 sec 72°C	+ 10 min 94°C 25 cycles + 10 min 72°C	Biometra TRIO-Thermoblock
RT1 - RT2	outer RT sequencing	0.2 µM	2 mM	15 sec 94°C 120 sec 65°C	40 cycles + 10 min 72°C	GeneAmp PCR System 9600 Biometra TRIO-Thermoblock
M13USPA35 - M13RSPNE(1)35	inner RT sequencing	0.4 µM	1.5 mM	30 sec 94°C 60 sec 65°C	30 cycles + 10 min 72°C	Biometra TRIO-Thermoblock
M13USP, M13RSP, AV36, AV44	RT sequencing			30 sec 96°C 15 sec 50°C 4 min 60°C	25 cycles	
AV150 - RT2	outer RVA, outer PRO sequencing	0.2 µM	2 mM	45 sec 95°C 30 sec 55°C 60 sec 72°C	40 cycles + 10min 72°C	GeneAmp PCR System 9600 Biometra TRIO-Thermoblock
IN5 - IN3	inner RT RVA	0.5 µM	4 mM	30 sec 94°C 30 sec 55°C 60 sec 72°C	30 cycles + 10 min 72°C	Biometra TRIO-Thermoblock
RVP5 - RVP3	inner PRO RVA	0.5 µM	3 mM	45 sec 95°C 30 sec 60°C 60 sec 72°C	30 cycles + 10 min 72°C	Biometra TRIO-Thermoblock
RVP5, RVP3	PRO sequencing			30 sec 96°C 15 sec 50°C 4 min 60°C	25 cycles	GeneAmp PCR System 9600
AV15 - AV2	outer RT sequencing	0.2 µM	1.5 mM	30 sec 95°C 30 sec 56°C 45 sec 72°C	35 cycles + 10 min 75°C	Biometra TRIO-Thermoblock
HP2080N - AV4	inner RT sequencing	0.4 µM	3 mM	90 sec 94°C 60 sec 37°C 2 min 72°C	25 cycles + 10 min 72°C	Biometra TRIO-Thermoblock
HP2080N, AV4, AV36, AV44	RT sequencing			30 sec 96°C 15 sec 50°C 4 min 60°C	25 cycles	GeneAmp PCR System 9600
AV1 - AV7	outer RT sequencing	0.2 µM	1.5 mM	30 sec 95°C 30 sec 56°C 45 sec 72°C	35 cycles + 10 min 72°C	Biometra TRIO-Thermoblock
AV3 - HP3797C	inner RT sequencing	0.4 µM	3mM	90 sec 94°C 60 sec 37°C 2 min 72°C	25 cycles + 10 min 72°C	Biometra TRIO-Thermoblock
AV3, NE(1)35	RT sequencing			30 sec 96°C 15 sec 50°C 4 min 60°C	25 cycles	

1. Excise the DNA fragment from the agarose gel with a clean, sharp scalpel. Weigh the gel slice in a tube. Add 300 µL of Buffer QX1 to 100 mg of gel.
2. Incubate at 50°C until the gel slice has completely dissolved. To help dissolve gel, mix by vortexing the tube every 2–3 min during the incubation. After the gel slice has dissolved completely, check that the color of the mixture is yellow. If the color of the mixture is orange or violet, add 10 µL of 3 *M* sodium acetate, pH 5.2, and mix.
3. Add 100 µL of isopropanol, for 100 mg gel, to the sample and mix. Place a QIAquick spin column in a provided collection tube. To bind DNA, apply the

sample to the QIAquick column, and centrifuge for 1 min at 13,000 rpm (15,000*g*). Discard flowthrough and place QIAquick column back in the same collection tube.

4. Add 500 µL of Buffer QX1 to QIAquick column and centrifuge for 1 min at 13,000 rpm (15,000*g*).
5. To wash, add 750 µL of Buffer PE to QIAquick column and let the column stand for 2–5 min, and then centrifuge for 1 min at 13,000 rpm (15,000*g*). Discard the flowthrough and centrifuge for an additional 1 min at 13,000 rpm (15,000*g*). Place the QIAquick column into a clean 1.5-mL microfuge tube.
6. To elute the DNA, add 50 µL of water to the center of the column, let it stand for 1 min, and centrifuge for 1 min.

5.1.3.4. Sequencing of the PCR Product

The strategy described below involves direct cycle sequencing of the PCR product, using the Dye Terminator technology for an ABI automated sequencer (ABI PRISM Dye Terminator Cycle Sequencing Core Kit, Perkin-Elmer).

1. Prepare the reaction premix by mixing per sample 4 µL of 5X sequencing buffer with 1 µL dNTP mix, 0.5 µL of each dye terminator, and 1 µL Ampli*Taq* DNA Polymerase, FS.
2. Add 8 µL reaction premix to approx 200 ng PCR product and 6 pmol primer (*see* **Table 7**). Adjust with water until a volume of 20 µL is reached.
3. Perform the cycling reaction according to **Table 8**.
4. Add 2 µL 3 *M* sodium acetate, pH 5.2, and 50 µL 95% ethanol in a microcentrifuge tube. Transfer the entire 20 µL of the reaction to the microcentrifuge tubes containing the ethanol solution. Vortex and place on ice for 10 min.
5. Pellet the DNA by centrifuging at 13,000 rpm (±15,000*g*) for 30 min. Carefully aspirate the ethanol solution with a micropipet. Remove as completely as possible; this supernatant contains unreacted dye terminators that may produce nonspecific bands in the sequencing run. If nonspecific bands seriously disturb the reading of the sequencing fragments, then next time perform this precipitation step twice by redissolving the pellet in water.
6. Rinse the pellet by adding 250 µL 70% ethanol. Centrifuge at 13,000 rpm (±15,000*g*) for 5 min. Carefully aspirate the whole alcohol solution with a micropipet. Air-dry the pellet.
7. Resuspend the pellet in 25 µL of template suppression reagent. Vortex and spin the sample. Heat the sample at 95°C for 2 min to denature. Vortex and spin the sample again. Place on ice until ready to use.
8. Load the sample on an ABI PRISM 310 (or another ABI sequencer).

5.2. ARMS Protocols

5.2.1. Experiment Outline

Selective PCRs for the detection of HIV-1 drug resistance mutations have first been described by Larder et al. (*3*), who called it amplification refractory

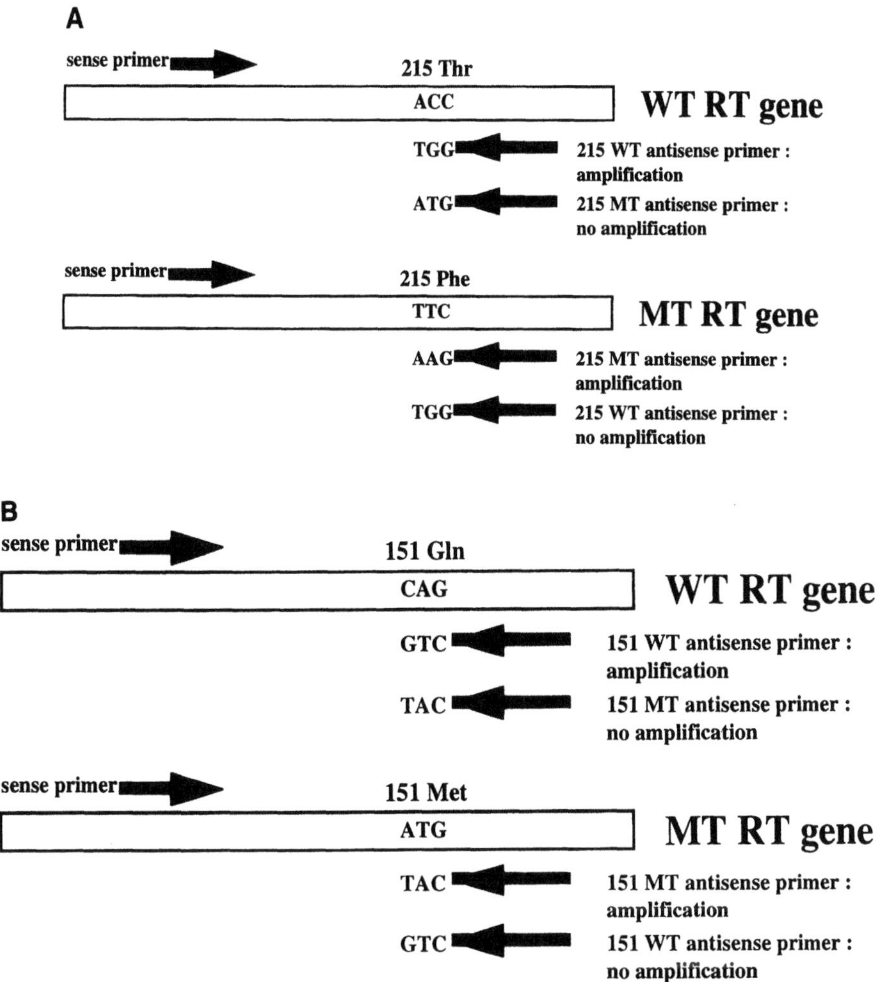

Fig. 2. Schematic representation of the ARMS principle.

mutation system (ARMS). The two ARMS protocols described here are based on a nested PCR of which the inner PCR is selective and performed separately with a wild-type (WT) and a mutant (MT) primer. Depending on which reaction scores positive, the template is judged WT, MT, or mixture (MX). The authors provide a protocol (adapted from **ref. *3***) for the 215 ARMS, with MT primers designed to score the AZT-related T215F mutation in the HIV-1 RT gene, but which also allows the detection of the more frequent AZT-related T215F mutation. A second protocol ***(15)*** describes the 151 ARMS, designed to detect the multinucleoside analog-related Q151M mutation ***(16)*** (*see* **Fig. 2**). The use of Ampli*Taq* Gold DNA polymerase, as described in the protocol, allows a clear discrimination of WT and MT strains. The method also works with Ampli*Taq* DNA polymerase, but then there is only a 10- to 100-fold discrimination between WT and MT strains, owing to primer leakage of MT primer on WT template or WT primer on MT template. The consequence is that correct scoring of mixtures requires a 10-fold dilution procedure of the outer PCR product with a repetition of the inner selective PCR to ensure that a scored mixture is a true mixture. Only when WT and MT signals disappear at the same dilution factor can the sample be scored as a mixture. Thus, a mixture with <10% WT or MT strain is diluted until it is resolved as MT or WT, respectively. In our hands, only a hot start with Ampli*Taq* Gold DNA polymerase allows the detection of mixtures with <10% WT or MT strains. because the performance of ARMS can depend on the specific conditions used in each lab, each lab should optimize these PCRs. The exact discriminatory power of the selective PCRs should then be judged using dilution series of viral RNA and proviral DNA using WT and MT strains. Tenfold serial dilutions of WT or MT virus particles in medium, tenfold serial dilutions of cells infected with pure WT or MT virus in uninfected cells, and dilutions of WT and MT virus particles together at different ratios should be prepared. To be able to judge the dilution series, the viral load of each virus stock used to make virus dilutions should be determined with a commercial HIV-1 viral load assay. The proviral copy number in the dilution series of the infected cells should be determined, e.g., by performing a PCR whose detection limit is known.

5.2.2. Materials

See **Subheading 5.1.**

5.2.3. Methods

5.2.3.1. Viral RNA Extraction and cDNA Synthesis; Proviral DNA Extraction

See **Subheadings 3.4.1.** and **3.4.2.**, but cDNA synthesis is with the reverse primer NE(1)35.

5.2.3.2. PCR and Detection of PCR Products

See **Subheadings 3.4.3.** and **3.4.4.**

1. Amplify 10 µL of cDNA or genomic DNA in a 50 µL outer PCR containing 10 m*M* Tris-HCl, pH 8.3, 50 m*M* KCl, 2.5 m*M* $MgCl_2$, 200 µ*M* dNTPs, 0.2 µ*M* primers (A35 and Ne(1)35), and 0.025 U/µL Ampli*Taq* DNA polymerase. The cycling conditions on a Perkin-Elmer 9600 thermocycler are 94°C for 15 s, 55°C for 15 s, and 72°C for 60 s for 40 cycles and a final extension step of 10 min at 72°C. This outer PCR product can be used for the inner PCR of both 151ARMS and 215ARMS. It can also be used for sequencing purposes.
2. Perform the 215ARMS inner PCR in a 50 µL mixture containing 10 m*M* Tris-HCl, pH 8.3, 50 m*M* KCl, 1.5 m*M* $MgCl_2$, 200 µ*M* dNTPs, 0.4 µ*M* primers (B and

215WT or 215MT), and 0.025 U/μL Ampli*Taq* Gold DNA polymerase. The cycling conditions on a Biometra cycler are 94°C for 30 s, 45°C for 30 s, and 72°C for 45 s for 25 cycles and a final extension step of 10 min at 72°C. A 10-min 94°C pre-PCR heat step is added to activate Ampli*Taq* Gold.

3. Use the same reaction buffer for the 151ARMS inner PCR (AV3 and 151WT or 151MT). The cycling conditions on a Biometra cycler are 94°C for 15 s, 45°C for 15 s, and 72°C for 30 s for 25 cycles and a final extension step of 10 min at 72°C. A 10-min 94°C pre-PCR heat step is added to activate Ampli*Taq* Gold.

Acknowledgments

The authors thank Christiane Callebaut for fine editorial assistance.

References

1. Dianzani, F., Antonelli, G., Turriziani, O., Riva, E., Simeoni, E., Signoretti, C., Set al. (1994) Zidovudine induces the expression of cellular resistance affecting its antiviral activity. *AIDS Res. Human Retroviruses* **10,** 1471–1478.
2. Zhang, H., Dornadula, G., Wu, Y., Havlir, D., Richman, D. D., and Pomerantz, R. J. (1996) Kinetic analysis of intravirion reverse transcription in the blood plasma of human immunodeficiency virus type 1-infected individuals: direct assessment of resistance to reverse transcriptase inhibitors in vivo. *J. Virol.* **70,** 628–634.
3. Larder, B. A., Darby, G., and Richman, D. D. (1989) HIV with reduced sensitivity to zidovudine (AZT) isolated during prolonged therapy. *Science* **243,** 1731–1734.
4. Larder, B. A., Chesebro, B., and Richman, D. D. (1990) Susceptibilities of zidovudine-susceptible and -resistant human immunodeficiency virus isolates to antiviral agents determined by using a quantitative plaque reduction assay. *Antimicrob. Agents Chemother.* **34,** 436–441.
5. Japour, A. J., Mayers, D. L., Johnson, V. A., Kuritzkes, D. R., Beckett, L. A., Arduino, J.-M., et al. (1993) Standardized peripheral blood mononuclear cell culture assay for determination of drug susceptibilities of clinical human immunodeficiency virus type 1 isolates. *Antimicrob. Agents Chemother.* **37,** 1095–1101.
6. Kellam, P. and Larder, B. A. (1994) Recombinant virus assay: a rapid, phenotypic assay for assessment of drug susceptibility of human immunodeficiency virus type 1 isolates. *Antimicrob. Agents Chemother.* **38,** 23–30.
7. Boucher, C. A. B., Keulen, W., van Bommel, T., Nijhuis, M., de Jong, D., de Jong, M., et al. (1996) Human immunodeficiency virus type 1 drug susceptibility determination by using recombinant viruses generated from patient sera tested in a cell-killing assay. *Antimicrob. Agents Chemother.* **40,** 2404–2409.
8. Maschera, B., Furfine, E., and Blair, E. D. (1995) Analysis of resistance to human immunodeficiency virus type 1 protease inhibitors by using matched bacterial expression and proviral infection vectors. *J. Virol.* **69,** 5431–5436.
9. Doyon, L., Croteau, G., Thibeault, D., Poulin, F., Pilote, L., and Lamarre, D. (1996) Second locus involved in human immunodeficiency virus type I resistance to protease inhibitors. *J. Virol.* **70,** 3763–3769.

10. Kaye, S., Loveday, C., and Tedder R. S. (1992) A microtitre format point mutaion assay: Application to the detection of drug resistance in human immunodeficiency virus type-1 infected patients treadted with zidovudine. *J. Med. Virol.* **37,** 241–246.
11. Stuyver, L., Wyseur, A., Rombot, A., Loruvagie, J., Scarcez, T., Verhofstede, C., Remland, D., Schinazi, R. F., and Rossau, R. (1997) Line probe assay for rapid detection of drug-selected mutations in the human immunodeficiency virus type 1 reverse transcriptase gene. *Antimicrob. Agents Chemother.* **41,** 284–291.
12. *ACTG Virology Manual for HIV Laboratories*, Division of AIDS, National Institutes of Allergy and Infectious Diseases, Version 2.0, Jan. 1993.
13. Pauwels, R., Balzarini, J., Baba, M., Snoeck, R., Schols, D., Herdewijn, P., Desmyter, J., and De Clercq, E. (1988) Rapid and automated tetrazolium-based colorimetric assay for the detection of anti-HIV compounds. *J. Virol. Methods* **20,** 309–321.
14. Reed, L. J. and Muench, H. (1938) A simple method of estimating fifty percent endpoints. *Am. J. Hyg.* **27,** 493–497.
15. Van Laethem, K., Van Vaerenbergh, K., Schmit, J. C., De Vroey, V., Schuurman, R., Sprecher, S., Hermans, P., De Clercq, E., Desmyter, J., and Vandamme, A. M. (1998) Selective PCR for the detection of HIV-1 drug resistance mutations in the follow-up of HIV-1 infected patients. ECEAR, Munich, Germany, February 28–March 3, abstract 154–P4.
16. Schmit, J.-C., Cogniaux, J., Hermans, P., Van Vaeck, C., Sprecher, S., Van Remoortel, B., Witvrouw, M., Balzarini, J., Desmyter, J., De Clercq, E., and Vandamme, A.-M. (1996) Multiple drug resistance to nucleoside analogues and nonnucleoside reverse transcriptase inhibitors in an efficiently replicating human immunodeficiency virus type 1 patient strain. *J. Infect. Dis.* **174,** 962–968.
17. Larder, B. A., Kellam, P., and Kemp, S. D. (1991) Zidovudine resistance predicted by direct detection of mutations in DNA from HIV-infected lymphocytes. *AIDS* **5,** 137–144.
18. Vandamme, A.-M., Debyser, Z., Pauwels, R., De Vreese, K., Goubau, P., Youle, M., Gazzard, B., Stoffels, A., Cauwenbergh, G. F., Anné, J., Andries, K., Janssen, P. A. J., Desmyter, J., and De Clercq, E. (1994) Characterization of HIV-1 strains isolated from patients treated with TIBO R82913. *AIDS Research and Human Retroviruses* **10,** 39–45.
19. Gu, Z., Gao, Q., Li, X., Parniak, M. A., and Wainberg, M. A. (1992) Novel mutation in the human immunodeficiency virus type 1 reverse transcriptase gene that encodes cross-resistance to 2',3'-dideoxyinosine and 2',3'-dideoxycytidine. *J. Virol.* **66,** 7128–7135.
20. Vandamme, A.-M. (1994) Polymerase chain reaction (PCR) as a diagnostic tool in HIV infection. V*erhandelingen van de Koninklijke Academie voor Geneeskunde van België*, LVI nr. **3,** 231–265.

20

Line Probe Assay for Detecting Mutations in HIV-1 Reverse Transcriptase

Lieven Stuyver, Ann Wyseur, Gonda Verpooten, and Rudi Rossau

1. Introduction

The human immunodeficiency virus type 1 (HIV-1) belongs to the family of positive-stranded, enveloped RNA viruses with a DNA intermediate step (retroviruses). Because of the lack of fidelity of the reverse transcriptase (RT), the replication is error-prone, and the infection is characterized by its quasispecies nature. Antiretroviral treatment with such compounds as zidovudine (AZT), zalcitabine (ddC), didanosine (ddI), stavudine (d4T), and lamivudine (3TC) select for quasispecies variants that are resistant to these compounds *(1)*. The detection of these variants is clinically important because they may affect the outcome of the treatment *(2)*.

To simultaneously detect most of the genetic changes that were selected on treatment, a reverse hybridization assay, called the Line Probe Assay (LiPA™) was developed at Innogenetics *(3)*. Using this approach, biotinylated polymerase chain reaction (PCR) fragments from the HIV-1 RT gene are hybridized against a panel of specific immobilized oligonucleotide probes. After a stringent hybridization, biotin groups are detected with a streptavidin-alkaline phosphatase-based colorimetric procedure. This LiPA technology for the detection of HIV-1 RT variants is now commercially available as a kit (LiPA HIV-1 RT) *(4)*. The complete methodology, including viral RNA extraction, cDNA synthesis, nested PCR, LiPA hybridization, and LiPA interpretation is described herein.

From: *Methods in Molecular Medicine, vol. 24: Antiviral Methods and Protocols*
Edited by: D. Kinchington and R. F. Schinazi © Humana Press Inc., Totowa, NJ

2. Materials

2.1. HIV-1 RT Amplification

2.1.1. Materials Not Included in the LiPA HIV-1 RT Kit

1. TRIzol LS Reagent (Gibco-BRL, Life Technologies, 10296-028).
2. High-pressure liquid chromatography (HPLC) or diethylpyrocarbonate-treated H_2O.
3. Avian myeloblastosis virus-RT (AMV-RT) (Stratagene, 600082).
4. AMV-RT buffer (1X): 50 m*M* Tris-HCl, pH 8.3, 40 m*M* KCI, 6 m*M* $MgCl_2$, 5 m*M* dithiothreitol (DTT).
5. dNTPs (each 10 m*M*) (Pharmacia Biotech).
6. Random Hexamer Primers $pd(N)_6$, prepare a 150-ng/µL solution (Pharmacia Biotech 27-2166-01).
7. Dextran T500, prepare a stock solution of 1 µg/µL (Pharmacia Biotech, 17-0320-01).
8. Human placental ribonuclease inhibitor (HPRI) (Amersham, E2310Z).
9. Ethanol.
10. Isopropanol.
11. Chloroform.
12. Pipets adjustable to deliver 1–20, 20–200, and 200–1000.
13. Microtube centrifuge at 4°C.
14. Water bath or dry heating block.
15. Vortex.
16. PCR thermal cycler (PE-480, Perkin Elmer).
17. *Taq* DNA polymerase (reaction buffer included; Stratagene, 600132).
18. Cotton-plugged tips.
19. Gloves (wear gloves at all stages).
20. Paraffin oil (Merck, 1.07174.2500).

2.1.2. Materials Included in the LiPA HIV-1 RT Kit

1. One tube with 300 µL mixture of the outer amplification primers, containing 0.01% NaN_3.
2. One tube with 300 µL mixture of the nested amplification primers, containing 0.01% NaN_3.
3. One tube containing 50 µL amplification control, containing 0.01% NaN_3. At the end of the amplification procedure, this amplification control should appear in a 2% agarose gel as a single band with a length of 640 bp (*see* **Notes 1** and **2**).

2.2. The LiPA HIV-1 RT Procedure

2.2.1. Materials Not Included in the Kit

1. Water bath with shaking platform, with inclined lid, temperature adjustable to 39 ± 0.5°C (Julabo SW21, Labortechnik, Seelbach, Germany), or the Innogenetics Auto-LiPA™.
2. An orbital or longitudinal shaker or rocker.

3. Aspiration device.
4. Distilled or deionized water.
5. Adjustable pipets.
6. Cotton-plugged tips.
7. Tweezers for manipulation of the strips.
8. Gloves.

2.2.2. Materials Included in the Kit

1. 20 LiPA HIV-1 RT strips.
2. Ready-for-use denaturation solution.
3. Ready-for-use hybridization solution.
4. Stringent wash buffer.
5. Concentrated conjugate (to be diluted l:100 in conjugate diluent before use).
6. Conjugate diluent.
7. Substrate buffer.
8. Concentrated substrate solution (NBT/BCIP: Nitroblue tetrazolium and 5-bromo-4-chloro-3-indolyl phosphate in dimethylformamide, to be diluted 1:100 in substrate buffer before use).
9. Concentrated rinse solution (to be diluted 1:5 in distilled H_2O before use).
10. Three incubation trays containing eight troughs each.
11. One plastic transparent reading chart for identification of positive lines.
12. One vial containing 50 µL LiPA control.

3. Methods

3.1. HIV-1 RT Amplification

3.1.1. RNA Isolation

1. Add 50 µL of plasma to 150 µL of TRIzol LS. Pipet up and down.
2. Incubate at room temperature for 5 min.
3. Add 40 µL of chloroform and shake by hand for 15 s.
4. Incubate for 2 min at room temperature.
5. Centrifuge for 15 min at 12,000*g* at 4°C.
6. Transfer the supernatant to a fresh tube, add 20 µL of Dextran T-500, and vortex.
7. Add 100 µL of isopropanol, vortex, and incubate for 10 min at room temperature.
8. Centrifuge for 10 min at 12,000*g* at 4°C.
9. Aspirate the supernatant, add 200 µL of ice-cold 75% ethanol, and centrifuge at 7500*g* for 5 min.
10. Aspirate supernatant and let the RNA pellet briefly dry.
11. RNA pellets can be stored at –20°C.

3.1.2. cDNA Synthesis

1. Dissolve the RNA pellet in 12 µL of mix (10 µL H_2O + 2 µL pd[N]$_6$).
2. Denature the RNA for 10 min at 70°C.

3. Cool immediately to 0°C (ice/water).
4. Prepare a cDNA mix containing 25 U of HPRI, 4 µL of 5X AMV-RT buffer, 1 µL of 10 m*M* dNTPs, and 8 U of AMV-RT, adjust with H_2O until reaching 8 µL. Add this cDNA mix to the 12 µL of RNA solution.
5. Incubate for 90 min at 42°C.
6. Freeze at –20°C or proceed to first amplification round.

3.1.3. First Amplification Round

This procedure is optimized for a Perkin-Elmer PE-480 amplification device. Other thermal cyclers can be used as well, but annealing, extension, and denaturation times need to be adapted for optimal amplification. Amplification mixtures are best prepared on ice.

1. Take 5 µL of cDNA reaction mixture and add 45 µL of a mix containing: 4.5 µL of 10X *Taq* buffer, 10 µL of outer HIV primers, 2 U of *Taq* polymerase, 0.25 µL of 10 m*M* dNTPs, add H_2O to 45 µL.
2. Add 50 µL of paraffin oil.
3. Start amplification procedure: Denature at 94°C for 1 min; 40X 94°C 1 min, 57°C 1 min, 72°C 1 min. Cool to 4°C until further use (*see* **Note 4**).

3.1.4. Second Amplification Round

1. Prepare a mix containing: 5 µL of *Taq* buffer, 10 µL nested HIV primers, 2 U of *Taq* polymerase, and 1 µL of 10 m*M* dNTPs, add H_2O to 48 µL (final concentration of $MgCl_2$ should be 1.5 m*M*).
2. Add 50 µL of liquid paraffin oil.
3. Add 2 µL of the first round PCR product (pipes through the paraffin oil).
4. Start amplification procedure: Denature at 94°C for 1 min; 35X 94°C 1 min, 57°C 1 min, 72°C 1 min.
5. Store the amplicons at –20°C.

3.1.5. Alternative Route

A protocol combining commercial kits for RNA extraction (Amplicor HIV Monitor test, Roche, 073 0246) and one-tube RT-PCR (Titan One-Tube RT" PCR system, Boehringer Mannheim, 1 855 476) was established. The procedure described herein is less sensitive than the one described in **Subheadings 3.1.1.–3.1.3.**, because positive amplification results were obtained only starting from 3000 copies/mL. The following protocol was used:

1. Take 25 µL of the RNA extraction.
2. Add 25 µL mix containing: 10 µL of Titan 5X RT-PCR buffer, 1 µL of 10 m*M* dNTPs, 10 µL of outer HIV primers, 2.5 µL of Titan DTT solution, 0.125 µL of HPRI, and 1 µL of Titan enzyme mix.
3. Add 50 µL of paraffin oil.
4. Incubate for 30 min at 50°C in a thermal cycler.

5. Start amplification cycle: Denature for 2 min at 94°C; 40X 94°C 1 min, 57°C 1 min, 68°C 1 min.
6. Nested PCR is carried out as described in **Subheading 3.1.4.**

3.1.6. Visualization of the Amplified Product

The presence of amplified product can be checked on a 2% agarose gel. Load 5 µL of the amplified product per slot. The second-round amplification product should appear as a single band with a length of 647 bp (**Fig. 1**).

3.2. LiPA HIV-1 RT Procedure

3.2.1. Test Principle

The LiPA HIV-1 RT typing test is based on the reverse hybridization principle. Biotinylated DNA material obtained during PCR is hybridized with specific oligonucleotide probes immobilized as parallel lines on membrane-based strips. After hybridization, streptavidin labeled with alkaline phosphatase is added and bound to any biotinylated hybrid previously formed. Incubation with BCIP/NBT chromogen results in a purple/brown precipitate.

With the LiPA HIV- 1 RT test, wild-type and drug selected variants at codon positions 41, 69, 70, 74, 184, and 215 of the HIV-1 RT gene can be detected *(3)*. These codon positions were previously found to be associated with genetic resistance to the antiretroviral drugs AZT, ddI, ddC, and 3TC *(1)*. The LiPA HIV-1 RT strip contains 20 lines, including the control lines for the conjugate binding and amplification (**Fig. 2**).

3.2.2. Manual Procedure

1. Heat the shaking water bath to 39°C. Check temperature using a calibrated thermometer. Prewarm the hybridization buffer in a 37°C water bath. Mix from time to time to dissolve the crystals that could be present. Do not proceed unless all crystals are dissolved.
2. Remove the required number of LiPA HIV-1 RT strips from their container (use tweezers). Include at least one negative and one positive control. The LiPA positive control included in the kit can be used.
3. Take the required number of test troughs and place them in the tray.
4. Pipet 10 µL of denaturation solution in the upper corner of each trough. Close the denaturation solution vial immediately after use.
5. Using cotton-plugged tips, add 10 µL of amplified product to the denaturation solution, and carefully mix by pipeting up and down. Allow denaturation to proceed for 5 min at room temperature.
6. Mix the prewarmed hybridization solution and add gently 2 mL to the denatured amplified product. Mix well by gentle shaking. Take care not to contaminate neighboring troughs.
7. Immediately place the strip into the trough with the marker line facing upward. The strip should be completely submerged in the hybridization solution.

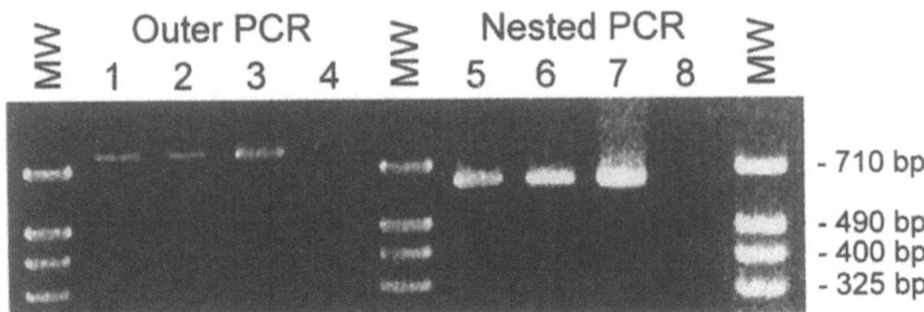

Fig. 1. Agarose gel (2%) showing the first- and second-round PCR product of the HIV- 1 RT gene. Lanes 1–3: first round PCR product of three samples with high viral load (more than 10^6 copies/mL). First-round PCR products (with low viral load) are, in general, PCR negative. Lane 4: negative control included in the first round amplification experiment. Lanes 5–8: nested round of PCR on the material shown in lanes 1–4, respectively. M.W.: molecular weight marker (in base pairs).

8. Place the tray into the shaking water bath, prewarmed to 39°C. Spilling of liquid over the edges of the troughs should be avoided. Therefore, adjust the water level between one-third and one-half of the height of the trough. Make sure that the troughs do not float on the water. The water should be in direct contact with the troughs. Close the lid and incubate for 30 min.
9. After hybridization, remove the tray from the water bath.
10. Hold the tray slightly inclined and aspirate the solution. Add 2 mL of prewarmed ready for-use stringent wash solution into each trough, and rinse by rocking the tray briefly (20 s) at room temperature. Aspirate the solution.
11. Repeat **step 10**.
12. Add 2 mL of prewarmed ready-for-use stringent wash solution, and incubate in the shaking water bath at 39°C for 10 min. Close the lid of the water bath.
13. Prepare the rinse solution and the conjugate solution.
14. Remove the tray from the water bath. Aspirate.
15. Wash the strips twice for 1 min using 2 mL of diluted rinse solution.
16. Add 2 mL of diluted conjugate to each trough and shake for 30 min at room temperature (20–25°C). To achieve homogeneous staining, strips should be completely submerged and move back and forth in the troughs. Select the shaker or rocker and the amplitude of the motion carefully. The amplitude should be as high as possible without spilling liquid over the edges of the troughs.
17. Dilute substrate just prior to the end of the conjugate incubation.
18. Wash the strips twice for 1 min using 2 mL of diluted rinse solution.
19. Wash the strips once with 2 mL of substrate buffer.
20. Add 2 mL of prepared substrate solution to each strip and shake for 30 min at room temperature
21. Wash the strips with 2 mL of distilled water by shaking for at least 5 min.

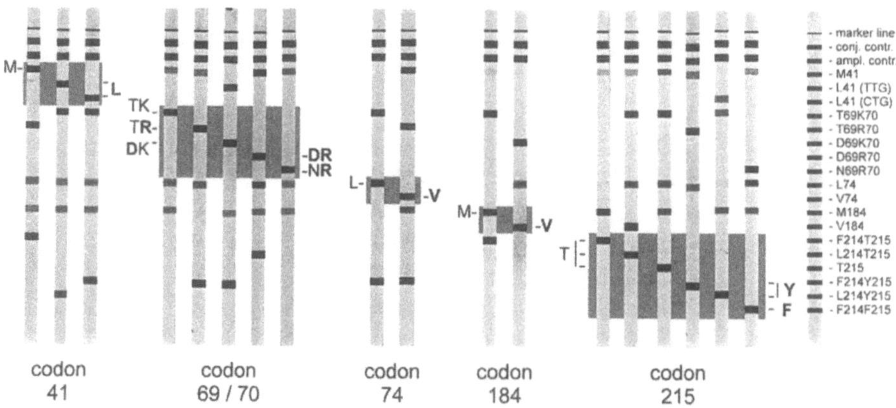

Fig. 2. The LiPA HIV-1 RT. The different possibilities for each codon are highlighted. The interpretation of each strip can be deduced from the information that is presented along the strips, or from the reading chart that is included on the extreme right.

22. Remove the strips from the troughs and let them dry on absorbent paper. Let dry completely before interpretation. Developed strips will retain color if stored dry and protected from light.

3.2.3. Automated Procedure Using the Auto-LiPA System

The Auto-LiPA procedure allows the automated processing of 30 strips in one run. After denaturation of the sample, the system proceeds automatically with the full procedure until final coloration of the strips. Manipulation errors are therefore excluded. One total run takes approx 2.5 h. The procedure allows highly standardized and reliable testing.

3.2.4. Interpretation of the Line Patterns

1. The uppermost pencil line is the marker line allowing correct orientation of the strip and positioning of the plastic reading chart.
2. The next line (line 1) is the conjugate control line. This line monitors proper performance of conjugate and substrate during the detection procedure.
3. Line 2 is the amplification control line. This line contains probes covering highly conserved regions of the HIV-1 RT region, and should be positive if the correctly amplified fragment from the HIV-1 RT gene is added and hybridization was not impaired. This line should not be visible in the negative control.
4. Color intensities between lines on one single strip may differ from one line to another.
5. The strip contains probes covering wild-type and drug-selected motifs for the following codon positions:

codon 41:	line 3: wild-type Met (ATG) **M41**
	line 4: mutant-type Leu (TTG) **L41**
	line 5: mutant-type Leu (CTG) **L41**

codon 69/70:	line 6: wild-type Thr/wild-type Lys **T641K70**
	line 7: wild-type Thr/mutant-type Arg **T69R70**
	line 8: mutant-type Asp/wild-type Lys **D69K70**
	line 9: mutant-type Asp/mutant-type Arg **D69R70**
	line 10: unknown-type Asn/mutant-type Arg **N69R70**
codon 74:	line 11: wild-type Leu **L74**
	line 12: mutant-type Val **V74**
codon 184:	line 13: wild-type Met **M184**
	line 14: mutant-type Val **V184**
codon 215:	lines 15–17: wild-type Thr **T215**
	lines 18, 19: mutant-type Tyr **Y215**
	line 20: mutant-type Phe **F215**

6. Reactivity at one of these lines is indicative for the presence of the corresponding motif in the isolate under investigation.
7. The motifs have been associated with resistance against the following antiviral compounds *(1)*:

	Wild-type	Mutant
AZT	M41	L41
	K70	R70
	T215	Y215, F215
ddI	L74	V74
ddC	T69	D69
3TC	M184	V184

8. If cloned and sequenced material is used to test the LiPA HIV-1 RT, single non-ambiguous reactivities are expected. If this is not the case, a more stringent compliance with the above conditions is a prerequisite. If a patient sample is used, and the LiPA result showed mixtures at different positions, under the described stringency conditions, the possibility of a mixture at those codon positions should be taken into consideration during the interpretation.
9. The LiPA control should show reaction on lines 1, 2, 3, 6, 11, 13, and 16. The LiPA control consists of biotinylated oligonucleotides complementary to the hybridization probes applied on these lines. Positive hybridization to these lines demonstrates satisfactory performance of the assay including hybridization, washing, and detection. The amplification control sample gives a clear positive signal on gel and on the strip on lines 1, 2, 3, 6, 11, 13, and 16.

4. Notes

1. NaN_3 is included as preservative. As this is a harmful solution, avoid contact with skin, eyes, and do not inhale or ingest. NaN_3 forms toxic gas when in contact with acids; and is explosive when in contact with copper or lead plumbing.
2. Store these reagents isolated from contaminating DNA at 2–8°C.
3. All these solutions contain 0.1% NaN_3 as preservative (LiPA control: 0.01%). Do not freeze these materials. Allow all materials to warm up to room temperature before use.

4. Include at least one positive and one negative control sample each time an amplification test is performed. An amplification positive control is included in the kit.
5. It is advisable to wear gloves at all stages of this procedure. Manipulate strips with tweezers. During hybridization, avoid splashing the water into the troughs.
6. The probes have been designed to be specific at the "one-nucleotide" level. This means that a difference of one nucleotide between the target sequence and the probe sequence will interfere with the hybridization, and hence the staining. Mixtures are in general accompanied with a strong probe reactivity at one probe line, and a weaker signal at another probe line of the same codon. Polymorphisms might sometimes result in weak hybridization signals, without affecting the interpretation of the resistance codons. In these cases, the stronger signal as observed in mixtures is not present.
7. Hybridization and stringent wash: Incubation at 39°C followed by the stringent wash are the most critical steps in avoiding false positive (temperature too low) and negative (temperature too high) results. For the manual procedure, a shaking water bath with inclined lid allows optimal temperature control when the lid is closed during incubation. Do not use hot air shakers for the hybridization or stringent wash, because heat exchange is too slow, and optimal hybridization cannot be reached within the indicated time span. Amplitude of the motion of the shaker or rocker is also critical and can lead to increased background staining.
8. Comparison with sequencing: Genotyping results have been compared with sequencing in several labs, including the authors' *(3)*. The consensus result of these studies is that more than 95% correlation exists between LiPA and sequencing. Studies to resolve the remaining ambiguities are ongoing. With respect to the detection of coinfections, LiPA was found to be much more sensitive. Comparison with other genotypic test systems, such as the point mutation assay *(5)* is also ongoing.

References

1. Schinazi, R. F., Larder, B. A., and Mellors, J. W. (1995) Mutations in retroviral genes associated with drug resistance. *Inter. Antiviral News* **4,** 95–107.
2. D'Aquila, R. T., Johnson, V. A., Welles, S. L., Japour, A. J., Kuritzkes, D. R., DeGruttola, V., Reichelderfer, P. S., Coombs, R. W., Crumpacker, C. S., and Kahn, J. O. (1995) Zidovudine resistance and HIV-1 disease progression during antiretroviral therapy. *Ann. Intern. Med.* **122,** 401–408.
3. Stuyver, L., Wyseur, A., Rombout, A., Louwagie, J., Scarcez, T., Verhofstede C., Rimland, D., Schinazi, R. F., and Rossau, R. (1997) Line Probe Assay for rapid detection of drug-selected mutations in the human immunodeficiency virus type 1 reverse transcriptase gene. *Antimicrobiol. Agents. Chem.* **41,** 284–291.
4. Stuyver, L., Wyseur, A., Rombout, A., Verhofstede, C., Rimland, D., Schinazi, R. F., and Rossau, R. (1997) Line Probe Assay (LiPA) for the detection of drug selected variants in the HIV-1 reverse transcriptase gene. *Inter. Antiviral News* **5,** 38–40.
5. Kaye, S., Loveday C., and Tedder, R. (1992) A microtitre format point mutation assay: application to the detection of drug resistance in human immunodeficiency virus type 1-infected patients treated with zidovudine. *J. Med. Virol.* **37,** 241–246.

21

RT-PCR for Amplification of Specific Fragments of HIV-1 Genome

Marie-Pierre de Béthune and Kurt Hertogs

1. Introduction

HIV, the etiologic agent of AIDS, is a retrovirus of the family *Lentiviridae*, first isolated in 1983 by the group of Luc Montagnier at the Pasteur Institute of Paris *(1)*. In the following years, much effort has been, and still is, focused on the search for antiviral drugs that would help to control the course of the disease in infected individuals. To assess the efficacy of those drugs, in vivo clinical markers of virus replication needed to be defined. These markers were for some years, surrogate, e.g., CD4 cell numbers, one of the main target cell types in the HIV replication cycle. More cumbersome methods were also used, such as the in vitro culture of plasma virus on donor peripheral blood lymphocytes (PBMC), with variable results. None of these techniques, however, could provide an accurate measure of virus replication. A major breakthrough in this field was the advent of methods that would allow for a direct quantification of circulating HIV. Viral load determinations soon proved to be an invaluable tool both in the clinical management of HIV-infected individuals and in the monitoring of therapeutic efficacy for commercially available or experimental antiviral drugs *(2)*.

Three commercial assays for viral load determination are currently available: Quantiplex® (Chiron), NASBA® (Organon-Teknika), and Amplicor® (Roche). Only the latter would fall into the topic of this chapter (*see* **Note 1**), because it is based on the RNA- or reverse transcriptase-polymerase chain reaction (RT-PCR) technique.

PCR was first described by Mullis et al. in 1985 *(3)*. Since its discovery, this technique has been used widely in all sorts of domains. In the field of HIV,

From: *Methods in Molecular Medicine, vol. 24: Antiviral Methods and Protocols*
Edited by: D. Kinchington and R. F. Schinazi © Humana Press Inc., Totowa, NJ

more precisely, its applications are numerous: besides its usefulness for viral load determination, as already mentioned, PCR can be used for amplifying particular sequences of the HIV genome to allow for the further characterization of the virus, both genotypically (subtyping, presence of drug resistance associated mutations) and phenotypically (drug-susceptibility profile of the circulating virus in treated individuals, Antivirogram™).

RT-PCR is performed in four steps, which will be described in this chapter: (1) extraction of HIV genomic RNA; (2) synthesis of cDNA; (3) PCR; and (4) analysis of PCR products.

A major drawback of PCR is the risk of contamination of samples to be analyzed by previously amplified material, yielding false positive results and/or ending in the amplification of genetic material from the wrong sample. To prevent this risk, special guidelines need to be strictly followed. These will be described in **Subheading 1.2.**

HIV, as already mentioned, is a retrovirus, i.e., the starting material submitted to amplification is RNA. This genetic material is very labile and can be efficiently hydrolyzed by RNases, which, on the contrary, are very stable and ubiquitous enzymes. Thus, special care must be taken to prevent contamination of the extraction area and equipment by these enzymes. This topic will be addressed in **Subheading 1.3.**

It is, of course, not possible to describe here all the PCRs that can be applied to HIV. A general procedure will be outlined, examplified by a reaction that yields a ±150-bp fragment in the *pol* gene of the virus. This reaction is able to detect one copy of viral RNA and is thus useful for the detection of HIV in unknown samples. Moreover it is able to detect all subtypes of HIV-1 *(4)*.

1.2. PCR Guidelines

Contamination of new samples by previously amplified genetic material can be a nightmare for people performing PCR routinely. Good organization of the laboratory and compliance to strict rules can prevent the occurrence of this contamination. It is better to be too hard on those, because once the contamination has happened, it is too late. Therefore, at least three different areas must be delimited in the laboratory, three separate rooms if this is possible:

1. A "nucleic acid isolation area," where new samples are stored and submitted to the extraction procedure.
2. A "pre-PCR area," where reaction mixes are prepared. This area can be a positive-pressure vertical laminar flow cabinet equipped with an ultraviolet (UV) lamp that is switched on for 20 min after use to destroy any possible contaminating DNA.
3. A "post-PCR area," where amplified products are analyzed and stored, if required. This area is best situated totally remote from the two other ones and, if possible, equipped with an interlock that can be UV-irradiated.

A fourth area must be defined if "nested-PCR," i.e., a second PCR with amplicons from a first PCR as starting material, needs to be performed. This "nested-PCR area" can be restricted to a negative-pressure laminar flow cabinet (type fume hood) equipped with an HEPA filter before the air exhaust and with a UV lamp that is switched on for 20 min after use to destroy any possible contaminating DNA.

Each of these areas must have its dedicated equipment (pipets, tube racks, ice buckets, centrifuges, vortex, freezers, refrigerators, and so on). A good way to prevent transfer of equipment from one area to another is the use of a color code (e.g., green for pre-PCR, white for the isolation area, and so on). A one-way flow is to be respected: pre-PCR area —> isolation area (—> nested-PCR area) —> post-PCR area. PCR tubes racks that must go from the pre-PCR area to the nested-PCR area and that eventually come back to the pre-PCR area need to be decontaminated by UV irradiation (20 min on each side) and/or with 10% bleach (overnight incubation).

Work in the different areas is preferentially performed with disposable protective clothing: gloves, overshoes, arm-sleeves—discarded each time an area is left. Lab coats should be renewed each week. Working with aerosol-tight tips ("filter tips") or, alternatively, with positive displacement pipets, is compulsory, to prevent contamination of the pipets and of the samples with material from other samples, amplified or not. Ice-making machine, pure water supply, chemicals, balances, pH meter, and other equipment required for preparation of solutions must be located in an area where no amplified material is allowed. Thermocyclers can be located in the nested-PCR area or in the post-PCR area, but never in the pre-PCR area or in the isolation area. Regarding the choice of a thermocycler, *see* **Note 2**. A laboratory where plasmids harboring HIV genomic sequences are purified must be considered a post-PCR area. A negative control should be included in the series of samples for each step of the entire procedure: RNA extraction, cDNA synthesis, PCR, nested-PCR, if applicable. This allows one to determine at which step a contamination took place, should one occur. To prevent carryover contamination, one can make use of a system based on an enzymatic hydrolysis of previously amplified material incorporated, e.g., in the Amplicor assay. This system is described in **Note 3**.

1.3. Working with RNA

As mentioned in **Subheading 1.**, RNA is a very labile molecule, and hence, the time between its extraction and its conversion to cDNA should be as short as possible. Extracted RNA should be stored at –80°C for no longer than 1 yr.

Ribonucleases (RNases) are ubiquitous enzymes, i.e., they are present on the operator's hands and in bacteria and molds that may be present on airborne dust particles. Always wear gloves and use proper microbiological sterile techniques when isolating RNA, to avoid hydrolysis of the extracted material by the enzyme. RNases are very solid enzymes that are difficult to inactivate. Use sterile disposable plastic ware, which is considered RNase-free, for handling RNA.

Glassware should be baked overnight at 200°C. Nondisposable plasticware should be rinsed thoroughly with 0.1 *N* NaOH, 1 m*M* ethylenediamine-tetra-acetic acid (EDTA), and then with RNase-free (diethylpyrocarbonate [DEPC]-treated) water. Alternatively, it can be treated with RNase AWAY™ (Molecular BioProducts), according to the manufacturer's instructions.

Water and in-house prepared solutions should be treated by the addition of 0.05% DEPC overnight at room temperature, followed by autoclaving for 30 min at 120°C, to remove any traces of DEPC. Tris buffers may not be treated with DEPC. For their preparation, use a dedicated Tris container, RNase-free weighing materials, and DEPC-treated water. Before and after extraction, wipe all working surfaces with denatured ethanol or 10% bleach or, for nonmetallic surfaces, with RNase AWAY.

1.4. Working with HIV

Samples should be stored at –80°C, if possible. The infectivity of HIV decreases rapidly at –20°C.

The first step of the extraction procedure, i.e., the denaturation of the sample with the lysis buffer, should be performed in a class II biosafety cabinet. The remainder of the procedure can be carried out on the bench, because the lysis buffer completely inactivates HIV.

It is recommended that aerosol-tight tips (filter tips) be used to prevent contamination of the pipets with HIV. Dispose of the tips that have been in contact with HIV in bleach, except if they have been used with a guanidine thiocyanate-containing buffer (*see* **Subheading 2.5.1.**). The remainder of the sample should be inactivated with bleach before being disposed of in an appropriate waste container.

2. Materials

2.1. Pre-PCR Area

1. Positive-pressure laminar flow cabinet equipped with a UV lamp.
2. Pipets for volumes up to 10, 200, and 1000 µL.
3. Corresponding aerosol-tight tips (filter tips).
4. 200-µL PCR tubes and racks.
5. Vortex.
6. Short-spin microcentrifuge.
7. Refrigerator and –20°C freezer, for storage of the reagents.

2.2. Nucleic Acid Isolation Area

1. Class II Biosafety cabinet.
2. Vortex.
3. Microcentrifuge.
4. Water bath.
5. Pipets for volumes up to 200 and 1000 µL.
6. Corresponding aerosol-tight tips (filter tips).
7. Disposable sterile plastic transfer (Pasteur) pipets.
8. Sterile 1.5-mL screw-cap tubes.
9. –80°C Freezer, for storage of the samples.
10. Refrigerator, for storage of the reagents.

2.3. Nested-PCR Area

1. Negative-pressure laminar flow cabinet (type fume hood) equipped with an HEPA filter before the air exhaust, and with a UV lamp.
2. Pipets for volumes up to 10 µL.
3. Corresponding aerosol-tight tips (filter tips).
4. Thermocycler.

2.4. Post-PCR Area

1. Thermocycler.
2. Equipment for agarose gel electrophoresis.
3. UV transilluminator.
4. Polaroid camera with UV-sensitive films.
5. Pipets for volumes up to 10, 200, and 1000 µL.
6. Corresponding aerosol-tight tips (filter tips).
7. Terasaki plates.
8. Refrigerator and –20°C freezer, for storage of the reagents.
9. –20°C Freezer, for storage of the PCR products.

2.5. Reagents

2.5.1. RNA Extraction

1. Lysis buffer: dissolve 120 g guanidine thiocyanate in 100 mL of 0.1 *M* Tris-HCl, pH 6.4, 22 mL of 0.2 *M* EDTA, pH 8.0, and 2.6 g of Triton X-100. Autoclave 20 min at 120°C and store at 4°C for no longer than 6 mo. **Warning:** Guanidine thiocyanate is a potent chaotropic agent and irritant. Do not bring any material that has contained this product (glassware, tips, pipets, and so on) in contact with acids (including bleach) because production of HCN would occur.
2. Wash buffer: dissolve 120 g guanidine thiocyanate in 100 mL of 0.1 *M* Tris-HCl, pH 6.4. Autoclave 20 min at 120°C and store at 4°C for no longer than 6 mo.
3. Silica suspension, prepared as follows: to a 2-L measuring cylinder containing ±100 mL DEPC-water, add 60 g SiO_2 and fill up to 500 mL with DEPC-water. Stir on a magnetic stirrer until all the silica is resuspended. Leave suspension overnight at room temperature, to allow the silica to sink to the bottom of the

cylinder. Carefully remove ±430 mL supernatant with a sterile pipet coupled to a vacuum aspirating device. Add DEPC-water up to 500 mL, slowly stir on a magnetic stirrer untill all the silica is resuspended, and leave at room temperature for 5 h. Carefully remove ±440 mL supernatant as described above. At no time allow the silica to dry. Homogenize the silica suspension by pipetting up and down several times. Adjust suspension pH to 2.0 with 32% HCl. Transfer suspension to a 250-mL bottle and autoclave 20 minutes at 120°C. Aliquot suspension in 1.5-mL screw-cap tubes and store at 4°C for no longer than 6 mo.

4. Freshly prepared 70% ethanol, using DEPC-water.
5. Acetone.
6. TE pH 8.0: 10 m*M* Tris-HCl, pH 8.0, 1 m*M* EDTA, pH 8.0. Autoclave 20 min at 120°C.
7. DEPC-water.

2.5.2. cDNA Synthesis

1. 10X PCR buffer: 100 m*M* Tris-HCl, 15 m*M* $MgCl_2$, 500 m*M* KCl, pH 8.3, at 20°C; stored at –20°C.
2. 25 m*M* $MgCl_2$ solution in DEPC-water, stored at 4°C (storage at –20°C might cause $MgCl_2$ to precipitate).
3. 50 μ*M* Random hexamers, stored at –20°C.
4. dNTPs mix, 2.5 m*M* each, in DEPC-water, stored at –20°C.
5. RNase inhibitor, 20 U/μL, stored at –20°C.
6. MuLV RT, 50 U/μL, stored at -20°C.
7. DEPC-water.

2.5.3. First or Outer PCR

1. 10X PCR buffer: 100 m*M* Tris-HCl, 15 m*M* $MgCl_2$, 500 m*M* KCl, pH 8.3, at 20°C; stored at –20°C.
2. 20 μ*M* of 5' outer primer (HPOL4235—CCCTACAATCCCCAAAGTCAAGG) in DEPC-water.
3. 20 μ*M* of 3' outer primer (HPOL4538—ACCTTTCCACTTCCCCGTCAT) in DEPC-water.
4. *Taq* DNA Polymerase, 5 U/μL. For the choice of the amplifying polymerase, *see* **Note 5**.
5. DEPC-water.

2.5.4. Second or Inner PCR

1. 10X PCR buffer: 100 m*M* Tris-HCl, 15 m*M* $MgCl_2$, 500 m*M* KCl, pH 8.3, at 20°C; stored at –20°C.
2. 25 m*M* $MgCl_2$ solution in DEPC-water, stored at 4°C (storage at –20°C might cause $MgCl_2$ to precipitate).
3. dNTPs mix, 2.5 m*M* each, in DEPC-water, stored at –20°C.
4. 20 μ*M* of 5' inner primer (HPOL4327—TAAGACAGCAGTACAAATGGCAG) in DEPC-water.

5. 20 µ*M* of 3' inner primer (HPOL4481—GCCCAAATAATGTCCCTGTCG) in DEPC-water.
6. *Taq* DNA polymerase, 5 U/µL.
7. DEPC-water.

2.5.5. Analysis of PCR Products

1. 10X TBE buffer: dissolve 100 g Tris base and 55 g boric acid in ±700 mL demineralized water, and 40 mL of 0.5 *M* EDTA (pH 8.0); adjust final volume to 1 L with demineralized water and store at room temperature.
2. Agarose (electrophoresis grade).
3. Ethidium bromide, 10 mg/mL, stored in the dark at 4°C. **Warning:** Ethidium bromide is a potent carcinogenic agent, always wear gloves while handling gels or solutions containing the dye. All solutions containing ethidium bromide should be disposed of as hazardous chemicals.
4. Sample loading buffer: 0.25% bromophenol blue, 0.25% xylene cyanol, 30% glycerol, in demineralized water, stored at 4°C.
5. Molecular weight markers, rendered ready-to-use by the addition of the appropriate volume of sample loading buffer, stored at 4°C.

3. Methods

3.1. RNA Extraction

The extraction procedure described below is by Boom et al. *(5)*. For alternative methods *see* **Note 4**.

1. Bring all reagents to room temperature. Crystals may have formed in the lysis and wash buffers on storage at 4°C. Incubate these at 37°C in a water bath until all crystals are dissolved and check for their homogeneity before use.
2. In all steps of the procedure, open and close tubes one at a time, and use a new tip or sterile disposable transfer pipet for each tube.
3. Label the required number of 1.5-mL screw-cap tubes and dispense 900 µL of lysis buffer to each of them.
4. Add 100 µL (or 200 µL) plasma to each tube and vortex vigorously for 3–4 s.
5. Check silica suspension carefully: if the silica is not entirely covered with water, discard tube and use a new one. Vortex silica suspension thoroughly (the suspension must be homogeneous), add 40 µL to each tube, and vortex vigorously. Vortex suspension between every two tubes to assure good homogeneity.
6. Incubate tubes 10 min at room temperature, vortexing them every 2 min to assure optimal binding of the RNA to the silica.
7. Spin tubes 1 min at 12,200*g* in the microcentrifuge.
8. Remove supernatant with a sterile disposable transfer pipet, taking care not to disturb the silica pellet.
9. Add 1 mL wash buffer to each tube and vortex vigorously to resuspend the silica pellet completely.

10. Spin tubes 1 min at 12,200*g* in the microcentrifuge.
11. Repeat **steps 8–10** once.
12. Remove supernatant with a sterile disposable transfer pipet taking care not to disturb the silica pellet.
13. Add 1 mL of 70% ethanol to each tube and vortex vigorously to resuspend the silica pellet completely.
14. Spin tubes 1 min at 12,200*g* in the microcentrifuge.
15. Repeat **steps 12–14** once.
16. Remove supernatant with a sterile disposable transfer pipet, taking care not to disturb the silica pellet.
17. Add 1 mL acetone to each tube and vortex vigorously to resuspend the silica pellet completely.
18. Spin tubes 1 min at 12,200*g* in the microcentrifuge.
19. Remove supernatant with a sterile disposable transfer pipet, taking care not to disturb the silica pellet. Remove as much acetone as possible.
20. Incubate tubes, open, at 56°C for 10 min in the water bath, to evaporate all the acetone. The pellet should have a white appearance when completely dry.
21. Add 50 µL TE buffer or DEPC-water to each tube and vortex vigorously to resuspend the silica pellet completely.
22. Incubate tubes, closed, at 56°C for 10 min in the water bath. Vortex tubes every 3 min, to assure optimal elution of the RNA from the silica.
23. Spin tubes 2 min at 12,200*g* in the microcentrifuge.
24. Transfer supernatant to a new 1.5-mL screw-cap tube and proceed immediately to cDNA synthesis or store at –80°C.

3.2. cDNA Synthesis

1. This reaction is carried out in a total volume of 20 µL.
2. All reagents and reaction mixes must be kept on ice until tubes are transferred to the thermocycler.
3. All reagents should be vortexed to assure proper homogeneity of solutions and shortly spinned down to avoid aerosol formation on opening of the vials.
4. Prepare cDNA reaction mix, described in **Table 1**, for $n + 2$ samples (n = number of RNA samples).
5. Dispense 16 µL cDNA reaction mix in n + 1200 µL PCR tubes.
6. Add 4 µL DEPC-water to the last tube (= negative control of cDNA synthesis).
7. Close all tubes and transfer them to the isolation area.
8. Spin RNA containing tubes 1 min at 12,200*g* to pellet traces of carried-over silica.
9. Add 4 µL of extracted RNA to the reaction tubes and close them tightly.
10. Incubate 10 min at room temperature to allow for annealing of the random hexamers to RNA.
11. Transfer tubes to the thermocycler and run following program: 42°C for 30 min; 99°C for 5 min; hold at 4°C.
12. Remove tubes from the thermocycler at any time during the last incubation (4°C) and proceed immediately to the first PCR, or store at –20°C.

Table 1
Composition of cDNA Reaction Mix

	Concentration			
Reagent	Unit	Stock	Final	Volume (μL) for 1 sample
DEPC H_2O				1.08
PCR buffer	X	10.00	1.00	2.00
$MgCl_2$	m*M*	25.00	3.50	2.80
dNTPs	m*M*	2.50	1.00	8.00
Random hexamers	m*M*	50.00	2.50	1.00
RNase inhibitor	U/μL	20.00	1.00	1.00
MuLV RT	U/μL	50.00	0.31	0.13
Total volume for cDNA mix				16.00
RNA				4.00
Total reaction mix				20.00

3.3. First or Outer PCR

1. This reaction is carried out in a total volume of 50 μL.
2. All reagents and reaction mixes must be kept on ice until tubes are transferred to the thermocycler.
3. All reagents should be vortexed to assure proper homogeneity of solutions and shortly spinned down to avoid aerosol formation on opening of the vials.
4. Prepare outer PCR mix, described in **Table 2**, for *n* + 3 samples (*n* = number of RNA samples).
5. Dispense 40 μL of outer PCR mix in *n* + 2200 μL PCR tubes.
6. Add 10 μL of cDNA to the corresponding outer PCR mix containing tubes, and store remainder of cDNA at –20°C.
7. Add 10 μL of DEPC-water to the last tube (=negative control of outer PCR).
8. Close all tubes tightly, transfer them to the thermocycler, and run following program: 94°C for 1 min, 50°C for 1 min, 72°C for 1 min, 35 cycles; 72°C for 10 min; hold at 4°C.
9. Turn on UV lamp of laminar flow cabinet for 20 min, to allow for destruction of any contaminating cDNA.
10. Remove tubes from the thermocycler at any time during the last incubation (4°C) and proceed immediately to the second PCR, or store at –20°C.

3.4. Second or Inner PCR

1. This reaction is carried out in a total volume of 50 μL.
2. All reagents and reaction mixes must be kept on ice until tubes are transferred to the thermocycler.
3. All reagents should be vortexed to assure proper homogeneity of solutions and shortly spinned down to avoid aerosol formation on opening of the vials.

Table 2
Composition of Outer PCR Mix

Reagent	Concentration Unit	Stock	Final	Volume (µL) for 1 sample
DEPC H_2O				32.75
PCR Buffer	X	10.00	1.00	5.00
HPOL4235	µ*M*	20.00	0.40	1.00
HPOL4538	µ*M*	20.00	0.40	1.00
Taq DNA polymerase	U/µL	5.00	0.025	0.25
Total volume for outer PCR mix				40.00
cDNA				10.00
Total reaction mix				50.00

4. Prepare inner PCR mix, described in **Table 3**, for *n* + 4 samples (*n* = number of RNA samples).
5. Dispense 48.50 µL of inner PCR mix in *n* + 3200 µL PCR tubes.
6. Add 1.5 µL DEPC-water to the last tube (=negative control of inner PCR).
7. Close all tubes and transfer them to the nested PCR area.
8. Add 1.5 µL of outer PCR DNA to the corresponding inner PCR mix containing tubes, and store remainder of outer PCR DNA at –20°C. This is the step in which risk for carryover of amplified material is the highest. When opening outer PCR tubes, avoid contact, by wearing gloves, with amplified material containing mix, which is often present on the inside of the tube lid. If spillage is suspected, change gloves immediately.
9. Close all tubes tightly, transfer them to the thermocycler and run following program: 94°C for 1 min, 50°C for 1 min, 72°C for 1 min, 25 cycles; 72°C for 10 min; hold at 4°C.
10. Turn on UV lamp of laminar flow cabinet for 20 min, to allow for destruction of any contaminating outer PCR DNA.
11. Remove tubes from the thermocycler at any time during the last incubation (4°C) and proceed immediately to the analysis of PCR products, or store at –20°C.

3.9. Analysis of PCR Products

1. Prepare a 1% agarose gel in 1X TBE.
2. Dispense 2 µL of sample loading buffer in *n* + 3 wells of a Terasaki plate (*n* = number of RNA samples).
3. Add 8 µL of each sample of the inner PCR to the wells and mix by pipeting up and down.
4. Load samples on the gel, with the appropriate molecular weight marker(s).
5. Run gel in 1X TBE at 200 V until the xylene cyanol dye is halfway.
6. Stain gel for 10 min in 1X TBE containing 0.5 µg/mL of ethidium bromide.
7. Destain gel for 5 min in tap water.

Table 3
Composition of Inner PCR Mix

Reagent	Concentration			Volume (µL) for 1 sample
	Unit	Stock	Final	
DEPC H_2O				34.25
PCR buffer	X	10.00	1.00	5.00
$MgCl_2$	m*M*	25.00	1.50	3.00
dNTPs	m*M*	2.50	0.20	4.00
HPOL4327	µ*M*	20.00	0.40	1.00
HPOL4481	µ*M*	20.00	0.40	1.00
Taq DNA polymerase	U/µL	5.00	0.025	0.25
Total volume for inner PCR mix				48.50
Outer PCR DNA				1.50
Total reaction mix				50.00

8. Visualize bands on the transilluminator and take a picture with the Polaroid camera to file of the results. Make sure no amplified material is observed in the lanes corresponding to the various negative controls.

4. Notes

1. It is not the aim of this chapter to describe the procedure for HIV-1 viral load determination using the Amplicor assay. The procedure for performing this assay is described well in the kit insert provided by the manufacturer.
2. Numerous suppliers sell thermocyclers to be used with 0.5-mL or 200-µL PCR tubes. Instruments with heated lids, mostly designed for work with 200-µL PCR tubes, are recommended. Indeed, they do not require the use of an oil overlay above the sample, which is cumbersome and a potential risk factor of crosscontamination of the samples.
3. The carryover prevention system is based on the incorporation of dUTP, instead of dTTP, in material produced during the PCR and the use of the enzyme uracil-*N*-glycosylase (UNG) ***(6)***. The latter catalyzes the cleavage of deoxyuridine containing DNA at deoxyuridine residues by opening the sugar ring at the C1 position. On heating at alkaline pH, conditions of the first step of PCR, the DNA chain breaks and becomes unamplifiable. UNG is inactive at temperatures above 55°C. A preliminary step must thus be included in the cycling program, i.e., an incubation at a temperature below 55°C, to allow for the hydrolysis of deoxyuridine containing contaminating amplicons by UNG, prior to amplification of the material of the new sample. At the end of the cycling program, the samples must be maintained at 72°C and removed from the thermocycler within 15 min. To prevent any degradation of the new deoxyuridine containing amplicons by residual or reactivated UNG, samples should be stored immediately at –20°C, or denatured (denaturing solution: 7 *M* urea, 20% saccharose,

0.01% bromophenol blue). There are several limitations to this method. First, the primers used for amplification should have an annealing temperature above 55°C to avoid degradation of newly synthesized deoxyuridine containing amplicons during PCR. This might complicate the choice of primers in the design of a new PCR, or result in the modification of the conditions of already existing PCRs, which, in turn, will need to be optimized again. Second, this carryover prevention method cannot be used in the case of nested-PCR, because the material synthetized in the outer PCR would be hydrolysed in the first step of the inner PCR. Third, the tubes need to be removed from the thermocycler almost immediately after the end of the cycling program, thus excluding the possibility to run PCRs overnight. Although deoxyuridine containing PCR products can be used for most applications (hybridization, dideoxy sequencing, cloning), UNG needs to be eliminated by phenol extraction or any other suitable method prior to further processing of the samples. Finally, PCR carryover prevention with UNG is expensive and renders the PCR procedure even more costly than it already is.

4. In a recent publication *(7)*, Verhofstede et al. have compared eight different extraction methods, some of which are commercial, for isolating HIV-1 RNA from plasma. From their results, it appears that the best method is that described by Chomczynski and Sacchi *(8)*, consisting of a guanidine thiocyanate treatment followed by three phenol-chloroform-isoamylalcohol extractions and an ethanol precipitation. However, phenol is a hazardous chemical that requires use under a fume hood. Moreover, the method implies several transfers to new tubes, which can be at risk for samples mix-up or cross-contamination if a large series of extractions is to be performed. The method by Boom et al. *(5)*, also used in the NASBA assay, gives good results too, and was therefore used in the procedure outlined in this chapter.
5. The choice of the polymerase used in the amplification reaction(s) is mainly oriented by the use that is made of the PCR product. Classically, *Taq* DNA polymerase is used with satisfactory results. More recently, however, much attention has been devoted to alternative enzymes that would be better suited for specific applications. For instance, besides its DNA-dependent DNA polymerase activity, *Tth* DNA polymerase *(9)* has the advantage of possessing, in the presence of Mn^{2+} ions, very efficient intrinsic RT activity, even at elevated temperatures, which allows problems associated with secondary structures often present in RNA to be overcome. It is the enzyme of choice for RT-PCR when the PCR products are not to be analyzed further, e.g., for sequencing, because the presence of Mn^{2+} ions can affect the fidelity of DNA synthesis. Other polymerases, such as *Pwo* and *Pfu* DNA polymerases, show an increased fidelity, owing to their 3'–5' exonuclease proofreading activity, a property lacked by *Taq* DNA polymerase. These enzymes also show a good processivity, which makes them useful for the amplification of larger fragments.

Acknowledgments

Tania Ivens and Hilde Azijn are gratefully acknowledged for their critical reading of the manuscript.

References

1. Barré-Sinoussi, F., Chermann, J. C., Rey, F., Nugeyre, M. T., Chamaret, S., Gruest, J., Dauguet, C., Axler-Blin, C., Brun-Vézinet, F., Rouzioux, C., Rozenbaum, W., and Montagnier, L. (1983) Isolation of a T-lymphotropic retrovirus from a patient at risk for acquired immunodeficiency syndrome. *Science* **220,** 868–871.
2. Mellors, J. W., Rinaldo, C. R., Gupta, P., White, R. M., Todd, J. A., and Kingsley, L. A. (1996) Prognosis in HIV-1 infection predicted by the quantity of virus in plasma. *Science* **272,** 1167–1170.
3. Saiki, R. K., Scharf, S., Faloona, F., et al. (1985) Enzymatic amplification of β-globin genomic sequences and restriction site analysis for diagnosis of sickle cell anemia. *Science* **230,** 1350–1354.
4. Fransen,K., Zhong, P., De Beenhouwer, H., Carpels, G., Peeters, M., Louwagie, J., Janssens, W., Piot, P., and van der Groen, G. (1995) Design and evaluation of new, highly sensitive and specific primers for polymerase chain reaction detection of HIV-1 infected primary lymphocytes. *Mol. Cell. Probes* **9,** 373.
5. Boom, R., Sol, C. J. A., Salimans, M. M. M., Jansen, C. L., Wertheim-van Dillen, P. M. E., and van der Noordaa, J. (1990) Rapid and simple method for purification of nucleic acids. *J. Clin. Microbiol.* **28,** 495–503.
6. Longo, M. C., Berninger, M. S., and Hartley, J. L. (1990) Use of uracil DNA glycosylase to control carry-over contamination in polymerase chain reactions. *Gene* **93,** 125–128.
7. Verhofstede, C., Fransen, K., Mariessens, D., Verhelst, R., van der Groen, G., Lauwers, S., Zissis, G., and Plum, J. (1996) Isolation of HIV-1 RNA from plasma: evaluation of eight different extraction methods. *J. Virol. Methods* **60,** 155–159.
8. Chomczynski, P. and Sacchi, N. (1987) Single step method of RNA isolation by acidic guanidinium thiocyanate-phenol-chloroform extraction. *Anal. Biochem.* **162,** 156–159.
9. Myers, T. W. and Gelfand, D. H. (1991) Reverse transcription and DNA amplification by a Thermus thermophilus DNA polymerase. *Biochemistry* **30,** 7661–7666.

22

Evaluation of Compounds Against Recombinant HIV Reverse Transcriptase

Jan Balzarini

1. Introduction

Reverse transcriptase (RT) has attracted particular attention as a target enzyme for AIDS chemotherapy, because the enzyme catalyzes a crucial step in the HIV replicative cycle. Effective inhibition of this enzyme prevents the formation of proviral DNA. RT is endowed with three independent enzymatic activities *(1,2)*. It has an RNA-dependent DNA polymerase (RDDP), DNA-dependent DNA polymerase (DDDP), and RNaseH activity. The first function catalyzes the polymerization of 2'-deoxynucleotides (2'-dNTPs) with viral genomic single-stranded RNA as template and an oligo DNA (or t-RNALys) as the primer. The second function of the enzyme hydrolyzes the RNA strand of the RNA-DNA hybrid (formed by the first function of the RT) to generate a single-stranded DNA chain. This will allow the third function of RT to happen, namely catalysis of the polymerization of 2'-dNTPs with single-stranded DNA as template and an oligo DNA as primer. The enzyme has, by that time, converted the viral single-stranded RNA genome to double-stranded DNA, which can now be circularized and incorporated into the host cell DNA by the virus-encoded integrase.

There are currently a variety of nucleoside analogs (i.e., AZT [zidovudine] *[3]*, DDC [zalcitabine] *[4]*, DDI [didanosine] *[4]*, D4T [stavudine] *[5]*, and 3TC [lamivudine] *[6]* [also designated NRTIs or nucleoside RT inhibitors]) and two nonnucleoside RT inhibitors (i.e., nevirapine [viramune] and BHAP [delavirdine] [also designated NNRTIs] *[7,8]*) officially approved for treatment of HIV-infected individuals. It should be noted that the NNRTIs are uniquely active against HIV-1, but not HIV-2 RT, whereas the NRTIs inhibit both HIV-1 and HIV-2 RTs. In addition, several other structural classes of

From: *Methods in Molecular Medicine, vol. 24: Antiviral Methods and Protocols*
Edited by: D. Kinchington and R. F. Schinazi © Humana Press Inc., Totowa, NJ

compounds have been reported to be inhibitory to HIV RT, including acyclic nucleoside phosphonates (i.e., PMEA, FPMPA, PMPA) ***(9–11)***, pyrophosphate analogs (i.e., PFA or foscarnet) ***(12,13)***, and a number of miscellaneous RT inhibitors. In this chapter, the authors will describe enzyme inhibition assays valuable for the testing of nucleoside analogs, nonnucleoside analogs, and other RT inhibitors. A detailed overview on the analysis of inhibition of retroviral RT by test compounds can be found in **refs. *14–16*.**

2. Materials

1. Radiochemicals: tritiated 2'-deoxythymidine 5'-triphosphate [*methyl*-^{3}H]dTTP, 2'-deoxyadenosine 5'-triphosphate [2,8-^{3}H]dATP, 2'-deoxyguanosine 5'-triphosphate [8-^{3}H]dGTP or 2'-deoxycytidine 5'-triphosphate [5-^{3}H]dCTP. The radiospecificities of the deoxynucleotides usually range between 15 and 30 Ci/mmol. They can be obtained from several companies such as Amersham (Buckinghamshire, UK), ICN (Costa Mesa, CA), NEN (DuPont Ltd., Hertfordshire, UK), Moravek Biochemicals (Brea, CA), and so forth. They can be used at 2 µCi/assay.
2. Template/primers:
   a. Premade template/primers: poly(C)·oligo($dG_{12–18}$); poly(dC)·oligo($dG_{12–18}$).
   b. Templates: poly(A); poly(C); poly(G); poly(I); poly(U).
   c. Primers: oligo $dT_{12–18}$; oligo $dC_{12–18}$; oligo $dA_{12–18}$; oligo $dG_{12–18}$.
   d. To prepare those homopolymeric template/primers that are only available as separate templates and primers, one may mix 0.15 m*M* poly(U), poly(A) and poly(I) with an equal volume of 0.0375 m*M* oligo(dA), oligo(dT), and oligo(dC), respectively.
   e. Heteropolymeric template/primer: the 16S and 23S *Escherichia coli* rRNA and the primer DNA oligomer complementary to positions 519–536 of 16S rRNA using the *E. coli* 16S rRNA deoxynucleotide numbering system can be obtained from Boehringer Mannheim.
3. Enzyme: recombinant HIV-1 RT.
4. Tris-HCl,pH 7.8; stock solution: 1 *M* in H_2O.
5. Dithiothreitol (DTT); stock solution: 100 m*M* in H_2O.
6. Glutathione; stock solution: 6 *M* in H_2O.
7. EDTA; stock solution: 10 m*M* in H_2O.
8. KCl; stock solution: 1 *M* in H_2O.
9. $MgCl_2$; stock solution: 100 m*M* or 160 m*M* in H_2O.
10. Bovine serum albumin; stock solution: 25 µg/mL in H_2O.
11. Triton X-100; stock solution: 1.2% in H_2O.
12. Inhibitor solution to be tested: prepare a 20-fold higher stock solution than the final inhibitor concentration that should be evaluated.
13. Calf thymus DNA: 150 µg/mL.
14. $Na_4P_2O_7$: 0.1 *M* in 1 *M* HCl.
15. Trichloroacetic acid: 10% (v/v) or 5% (v/v) in water.
16. Ethanol (95%).
17. Milli-Q water.

18. Plastic Eppendorf tubes.
19. Shaking water bath at 37°C.
20. Micropipets.
21. Ice bath.
22. Multifilter manifold apparatus and 2.5-cm Whatman 3M filter disks.
23. Liquid scintillation (β) counter.

3. Methods

3.1. RT Assay in the Presence of Artificial Template/Primer

1. The reaction mixture (50 µL) contains following ingredients:
   a. 2.5 µL Tris-HCl (pH 7.8) 1 *M*; final concentration: 50 m*M*.
   b. 2.5 µL dithiothreitol 100 m*M*; final concentration: 5 m*M*.
   c. 2.5 µL glutathione 6 *M*; final concentration: 300 m*M*.
   d. 2.5 µL EDTA 10 m*M*; final concentration: 500 µ*M*.
   e. 2.5 µL KCl 3 *M*; final concentration: 150 µ*M*.
   f. 2.5 µL $MgCl_2$ 100 m*M*; final concentration: 5 m*M*.
   g. 2.5 µL bovine serum albumin 25 µg/mL; final concentration: 1.25 µg.
   h. 2.5 µL labeled of either dTTP, dGTP, dCTP, or dATP substrate containing 2 µCi/assay. Nonradiolabeled substrate can be added to reach a final substrate concentration of 5, 7.5, 10, 12.5, 15, 20, 25, or 30 µ*M*.
   i. 2.5 µL fixed concentration of template/primer poly(A).oligo(dT) (0.3 m*M*); poly(C). oligo(dG) (2 m*M*); poly(I).oligo(dC) (0.3 m*M*); poly(U).oligo(dA) (0.3 m*M*); final concentration of template primer: 0.015 or 0.1 m*M*.
   j. 2.5 µL Triton X-100 (1.2%); final concentration: 0.06%.
   k. 10 µL inhibitor solution (containing various concentrations of the compound).
   l. 14 µL H_2O.
   m. 1 µL RT preparation.
2. The reaction will be started by the addition of the enzyme. The reaction mixtures are incubated at 37°C for 15, 30, or 60 min (depending on the linearity of the reaction), at which time 100 µL of calf thymus DNA (150 µg/mL), 2 mL of $Na_4P_2O_7$ (0.1 *M* in 1 *M* HCl), and 2 mL of trichloroacetic acid (TCA) (10% v/v) are added in this sequential order. The solutions are kept on ice for 30 min to allow efficient (radiolabeled) DNA precipitation and then brought onto filter disks mounted on a manifold apparatus. The acid-insoluble material on the filters is washed with 2 × 5 mL of TCA 10%; 2 × 5 mL of TCA 5% and 2 × 2 mL of ethanol (to remove radiolabel that is not incorporated into the template/primer) and analyzed for radioactivity in a liquid scintillation counter (β counter).
   a. For the experiments in which the 50% inhibitory concentration (IC_{50}) of the test compounds has to be determined, fixed concentrations of [^{3}H]dTTP, [^{3}H]dGTP, [^{3}H]dATP, or [^{3}H]dCTP are used. The concentration may vary from 1.25 to 2.5 µ*M*, depending on the radiospecificity of the compounds. If similar substrate concentrations need to be compared, one can either lower or increase the radiolabel, or, preferably, add nonradiolabeled substrate to the reaction mixture to adjust the radiolabeled substrate concentration.

b. For the experiments in which the IC_{50} and K_i values of the test compounds have to be determined with respect to the natural substrates, appropriate concentrations of the natural substrate and a fixed concentration of template/primer will be used (as indicated in **step 1h** and **step 1i**).
c. For the experiments in which the K_i values of the test compounds has to be determined with respect to the template/primers, appropriate concentrations of the template/primers will be used in the presence of a fixed concentration of 1.25 μ*M* [^{3}H]dTTP, 2.5 μ*M* [^{3}H]dGTP, 1.75 μ*M* [^{3}H]dATP, or 2.5 μ*M* [^{3}H]dCTP. The latter concentrations has preferably to exceed at least fivefold the K_m values of the enzyme for the dNTP substrates.
d. For the experiments in which the (ir)reversible inhibition of the test compound has to be evaluated, a 25, 50, and 75% inhibitory concentration of test compound is exposed to serial dilutions of the enzyme in the presence of a fixed concentration of [^{3}H]dGTP (2.5 μ*M*) and 0.1 m*M* poly(C).oligo(dG) or [^{3}H]dTTP (1.25 μ*M*) and 0.025 m*M* poly(A)·oligo(dT). The enzyme dilutions may represent 100% (undiluted enzyme, resulting in, preferably, 200,000 dpm of reaction product), 80, 60, 40, 20, and 10% of the enzyme activity. For reversible enzyme inhibition by the compound, the activity values can be plotted on a line that will dissect in the zero-point of a velocity (*y*-axis) versus enzyme concentration (*x*-axis) graph (as also control values [without inhibition] do). For irreversible enzyme inhibition by the compound, the activity values can be plotted on a line for which the slope will be parallel to that of the control line (without inhibition), and will dissect somewhere on the *x*-axis (right of the zero intersection point), because a constant amount of enzyme is irreversibly inactivated by the compound and thus not available anymore to catalyze the reaction. By diluting the enzyme, a certain enzyme dilution will be completely inactivated by the compound, resulting in lack of any enzyme reaction (dissection point on the *x*-axis). Lower enzyme concentrations are obviously fully inactivated by the inhibitor as well, resulting in no reaction (data points located on the *x*-axis).

3.2. RT Assay in the Presence of Heteropolymeric Template/Primer

1. The reaction mixture (50 μL) contains following ingredients:
   a. 2.5 μL Tris-HCl (pH 7.8) 1 *M*; final concentration: 50 m*M*.
   b. 2.5 μL DTT 100 m*M*; final concentration: 5 m*M*.
   c. 2.5 μL glutathione 6 *M*; final concentration: 300 m*M*.
   d. 2.5 μL EDTA 10 m*M*; final concentration: 500 μ*M*.
   e. 2.5 μL KCl 1 *M*; final concentration: 50 m*M*.
   f. 2.5 $MgCl_2$ 160 m*M*; final concentration: 8 m*M*.
   g. 2.5 μL bovine serum albumin 25 μg/mL; final concentration: 1.25 μg.
   h. 2.5 μL radiolabeled (dTTP) substrate (2 μCi/assay); final concentration: 1.25 μ*M*.
   i. 2.5 μL nonradiolabeled dATP 12.8 m*M*; final concentration: 640 μ*M*.
   j. 2.5 μL nonradiolabeled dCTP 12.8 m*M*; final concentration: 640 μ*M*.
   k. 2.5 μL nonradiolabeled dGTP 12.8 m*M*; final concentration: 640 μ*M*.

l. 2.5 µL primed rRNA 66.6 µg/mL; final concentration: 3.33 µg/mL.
m. 2.5 µL Triton X-100 1.2%; final concentration: 0.06%.
n. 2.5 µL inhibitor solution (20-fold higher concentration than the final concentration requested).
o. 13 µL H_2O.
p. 2 µL RT preparation.

2. The reaction mixture is incubated at 37°C for 20 min (or longer time periods depending the linearity of the reaction) in a shaking water bath or at a thermoblok that may fit Eppendorf tubes, and the reaction is stopped by adding 100 µL of calf thymus DNA (150 µg/mL), 2 mL of $Na_4P_2O_7$ (0.1 *M* in 1 *M* HCl), and 2 mL of TCA in this sequential order. Acid-insoluble material is washed and analyzed for radioactivity as described in **Subheading 3.1., step 2.**

4. Notes

1. All solutions should be made in water of the highest purity because trace amounts of impurities in the water can affect the enzyme reaction. Milli-Q water used to prepare solutions for HPLC analysis is of sufficiently good quality.
2. Make sure all recipients in which buffers or solutions are prepared are carefully washed and cleaned for the same reasons as mentioned in **Note 1.**
3. Lipophylic inhibitors should be dissolved in dimethyl sulfoxide (DMSO). To avoid precipitation in the aqueous (polar) reaction mixture and to avoid different DMSO concentrations in the reaction mixture depending on the inhibitor concentration present, it is highly advisable to keep the DMSO concentrations constant in all reaction tubes, including the control tubes without inhibitor. DMSO may inhibit the RT reaction at varying degrees, depending on the nature of the RT enzyme. Ten percent DMSO is probably the maximum concentration that should be present in the reaction mixture (it may inhibit up to 50% of the reaction). It has been observed that lower concentrations of DMSO can even stimulate the RT reaction!
4. A preliminary experiment should always be carried out first to define the linearity of the enzyme reaction. The enzyme mixture should be incubated for different time periods (10, 20, 30, 40, 50, 60, 90, 120 min), and the inhibition experiments should be carried out for a time period at which the enzyme reaction is still proceeding linearly in time.
5. The reaction is started by the addition of enzyme. The enzyme should be kept on ice, whereas the reaction mixture can be brought shortly at room temperature or even at 37°C before starting the reaction. Enzyme will be added to each tube individually and the reaction started at time intervals of 15, 20, or 30 s. Since each tube has to be incubated for an identical time period at 37°C, the reaction has to be stopped in each tube individually at the same time intervals as those at which the reactions in the different test tubes were initiated.
6. The control reaction should preferably have 20,000–200,000 dpm of radiolabel incorporated into the TCA-insoluble material. If too low values are obtained, they can be increased by increasing the amount of radiolabel input (expensive!), and/or by increasing the enzyme concentration, and/or by prolonging the incuba-

tion time of the reaction mixture. In blank samples (without enzyme), no more than 5–10% of radiolabel should remain on the filters. Too high blank values may be owing to insufficient washing of the filters.

7. The water added to the reaction mixture can be (partially) replaced by other components that should be added to the reaction mixture. It will allow some flexibility in changing or adding other components to the reaction mixture without changing the concentrations of the obligatory constituents of the mixture.
8. Usually, the constituents of the reaction mixture (in 2.5-µL values) should not be added individually to the reaction tubes. Instead, premixes should be made containing several constituents together, allowing addition of higher volumes to the reaction tubes, which will save time and increase homogeneity in the reaction.

References

1. Steitz, T. A. (1993) DNA- and RNA-dependent DNA polymerases. *Curr. Opin. Struct. Biol.* **3,** 31–38.
2. Verma, I. M. (1977) The reverse transcriptase. *Biochim. Biophys. Acta* **473,** 1–38.
3. Mitsuya, H., Weinhold, K. J., Furman, P. A., St. Clair, M. H., Nusinoff Lehrman, S., Gallo, R. C., Bolognesi, D., Barry, D. W., and Broder, S. (1985) 3'-Azido-3'-deoxythymidine (BW A509U): an antiviral agent that inhibits the infectivity and cytopathic effect of human T-lymphotropic virus type III/lymphadenopathy-associated virus *in vitro*. *Proc. Natl. Acad. Sci. USA* **82,** 7096–7100.
4. Mitsuya, H. and Broder, S. (1986) Inhibition of the *in vitro* infectivity and cytopathic effect of human T-lymphotropic virus type III/lymphadenopathy-associated virus (HTLV-III/LAV) by 2',3'-dideoxynucleosides. *Proc. Natl. Acad. Sci. USA* **83,** 1911–1915.
5. Baba, M., Pauwels, R., Herdewijn, P., De Clercq, E., Desmyter, J., and Vandeputte, M. (1987) Both 2',3'-dideoxythymidine and its 2',3'-unsaturated derivative (2',3'-dideoxythymidinene) are potent and selective inhibitors of human immunodeficiency virus replication *in vitro*. *Biochem. Biophys. Res. Commun.* **142,** 128–134.
6. Soudeyns, H., Yao, X.-J., Gao, Q., Belleau, B., Kraus, J.-L., Nguyen-Ba, N., Spira, B., and Wainberg, M. A. (1991) Anti-human immunodeficiency virus type 1 activity and *in vitro* toxicity of 2'-deoxy-3'-thiacytidine (BCH-189), a novel heterocyclic nucleoside analog. *Antimicrob. Agents Chemother.* **35,** 1386–1390.
7. Merluzzi, V. J., Hargrave, K. D., Labadia, M., Grozinger, K., Skoog, M., Wu, J., Shih, C.-K., Eckner, K., Hattox, S., Adams, J., Rosenthal, A. S., Faanes, R., Eckner, R. J., Koup, R. A., and Sullivan, J. L. (1990) Inhibition of HIV-1 replication by a nonnucleoside reverse transcriptase inhibitor. *Science* **250,** 1411–1413.
8. Romero, D. L., Busso, M., Tan, C.-K., Reusser, F., Palmer, J. R., Poppe, S. M., Aristoff, P. A., Downey, K. M., So, A. G., Resnick, L., and Tarpley, W. G. (1991) Nonnucleoside reverse transcriptase inhibitors that potently and specifically block human immunodeficiency virus type 1 replication. *Proc. Natl. Acad. Sci. USA* **88,** 8806–8810.
9. Balzarini, J., Hao, Z., Herdewijn, P., Johns, D. G., and De Clercq, E. (1991) Intracellular metabolism and mechanism of anti-retrovirus action of 9-(2-

phosphonylmethoxyethyl)adenine, a potent anti-human immunodeficiency virus compound. *Proc. Natl. Acad. Sci. USA* **88,** 1499–1503.

10. Balzarine, J., Holý, A., Jindrich, J., Dvorakova, H., Hao, Z., Snoeck, R., Herdewijn, P., Johns, D. G., and De Clercq, E. (1991) 9-[(2RS)-3-fluoro-2-phosphonylmethoxypropyl] derivatives of purines: a class of highly selective antiretroviral agents *in vitro* and *in vivo*. *Proc. Natl. Acad. Sci. USA* **88,** 4961–4965.
11. Balzarini, J., Holý, A., Jindrich, J., Naesens, L., Snoeck, R., Schols, D., and De Clercq, E. (1993) Differential antiherpes virus and antiretrovirus effects of the (S) and (R) enantiomers of acyclic nucleoside phosphanates: potent and selective *in vitro* and *in vivo* antiretrovirus activities of (R)-9-(2-phosphonomethoxypropyl)-2,6-diaminopurine. *Antimicrob. Agents Chemother.* **37,** 332–338.
12. Sundqvist, B. and Öberg, B. (1979) Phosphonoformate inhibits reverse transcriptase. *J. Gen. Virol.* **45,** 273–281.
13. Vrang, L. and Öberg, B. (1986) PPi analogs as inhibitors of human T-lymphotropic virus type III reverse transcriptase. *Antimicrob. Agents Chemother.* **29,** 867–872.
14. Segel, I. H. (1976) *Biochemical Calculations*, 2nd ed. Wiley, New York, p. 208.
15. Balzarini, J. and De Clercq, E. (1996) Analysis of inhibition of retroviral reverse transcriptase. *Methods Enzymol.* **275,** 472–502.
16. Balzarini, J., Pérez-Pérez, M.-J., San-Félix, A., Camarasa, M.-J., Bathurst, I. C., Barr, P. J., and De Clercq, E. (1992) Kinetics of inhibition of human immunodeficiency virus type 1 (HIV-1) reverse transcriptase by the novel HIV-1-specific nucleoside analogue 1-[2',5'-bis-O-(*tert*-butyldimethylsilyl)-β-D-ribofuranosyl]-3'-spiro-5"-[4"-amino-1",2"-oxathiole-2",2"-dioxide]-thymine (TSAO-T). *J. Biol. Chem.* **267,** 11,831–11,838.

23

Ultrasensitive Detection of Reverse Transcriptase Activity by the Amp-RT Assay

Applications to the Measurement of Virus Loads and Phenotypic Drug Resistance

J. Gerardo García Lerma and Walid Heneine

1. Introduction

Retroviruses are widely prevalent among vertebrates and are the causative agents of a variety of diseases in humans and animals including immunodeficiences, leukemias, and lymphomas *(1)*. The retrovirus family is characterized by the presence of virion-associated reverse transcriptase (RT), an enzyme that transcribes the viral genomic RNA into a double-stranded DNA copy. This feature has led to studies of the unique enzymatic function of RT for two main applications. First, RT is a good diagnostic tool for the generic detection of the presence of retroviruses. Second, the RT enzyme constitutes a primary target for antiviral drug therapy *(1,2)*.

The authors describe an ultrasensitive method that measures RT activity. The assay adopts polymerase chain reaction (PCR) amplification for detecting the cDNA product of the reaction, and therefore was named Amp-RT *(3,4)*. Amp-RT measures the ability of a sample to produce a DNA copy of a known heteropolymeric RNA template by extending a complementary DNA oligoprimer. The RNA template used in Amp-RT is a sequence from the genome of the encephalomyocarditis virus. This chapter describes in detail the Amp-RT method and its use as (1) a qualitative assay for the generic detection of retroviruses, (2) a quantitative method to measure virus loads of the human immunodeficiency virus type 1 (HIV-1), and (3), a screening method for susceptibility of HIV-1 to RT inhibitors.

From: *Methods in Molecular Medicine, vol. 24: Antiviral Methods and Protocols*
Edited by: D. Kinchington and R. F. Schinazi © Humana Press Inc., Totowa, NJ

2. Materials

1. Encephalomyocarditis plasmid DNA (1 ng/25 µL, Novagen, cat. no. 691781).
2. Large-scale T7 transcription kit (Novagen, cat. no. 692561).
3. RNase inhibitor (RNasin, 40,000 U/mL, Promega, cat. no. N211B).
4. RNase-free DNase (RQI, 1000 U/mL, Promega, cat. no. M6101).
5. Sense T7-EmcF1 primer (5'-GGTACCTAATACGACTCACTATAGGGAGAC ATTAG CCATTT CAACCCAT-3') (T7 promoter sequence underlined).
6. Antisense EmcR2 primer (5'-GTTCATGACAGGCCGATACAGAGG-3').
7. 5'-biotin-labeled EmcR2 antisense primer.
8. Sense EmcF1 primer (5'-CTCCCATCAGGTTGTGCAGCGACC-3').
9. ^{32}P-labeled EmcP1 probe (5'-TGCTCTCACCTTATCAAAATCCAAT-3').
10. Digoxigenin-labeled EmcP1 probe (5'-ATTGGATTTTGATAAGGTGAG AGCA-3').
11. Recombinant HIV-1 RT (rHIV-1 RT, NEN-DuPont, cat. no. NEI-490).
12. Deoxynucleoside triphosphate (dNTP) kit (high-performance liquid chromatography [HPLC] purified, USB, cat. no. US 77100).
13. Native *Taq* DNA polymerase (5000 U/mL, Perkin-Elmer Corp., cat. no. 5600-11/92).
14. 10X PCR buffer (Perkin-Elmer Corp., cat. no. 55690-1/93).
15. 1.5-mL-polyallomer microfuge tubes (Beckman, Inc., USA, cat. no. 357448).
16. DIG-detection ELISA (TMB, Boehringer Mannheim, cat. no. 1603 434).

3. Methods

3.1. Preparation of the RNA Template from the Encephalomyocarditis Virus Genome

The exogenous RNA template (350 bp) used in the Amp-RT assay is prepared from a plasmid-cloned sequence of the encephalomyocarditis virus (EMCV) (positions 7114-7516, GenBank accession number M81861), and is generated by in vitro transcription of a T7-tagged PCR product by using T7 bacteriophage RNA polymerase.

3.1.1. Generation of T7-Tagged EMCV DNA Sequence for In Vitro Transcription

The EMCV sequence is first PCR amplified from the EMCV plasmid by using EmcR2 and an T7-EmcF1 primer that contains the promoter sequence of T7 at the 5' end necessary for in vitro transcription. The PCR reaction is prepared as follows:

1. Add 25 µL of EMCV plasmid DNA (1 ng/25 µL) to a PCR cocktail containing 10 µL of 10X PCR buffer, 0.5 µL of T7-EmcF1 (200 ng/µL), 0.5 µL of EmcR2 (200 ng/µL), 2 µL of dNTP mixture (10 m*M* each), 61.5 µL of water, and 0.5 µL of *Taq* DNA polymerase (5000 U/mL).
2. The conditions for PCR are 35 cycles at 95°C for 1 min, 55°C for 1 min, and 72°C for 1 min.

3. Check the PCR products by electrophoresis in 1.8% agarose gels. The band is visualized by staining with ethidium bromide. The amplified product is 401 bp in size.
4. Purify the DNA from the PCR reaction by standard phenol:chloroform extraction and isopropanol precipitation.
5. Calculate the concentration of DNA by measuring the absorbance at 260 nm. Ensure a good quality of the DNA preparation by having a ratio of A_{260}/A_{280} between 1.8 and 2.0.

3.1.2. In Vitro Transcription of the T7-Tagged EMCV DNA Sequence

The large-scale T7 transcription kit is used according to the manufacturer's instructions. Briefly,

1. Prepare the transcription cocktail containing 5 µg of purified T7-EMCV PCR product, 20 µL of 5X transcription buffer, 10 µL of 20 m*M* dATP, 10 µL of 20 m*M* dCTP, 10 µL of 20 m*M* dGTP, 10 µL of 20 m*M* dUTP, 1 µL of 1 *M* dithiothreitol (DTT), 1 µL of 40 U/µL RNasin, RNase-free water to 99 µL, and 1 µL of T7 RNA polymerase. Incubate for 2 h at 37°C.
2. Add 5 U of RNase-free DNase I, mix well, and incubate for 30 min at 37°C.
3. Repeat the DNase digestion step.
4. Purify the in vitro-transcribed RNA by phenol:chloroform extraction and isopropanol precipitation, and resuspend the pellet in 200 µL of RNase-free water.
5. Calculate the concentration of RNA by measuring the absorbance at 260 nm. One A_{260} unit equals 40 µg/mL RNA. The value of A_{260}/A_{280} should be between 1.8 and 2.0.

3.1.3. Assessment of Quality of the RNA Template

It is extremely important to control the quality of the two DNase digestions to ensure that the RNA template is free of residual EMCV plasmid DNA. Presence of EMCV DNA would result in false-positive results or background Amp-RT signal. To check for absence of EMCV DNA, the RNA template is subjected to PCR amplification and probing by Southern blot hybridization to ^{32}P-labeled EmcP1 probe.

1. Set up PCR reactions according to the protocol described in **Subheading 3.1.1.** with the primer pair EmcF1/EmcR2. Test 10, 20, and 40 ng of RNA template.
2. If positive results are seen after probing, repeat the digestion by DNase. Add 10 µg of RNA template to a solution containing 20 U of RNase-free DNase, 1.5 U of RNasin, 50 m*M* of $MgCl_2$, 5 m*M* of DTT, and 2 m*M* of ethylene glycol-bis (3'-aminoethyl ether)-*N,N,N',N'*-tetra-acetic acid (EGTA). Mix well and incubate for 60 min at 37°C.
3. Incubate for 15 min at 70°C to inactivate the DNase.
4. Check again for the absence of EMCV DNA by repeating the PCR testing. If negative PCR results are seen, proceed to check the functional quality of the template.

For testing the function of the synthesized RNA template, run Amp-RT reactions with 10 ng of RNA template and 10-fold dilutions of rHIV-1 RT from 10^{-6} to 10^{-11} units. Alternatively, HIV-1 virions can be used as a source of RT at concentrations equivalent to 0.2–0.00002 pg of p24 antigen (measured by the Coulter HIV-1 p24 antigen assay). The dilutions should be made in 1X RT buffer C (50 m*M* Tris-HCl, pH 8.3, 50 m*M* KCl, 10 m*M* $MgCl_2$).

A good RNA template should support Amp-RT reactions at a minimum sensitivity of 10^{-9} or 10^{-10} U of rHIV-1 RT (with a specific activity of 1890 U/mg), or HIV-1 virions corresponding to 0.002 or 0.0002 pg of p24 antigen.

3.2. The Amp-RT Assay

3.2.1. Sample Preparation

3.2.1.1. Culture Supernatant

No sample preparation or processing is needed for testing culture supernatants. Typically, 10 µL is applied to the RT buffer A, which can be prepared without the addition of NP-40 and therefore has no NP-40 (the final concentration of NP-40 in the RT reaction will be 0.06%). Culture supernatants should be cell-free because contamination with cellular DNA polymerases may produce false positive results.

3.2.1.2. Serum or Plasma Samples

For serum/plasma samples, the final concentration of NP-40 in the RT reaction is 0.6%. The Amp-RT testing can be made in one of two protocols. The first does not require processing and involves direct testing of 2 µL of serum/plasma. The use of a 2-µL pipet (Gilson, France) is recommended to minimize variability in sampling. Heparinized plasma is avoided for possible risks of inhibition of *Taq* DNA polymerase by heparin in the PCR component of the test. This protocol can be used as a rapid qualitative screening for RT activity. The second protocol uses virus pellets prepared by ultracentrifugation of plasma/serum at 99,000*g* for 1 h at 4°C in 1.5-mL-polyallomer microfuge tubes. The pellet is resuspended in 1X RT buffer C. Typically, pellets from 10 to 25 µL of plasma/serum are tested. This protocol may be used for qualitative or quantitative detection of RT in cell-free retroviruses. The use of plasma/serum-free virus pellets eliminates the possibility of inhibition of RT by anti-RT antibodies.

3.2.2. RT Reaction of Amp-RT

1. Add two drops of mineral oil to 250-µL PCR tubes.
2. Add 40–48 µL of RT buffer A depending on the volume of sample to be tested.
3. Add 2–10 µL of sample to make up the final volume to 50 µL. Give a quick spin in a microfuge.

a. RT buffer A /reaction: 20 µL of RT buffer B *(see below)*, 13.5 µL of NP-40 (2%), 0.25 µL of RNasin (40,000 U/mL), 0.5 µL of EMCV RNA template (20 ng/µL), 0.5 µL of biotin-labeled EmcR2 (200 ng/µL), and 5.25–13.25 µL diethyl pyrocarbonate (DEPC)-water (total volume/reaction: 40–48 µL).
b. RT buffer B: 10 µL of 5X RT buffer C, 2 µL of dNTP (10 m*M* each), 5 µL of EGTA (10 m*M*), 1.5 µL of NP-40 (2%), 1 µL of DTT (100 m*M*), and 0.5 µL of DEPC-water (total volume/reaction: 20 µL).
c. 5X RT buffer C: 250 m*M* Tris-HCl, pH 8.3, 250 m*M* KCl, 50 m*M* $MgCl_2$.
4. Incubate RT reactions for 2 h at 37°C.
5. Denature the RT by heating the tubes at 95°C for 5 min, chill on ice or store at –70°C.

3.2.3. PCR Amplification of RT Products

1. Prepare the PCR cocktail by adding 10 µL of 10X PCR buffer, 0.5 µL of EmcF1 primer (200 ng/µL), 0.5 µL of *Taq* DNA polymerase (5000 U/mL), and 39 µL of water. The final volume per sample is 50 µL.
2. Add 50 µL of PCR cocktail to each tube. Give a quick spin in a microfuge.
3. The conditions for PCR are 35 cycles of 95°C for 1 min, 55°C for 1 min, and 72°C for 1 min.

3.3. Qualitative Detection of Amp-RT Products by Southern Blot Hybridization or Enzyme-Linked Immunosorbent Assay (ELISA)

For qualitative detection, 20 µL of the PCR reaction product is electrophoresed in 1.8% agarose gels, and Southern blot hybridized to a ^{32}P-end-labeled internal probe (EmcP1) following standard procedures. Blots can be exposed for 3–24 h. Alternatively, a nonradioactive ELISA-based detection system may be used as described in **Subheading 3.4.**

3.4. Quantitative Amp-RT Assay

A quantitative Amp-RT assay is a useful laboratory tool for several applications, including the determination of HIV-1 levels in culture supernatant or biological fluids (e.g., plasma and serum), and the study of HIV-1 RT susceptibility to RT inhibitors. The authors describe a quantitative Amp-RT assay for measuring RT activity of HIV-1. Quantitation is based on a calibration curve made by external standards. The standards used can be known numbers of HIV-1 particles (from 10,000 to 1) or known numbers of HIV-1 RT molecules. Virion numbers of an HIV-1 stock can be easily determined from the concentration of p24 antigen on the basis of 10^{-4} pg of p24 antigen per virion as previously estimated ***(5)***. Alternatively, the virion numbers can be determined by RT-PCR analysis or by electron microscopy. HIV-1 RT with a well-characterized specific activity and known p66/p51 protein content can also be used to generate standard curves with known numbers of RT molecules. Commercially available rHIV-1 RT is a good source (e.g., NEN-DuPont). If levels of RT activity in samples are needed with no relevance to virus counts, the Amp-RT results can be expressed as units of enzymatic activity from a standard curve of HIV-1 RT. **Figure 1** shows the dynamic range of Amp-RT, which extends over 4 $\log_{10}$. Identical linearities are seen when HIV-1 virions or rHIV-1 RT are used.

For quantitation of HIV-1 virus load in serum/plasma samples, testing samples in duplicate is recommended. Samples are considered positive and are quantifiable when duplicate test results are positive. Samples with negative or discordant duplicate results are considered Amp-RT negative. Quantitative detection of Amp-RT PCR amplicons is made by an ELISA-based, nonradioactive oligoprobing system. The system uses streptavidin-coated microtiter wells that capture the biotin-labeled PCR product (DIG-detection ELISA). The protocol for the ELISA is as follows:

1. Add 180 µL of 1X hybridization buffer (5X SSC [1X SSC is 0.15 *M* of NaCl plus 0.015 *M* of sodium citrate], 20 m*M* of HEPES, 2 m*M* of EGTA, pH 8.0, 0.1% Tween-20) to the streptavidin-coated microtiter wells.
2. Add 20 µL of Amp-RT product per well. Include probe only wells as a control for nonspecific binding, and substrate-only wells to determine the optical density value of pure peroxidase substrate. Incubate for 30 min at 37°C.
3. Wash the plate six times with phosphate-buffered saline (PBS), 0.05% Tween-20, and 2 m*M* of EGTA.
4. Add 250 µL of denaturing solution (0.4 *N* NaOH, 0.6 *M* NaCl) to each well, and incubate for 15 min at room temperature.
5. Wash the plate as in **step 3**.
6. Add 40 ng of digoxigenin-labeled EmcP1 probe per well in 200 µL of 1X hybridization buffer, and incubate for 1 h at 37°C.
7. Wash the plate as in **step 3**.
8. Incubate the plate for 1 h at 37°C with 200 µL of a peroxidase-labeled antidigoxigenin antibody (4 mU/mL; stock solution diluted 1/5000 in PBS, 1% gelatin).
9. Wash the plate as in **step 3**.
10. Add 200 µL of tetramethylbenzidine substrate and incubate for 30 min at room temperature protected from light.
11. Measure the absorbance at 450 nm with a reference filter at 630 nm.

3.5. Other Applications of the Amp-RT Assay

3.5.1. Analysis of Susceptibility of HIV-1 RT to Nonnucleoside RT Inhibitors

Amp-RT can be used for the study of drug susceptibility of HIV-1 RT to RT inhibitors, including nucleoside analogs and nonnucleoside RT inhibitors. The authors describe the use of Amp-RT to study the resistance of HIV-1 RT to nevirapine (NVP), a nonnucleoside RT inhibitor.

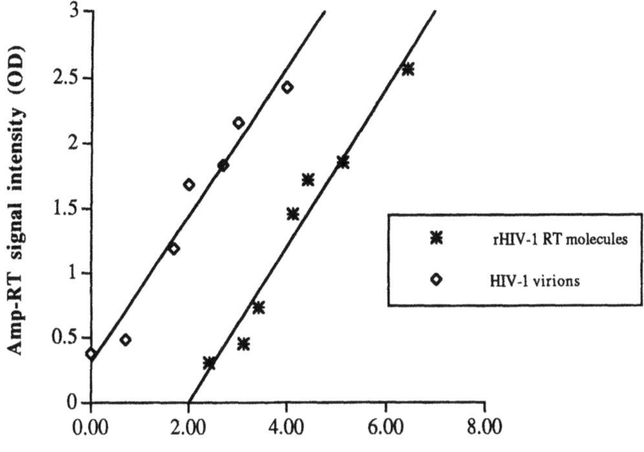

Fig. 1. Linearity analysis of a quantitative Amp-RT assay by using rHIV-1 RT or HIV-1 virions as standards.

Figure 2 illustrates the inhibition of Amp-RT by NVP in a sensitive HIV-1 strain (50% inhibitory concentration [IC_{50}] = 0.038 μ*M*), and in several resistant strains with IC_{50} values ranging from 20 to >100. The protocol used in this Amp-RT application is similar to that described in **Subheading 3.2.**, with the exception that final drug concentrations from 0 to 1000 μ*M* are added to RT buffer A. The results in **Fig. 2** show that at a concentration of 100 μ*M* NVP, Amp-RT can reliably differentiate between NVP-sensitive and -resistant virus. Virus mixtures containing 25% resistant virus may also be differentiated from sensitive virus, as shown in **Fig. 3**. These results have implications on screening for phenotypic drug resistance by the Amp-RT assay by direct analysis of HIV-1 virus from culture supernatant or from plasma of HIV-1-infected persons.

3.5.2. Detection of Novel or Variant Retroviruses

Because Amp-RT is a generic test, it has the advantage of detecting all retroviruses. This makes it an ideal tool to detect novel retroviruses or variants of known retroviruses, such as the divergent group O of HIV-1 *(3,4)*. However, despite the generic character of Amp-RT, the assay can be modified to become more specific for individual retroviruses. This can be achieved by using virus-specific RT inhibitors or virus-specific anti-RT antibodies that can block RT activity.

4. Notes

1. Occasionally, some lots of RNasin may have low levels of RT activity. Therefore, testing for the presence of residual activity in a new lot of RNasin is recommended.

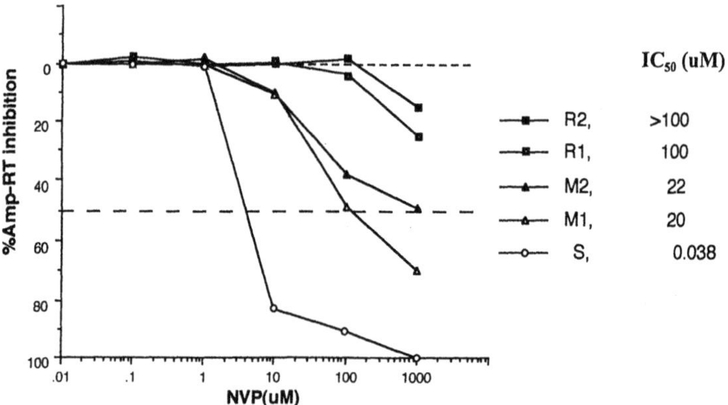

Fig. 2. Differentiation between NVP-sensitive and NVP-resistant HIV-1 virus isolates by analysis of RT inhibition by NVP in the Amp-RT assay.

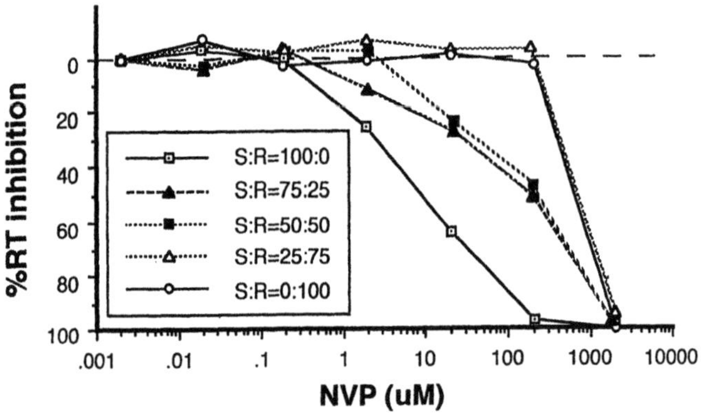

Fig. 3. Inhibition of RT activity of HIV-1 by NVP in the Amp-RT assay. Comparison among a sensitive strain (S), an NVP-resistant strain (R), and different ratios of sensitive to resistant virus.

2. Large volumes of RT cocktail may be prepared and stored at –80°C in aliquots.
3. To minimize the risk of PCR contamination, PCR tubes and pipets can be exposed to ultraviolet (UV) irradiation (UV Stratalinker 2400, Stratagene) to inactivate contaminating DNA.
4. Long-term storage of the RNA template is in liquid nitrogen in aliquots of 25 µL at 400 ng/µL. Working solutions (20 ng/µL) are prepared by dilution in DEPC-water to a final concentration of 20 ng/µL. These aliquots can be stored at –80°C.

Acknowledgment

The authors are grateful to Shinji Yamamoto and William M. Switzer for their contributions.

References

1. Coffin, J. M. (1990) Retroviridae and their replication, in *Fields' Virology*, 2nd ed. (Fields, B. N., Knipe, D. M., Chanock, R. M., et al., eds.), Raven, New York, pp. 1437–1500.
2. Schinazi, R. F., Mead, J. R., and Feorino, P. M. (1992) Insights into HIV chemotherapy. *AIDS Res. Human Retroviruses* **8,** 963–990.
3. Heneine, W., Yamamoto, S., Switzer, W. M., Spira, T. J., and Folks, T. M. (1995) Detection of reverse transcriptase by a highly sensitive assay in sera from persons infected with human immunodeficiency virus type 1. *J. Infect. Dis.* **171,** 1210–1216.
4. Yamamoto, S., Folks, T., M., and Heneine, W. (1996) Highly sensitive qualitative and quantitative detection of reverse transcriptase activity: Optimization, validation, and comparative analysis with other detection systems. *J. Virol. Meth.* **61,** 135–143.
5. Bourinbaiar, A. S. (1991) HIV and *gag*. *Nature* **349,** 111.

24

Reverse Transcriptase Assay Based on Product Enhancement for Assessing the Drug Susceptibility of Retroviruses

Jürg Böni and Jörg Schüpbach

1. Introduction

All replication-competent retroviruses possess a characteristic enzyme, reverse transcriptase (RT), which is present at 20–70 mol/virus particle ***(1–3)***. The enzyme is cleaved, and thereby activated, from an inactive precursor by the action of another retroviral enzyme, the viral protease. All RTs possess three distinct enzymatic activities: (1) an RNA-dependent DNA polymerase, which is the RT in the strict sense of the word, (2) an RNase H, and (3) a DNA-dependent DNA polymerase. After infection of a new host cell, these different activities serve in turn to synthesize a cDNA of the viral RNA, to degrade RNA from the cDNA-RNA heteroduplex, and to duplicate the cDNA strand (reviewed in **ref. *4***).

Being indispensable for retroviral replication, RT is a key target for antiretroviral treatment. Particle-associated RT activity is, on the other hand, also a unique marker of infectious retrovirus particles. Measuring particle-associated RT activity with a sensitive procedure can thus be used as a screening test for retroviruses of any kind, to measure the virus load in individuals with verified infection to assess the need for antiretroviral treatment, and to monitor the effects of antiretroviral treatment.

All of these tasks can now be addressed with a family of novel tests collectively named product-enhanced reverse transcriptase (PERT) assays. PERT assays combine the broad detection range of RT tests with the high sensitivity of nucleic acid amplification procedures. PERT assays are based on the selective enhancement, by polymerase chain reaction (PCR) or one of the various

From: *Methods in Molecular Medicine, vol. 24: Antiviral Methods and Protocols*
Edited by: D. Kinchington and R. F. Schinazi © Humana Press Inc., Totowa, NJ

other nucleic acid amplification methods, of the cDNA product synthesized by the test sample's RT activity from an RNA template. An overview of these diverse procedures has been published ***(5)***. Assays based on this principle were also established by others (***6,7***; *see also* Chapter 20).

Figure 1 summarizes the PERT assay procedure currently used in the authors' laboratory and described in detail in **Subheadings 2.–4.** Initial evaluation showed that the assay is 10^6–10^7 times more sensitive than a conventional RT test based on the incorporation of labeled deoxynucleoside triphosphates into a homopolymeric template-primer combination. The assay detected a variety of different retroviruses or RTs at a concentration corresponding to 1 nU RT activity in the case of murine leukemia virus, which corresponds to 2.1×10^2 enzyme molecules or 3–11 particles ***(8)***. The assay, in fact, detects retroviruses at least as sensitively as PCR for viral RNA, as demonstrated in the model of HIV-1. Testing of serial dilutions of HIV-1 by PERT assay and PCR for viral RNA indicated a detection level of five particles. With a 100-µL sample, all of 30 untreated patients at different stages of HIV-1 infection were positive. In HIV-1 seroconversion panels, the PERT assay detected more positives than any other method, including PCR for viral RNA. Most important, the test's high sensitivity is not compromised by an unacceptably low specificity; the prevalence of elevated RT activity among 160 unselected blood donors was only 1.9% ***(9)***. Because the cause of RT in these cases has not been established, a precise figure for the PERT assay's specificity cannot yet be given. However, in at least two fluids that were positive for RT only by PERT assay and that the authors have further analyzed, relevant retroviral sequences were found (***10,11***, and unpublished data). In another case, the RT activity could repeatedly be passaged to fresh leukocytes in vitro, thus suggesting a replication-competent agent, which the authos have not yet identified ***(12)***. Futhermore, successful application of the PERT assay for the identification of new retroviruses have also been reported by other researchers (*see*, e.g., **ref.** ***13***).

A recent study has shown that the PERT assay can be used to monitor the effect of antiretroviral treatment of HIV-1 infected patients. In this study, HIV RNA by the Roche HIV Monitor assay (Roche Diagnostic Systems, Inc., Branchburg, NJ) became undetectable in 33 of 125 samples (26.4%) from 23 patients treated with an antiretroviral combination therapy. Particle-associated RT correlated well with the values of viral RNA, but remained above the detection limit of the PERT assay, even in samples that were negative by both PCR for viral RNA and a p24 antigen detection procedure shown to be as sensitive as PCR ***(14)***. Moreover, the susceptibility to RT inhibitors of virus populations taken from biological fluids ex vivo can be directly assessed in vitro, without a need to first amplify the virus in cell culture. Thus, the RT activity

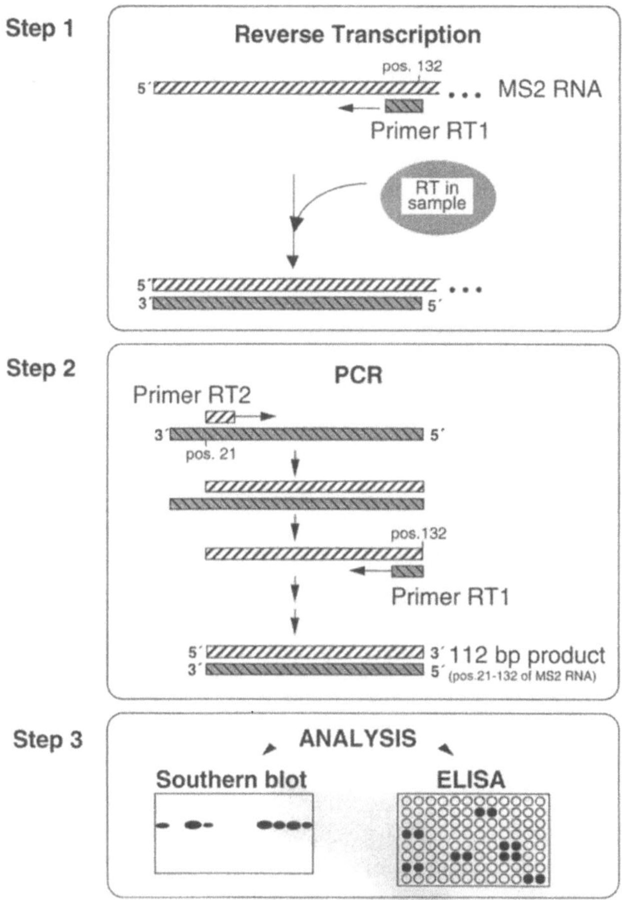

Fig. 1. Schematic representation of the described ultrasensitive reverse transcriptase assay, using PCR for product enhancement.

associated with a defective endogenous avian retrovirus found in chicken-cell–derived, live attenuated virus vaccines was susceptible to AZT triphosphate, as well as dideoxythymidine triphosphate, whereas a recombinant murine leukemia virus RT added as a control was completely resistent to both drugs *(15)*. Susceptibility of virus to nonnucleoside RT inhibitors should also be testable in this way.

Taken together, PERT assays can be used to detect and quantitate retroviruses. The advantages compared with amplification procedures for specific viral sequences are obvious: one test fits all existing retroviruses, and there is no impediment to sensitivity owing to sequence variation, which is a documented drawback of viral load measurements by PCR *(16)*.

Before starting, a word of caution. Be aware that working with blood from infected individuals or material derived from it means handling infectious material. Always work with special lab coats and gloves in a sterile workbench that is specifically designed for this kind of work. Do not use glass or any other materials that could inflict skin lesions. For centrifugation, use aerosol-resistant containers or centrifuges that can prevent laboratory contamination in case of vessel breakage or any other reason of spillage.

2. Materials

2.1. Sample Pretreatment

2.1.1. Preparation of Plasma

1. 15-mL Polypropylene centrifuge tube (e.g., Falcon from Becton-Dickinson, Nunc from Gibco-BRL, Life Technologies, Gaithersburg, MD) (*see* **Note 1**).
2. 5-mL Syringe with a long, reusable, blunt point medical needle (*see* **Note 2**).
3. Disposable syringe disk filter holders: 0.8 µm, 0.2 µm (e.g., *Minisart* from Sartorius GmbH, Göttingen, Germany).
4. Tabletop centrifuge with aerosol resistant containers accomodating 15-mL centrifuge tubes.

2.1.2. Preparation of Virus Particles (See **Note 3**)

1. Sterile 1X PBS: 136 m*M* NaCl, 3 m*M* KCl, 8 m*M* Na_2HPO_4, 1.5 m*M* KH_2PO_4 (e.g., from Gibco-BRL).
2. Virus resuspension buffer: 50 m*M* KCl, 25 m*M* Tris-HCl, pH 7.5, 0.25 m*M* Na_2EDTA, 5 m*M* dithiothreitol (DTT), 50% glycerol. Store at –80°C for up to 3 mo (DTT).
3. 5-mL Syringe with a blunt point medical needle as in **Subheading 2.1.1., item 2**.
4. 0.2-µm Disposable syringe disk filter holder as in **Subheading 2.1.1., item 3**.
5. Ultracentrifuge, rotor, and tubes (*see* **Note 4**).

2.2. PERT Assay (See Note 5)

2.2.1. Reverse Transcription (See **Note 6**)

1. 10 µ*M* Reverse transcription primer: 5'-CATAGGTCAAACCTCCTAGGAATG-3' (RT-1). Store at –20°C.
2. Template RNA: bacteriophage MS2-RNA at 0.8 µg/µL (Boehringer Mannheim, Germany).
3. 10X RT buffer: 0.5 *M* KCl, 80 m*M* $MgCl_2$, 0.5 *M* Tris-HCl, pH 8.3, 1.2 mg/mL BSA (molecular biology grade), 100 m*M* DTT. Store frozen in tightly sealed tubes at –80°C for up to 3 mo (DTT).
4. 5 m*M* dNTP mixture (dATP, dGTP, dCTP, TTP). Store frozen at –20°C.
5. 10% Triton X-100 in distilled water.
6. Recombinant human placental RNase inhibitor (RNasin from Promega, Madison, WI) (*see* **Note 7**).
7. Mineral oil.

2.2.2. PCR Amplification

1. 10X differential amplification buffer for PERT assay: 13.3 m*M* Tris-HCl, pH 8.3, 500 m*M* KCl, 0.013% gelatin. Store frozen at –20°C.
2. 25 m*M* Na_2-EDTA, pH 8.0.
3. 10 µ*M* PCR primers: RT-1 as in **Subheading 3.2.1., step 1**; 5'-TCCTGCTCAAC TTCCTGTCGAG-3' (RT-2). Store frozen at –20°C.
4. 80 ng/µL RNase A in 50 m*M* sodium acetate, 0.3 m*M* EDTA, 50% glycerol (Amersham International, Bucks, UK). Store at 4°C (*see* **Note 8**).
5. *Taq* DNA polymerase at 5 U/µL.
6. Thermal cycling machine.

2.2.3. Detection of Amplified DNA by Enzyme-Linked Immunosorbent Assay (ELISA)

2.2.3.1. Preparation of Microtiter Plate for ELISA

1. 96-well flat bottomed microtiter plate (e.g., Immulon-2, from Dynatech Laboratories, Chantilly, VA, or Nunc, Gibco-BRL).
2. Coating buffer: 100 m*M* Tris-HCl, pH 7.4, 200 m*M* NaCl.
3. 10 mg/mL avidin (e.g., Boehringer Mannheim): Dissolve avidin in PBS at 20 mg/mL, then add an identical volume of glycerol and mix completely. Store at –20°C.
4. Blocking buffer: Coating buffer containing 0.05% Tween-20, 5% bovine serum albumine (BSA) and 20% heat inactivated serum (*see* **Note 9**).
5. Wash solution: Coating buffer containing 0.3% Tween-20.
6. Microplate shaker.

2.2.3.2. Detection of Amplified DNA Products

1. 10X PCR buffer: 500 m*M* KCl, 100 m*M* Tris-HCl, pH 8.3, 15 m*M* $MgCl_2$, 0.01% gelatin. Store frozen at –20°C.
2. 5'-labeled oligonucleotide probes: 5'-biotin-TTAATGTCTTTAGCGAGACGC-3' (RT-3-BIO) at 0.3 µ*M* and 5'-digoxigenin-ATGGCTATCGCTGTAGGTAGC-3' (RT-5-DIG) at 1.0 µ*M*. Store frozen at –20°C.
3. 100 m*M* Na_2-EDTA, pH 8.0.
4. Anti-digoxigenin Fab fragments, alkaline phosphatase labeled, 150 U/mL (Boehringer Mannheim).
5. Substrate buffer: 100 m*M* diethanolmine, pH 9.5, 0.5 m*M* $MgCl_2$.
6. Substrate tablets: 5 mg tablets of disodium p-nitrophenyl phosphate (PNPP) (e.g., Amresco, Solon, OH, or Pierce Chemical, Rockford, IL) (*see* **Note 10**).
7. Microplate reader at 405 nm.
8. Mineral oil, blocking buffer, wash solution, and microplate shaker as above.

3. Methods

3.1. Sample Pretreatment

3.1.1. Preparation of Plasma

1. Add 10 mL of EDTA-anticoagulated whole blood to a 15 mL centrifuge tube and spin the tube with 1500*g* at 4°C for 30 min (*see* **Note 11**).

2. Aspirate the plasma carefully, avoiding thrombocytes and any white blood cells, with a 5-mL syringe fitted with a long, blunt point medical needle.
3. Remove the needle and mount a 0.8 μ*M* followed by a 0.2-μm syringe disk filter holder.
4. Mix the contents by inverting the syringe and then slowly filter the plasma in a new 15-mL centrifuge tube.
5. Distribute 0.5-mL aliquots in 1.5-mL microfuge tubes and store at –80°C (*see* **Note 12**).

3.1.2. Preparation of Virus Particles (See Note 3)

1. Thaw frozen plasma, invert the tube several times to homogenize the plasma, and spin down aggregates at full speed for 10 min to clear plasma.
2. In a 5-mL syringe equipped with a long, blunt point medical needle, aspirate first 4.5 mL PBS and then the cleared plasma without disturbing the pellet.
3. Remove the needle and mount a 0.2-μm syringe disk filter holder.
4. Mix the contents by inverting the syringe and then slowly filter the diluted plasma in an ultracentrifuge tube.
5. Weigh the closed tube and, if necessary, add sterile PBS to adjust for weight difference with a balancing tube.
6. Spin down virus in the ultracentrifuge at 4°C with 70,000*g* for 90 min.
7. Remove supernatant completely without disturbing the (often invisible) virus pellet (*see* **Note 13**).
8. Add 50 μL of virus resuspension buffer to the tube, vortex repeatedly, and transfer the resuspended virus to a microfuge tube (*see* **Note 14**).
9. Proceed directly to the PERT assay or, if necessary, store sample at –80°C.

3.2. PERT Assay (See Note 15)

3.2.1. Reverse Transcription

1. Mix in a microtube for each reaction: 0.9 μL of reverse transcription primer RT-1 (9 pmol) and 0.4 μL of MS-2 template RNA (0.28 pmol).
2. Heat tube at 95°C for 5 min, then incubate at 37°C for 30 min to allow annealing of the primer. Cool on ice before adding primer-template to the reaction mixture.
3. Mix on ice for each reaction in a total volume of 18.7 μL the following: RNase free water, 3.0 μL of 10X RT buffer, 6.0 μL of 5 m*M* dNTP mixture, 1.2 μL of 10% Triton X-100, RNase Inhibitor to 1 U/μL (*see* **Note 16**).
4. Add 1.3 μL of primer-template. The volume for each reaction should now be 20 μL.
5. Transfer 20 μL of the reaction mixture to a PCR tube and overlay with 50 μL of mineral oil (*see* **Note 17**).
6. Add 10 μL of virus supension to each tube (*see* **Note 18**).
7. Incubate at 37°C for 90 min.
8. Heat-inactivate RT and RNase inhibitor at 95°C for 5 min.
9. Proceed directly to PCR amplification or store the tubes frozen at –20°C.

3.2.2. PCR Amplification

1. Mix for each reaction: 17.3 µL of water, 2.5 µL of 10X differential amplification buffer for PERT assay, 2.6 µL of 25 m*M* Na_2-EDTA (*see* **Note 20**), 0.475 µL of primer RT-1 (4.75 pmol), 1.375 µL of primer RT-2 (13.75 pmol), 0.5 µL of 80 ng/µL RNase A (*see* **Note 19**).
2. Add for each reaction 0.25 µL of *Taq* DNA polymerase and mix well.
3. Add 25 µL of this mixture to each PCR tube and spin the tubes briefly in a microfuge.
4. Amplify the DNA for 25 cycles with a cycle profile of 94°C for 30 s, 55°C for 1 min, and 72°C for 1 min (*see* **Note 21**).

3.2.3. Detection of Amplified DNA by ELISA (See **Note 22**)

3.2.3.1. Preparation of Microtiter Plate for ELISA

1. Prepare coating solution by adding 5 µL of 10 mg/mL avidin to each milliliter of coating buffer required (final concentration 50 µg/mL).
2. Add 50 µL of coating solution per well, stir briefly on a microplate shaker, and incubate at 4°C overnight (*see* **Note 23**).
3. Aspirate coating solution, add 200 µL of blocking buffer, stir briefly on microplate shaker, and incubate at 37°C for at least 1 h.
4. Before adding the hybridized DNA (*see* **Subheading 3.2.3.2.**), remove blocking buffer and wash wells once with 200 µL of wash solution (*see* **Note 24**).

3.2.3.2. Detection of Amplified DNA Products (*See* **Note 25**)

1. Prepare the hybridization mixture by adding for each analysis: 13.5 µL of sterile water, 2.5 µL of 10X PCR buffer, 1.0 µL of each labeled oligonucleotide probe (corresponding to 0.3 pmol of RT-3-BIO and 1 pmol of RT-5-DIG), 7.0 µL of 100 m*M* Na_2-EDTA (*see* **Note 26**).
2. Add 10 µL of amplified DNA in a PCR tube (*see* **Note 27**).
3. Add 25 µL of the hybridization mixture and overlay with 25 µL of mineral oil.
4. Denature DNA at 95°C for 5 min and hybridize on thermal cycler at 45°C for 15–30 min (*see* **Note 25**).
5. Transfer the contents of the tube to a well of the coated and blocked microtiter plate (*see* **Note 28**).
6. Allow binding of the hybrids on a microplate shaker at room temperature for 15–30 min (*see* **Note 25**).
7. Aspirate the contents and wash the wells twice with 200 µL of wash solution (*see* **Note 24**).
8. Dilute the alkaline phosphatase labeled antidigoxigenin Fab fragments 1:625 (i.e., 16 µL in 10 mL) in blocking buffer and add 100 µL per well.
9. Stir briefly on the microplate shaker and incubate at 37°C for 30 min (*see* **Note 25**).
10. During antibody incubation dissolve one 5 mg tablet of PNPP in substrate buffer (*see* **Note 29**).

11. Aspirate the antibody and wash wells four times with 200 µL of wash solution (*see* **Note 24**).
12. Flick plate inversely on a dry towel to remove all residual drops of wash solution.
13. Add 50 µL of PNPP substrate solution, stir briefly on microplate shaker, and incubate at 37°C for 20 min.
14. To stop the reaction add 50 µL of 100 m*M* Na_2-EDTA, pH 8.0, stir on microplate shaker, and read absorbance with a microplate reader at 405 nm (*see* **Note 30**).

4. Notes

1. Do not use tubes of glass, polystyrene, or any material that might break during centrifugation.
2. For safety reasons, do not use sharp needles! After use, the blunt point needles are decontaminated in 1% sodium hypochlorite, rinsed with distilled water, and autoclaved.
3. Virus particles from blood plasma are concentrated by ultracentrifugation. Carry out ultracentrifugation only if you are familiar with this technique or if you have been carefully instructed how to do it. Take any precaution to avoid a laboratory disaster because of mishandling or a mishap (e.g., breakage of a tube).
4. Use an ultracentrifuge that is equipped with a sterile filter connected to the vacuum pump and that allows decontamination of the chamber by gas before the chamber has to be opened. Use a fixed angle rotor and thick walled centrifuge tubes with screw caps and O-rings. Make sure they can withstand the applied *g*-forces, even if they are only partially filled. After collecting the virus pellet, decontaminate the tubes, caps, and O-rings with a suitable disinfectant (e.g., sodium hypochloride) before washing them.
5. All reagents used for the PERT assay must be free of any contaminating MS2-DNA. To avoid carryover contamination, set up at least two different rooms for work with materials before and after PCR. Use different sets of equipment, chemicals, and disposables. If possible, avoid the use of pH probes and spatula. If glass ware is used, do not have them washed in a central facility (where it can get contaminated), wash and bake it personally (at 240°C for 5 h). It may be a good idea to have a friend at a different location (where no work with MS2 is carried out) who can prepare solutions. Use only positive displacement pipetes or pipet tips with filters especially for PCR. The published recommendations in **ref.** ***17*** are useful.
6. All solutions used for reverse transcription must be free of RNase. If all solutions are prepared with RNase-free water in disposable plastics and no contact with RNase-contaminated spatula or pH probes has occurred, the solutions need not be treated any further. Otherwise, to decontaminate the solutions add diethyl pyrocarbonate (DEPC) (e.g., Sigma, St. Louis, MO) to the solution to a final concentration of 0.1%, shake, let sit overnight with loosened caps, and then autoclave for 15 min. Note that DEPC might be carcinogenic and that solutions containing Tris cannot be decontaminated with DEPC, but must be prepared with special caution to prevent any RNase contamination.

7. The right choice of RNase inhibitor is crucial for achieving a low detection limit because it contains some contaminating RT activity. To get optimal results, test several lots before choosing the one with the lowest activity. The authors have found recombinant RNase inhibitor to be superior to the native protein.
8. Some RNase A preparations have been found to be inhibitory to PCR at comparable concentrations. This particular enzyme works fine. However, there may also be other suitable products.
9. Prepare the solution fresh each time or store aliquots frozen at –20°C. As serum for blocking nonspecific binding sites, normal goat or lamb serum can be used. Check out several batches of serum and choose the one with the best signal-to-background ratio.
10. Store tablets at –20°C. Do not touch them with bare hands.
11. If blood volumes smaller than 10 mL are handled, blood may be distributed to several microfuge tubes and the cells sedimented with 4000*g* at 4°C for 10 min.
12. If you want to proceed without freezing plasma, transfer plasma directly to 4.5 mL of PBS in an ultracentrifuge tube and go on with **step 5** in **Subheading 3.1.2.**
13. Mark the tubes before the ultracentrifugation on the outside where the pellet is expected to locate, in case the pellet remains invisible.
14. To obtain an accurate value of the RT activity, resuspend the pellet as homogeneously as possible. This will take some time.
15. In the procedure described below, the amplified DNA is detected by an ELISA. The detection limit for RT is slightly above the background of this ELISA. It must be realized that the generated signal is dependent on several variables, including incubation time or temperature for reverse transcription, the number of amplification cycles, or the source and properties of enzymes and cofactors. Therefore, to fit signals into the window provided by the ELISA, it will be necessary to adjust some of these variables.

    Like all laboratory procedures, the PERT assay requires adequate controls to assure the quality of the entire detection procedure. Negative and positive controls must be included for each step of the procedure (i.e., sample preparation, reverse transcription, PCR amplification, and detection of amplified product). In addition, to quantify RT, the PERT assay requires an activity standard.

    The authors have used two different activity standards: virus and RT standards. They have tested several viruses, but not all of them are suitable. For optimal results, make a dilution series of HIV-1 containing culture supernatant in plasma, with RNA equivalents ranging from 1 to 0.1, and 0 copies/mL. Prepare aliquots and store them at –80°C. Run a set of these dilutions with each preparation of virus particles, as described in **Subheading 3.1.2.** These samples also serve as positive and negative sample preparation controls. To prepare RT standards, commercially available RTs from Moloney murine leukemia virus, avian myeloblastosis virus, or HIV-1 can be used. Dilute the RT down to about 10^{-5} U/µL using positive displacement pipets and with the greatest possible care. Store aliquots at –80°C. The more aliquots are made, the longer the RT standard will last. For each run of the PERT assay, make a dilution series of RT ranging from approx 10^{-6} U/µL to 10^{-11} U/µL in virus resuspension buffer.

To achieve accurate results, duplicate testing of samples is highly recommended. In addition, it will be necessary to dilute resuspended virus with high levels of RT activity because the ELISA method provides only a limited dynamic range. In some specimens, the resuspended virus contains inhibitors of the assay. To identify these specimens and to avoid significant underestimates of RT activity, a second set of reactions is run to which a defined amount of purified RT is added.

16. This mixture, without the RNase inhibitor, can be prepared in advance and stored at –80°C for at least 3 mo.
17. As an alternative, heat-resistant microtiter plates and corresponding thermal cycling machines can be used. This increases the capacity of reactions that can be analyzed and allows easy transfer of samples with a multichannel pipet after amplification.
18. Virus is added last to prevent contamination from one sample to the next. If this can be ruled out, virus may be added first, followed by the reaction mixture and mineral oil.
19. This mixture, without *Taq* DNA polymerase, can be prepared in advance and stored at –80°C for at least 6 mo. *Taq* DNA polymerase is added immediately before dispensing.
20. The concentration of free magnesium is adjusted to 1 m*M*.
21. The holding times of this cycle profile are not optimized, but can be shortened. Optimal holding times are dependent on the type of temperature (external or internal thermal probes) and time control (the clock usually starts below or above the holding temperature and the exact temperature difference varies among different models of the thermal cycling machines).
22. Amplified DNA is identified by solution hybridization of two nonisotopically labeled oligonucleotides to one strand of the amplified DNA. Following hybrid formation DNA is bound to a solid phase and detected by enzyme-labeled specific antibodies. Because only one strand is used for detection, the other one is washed off and constitutes the main source of laboratory contamination and carryover. Take precautions to avoid the spread of these molecules to other rooms (e.g., work in a chemical fume hood, decontaminate used wash buffer with acid or sodium hypochloride, and so on).
23. Wells can also be coated at 37°C for 1 h.
24. All wash steps are performed manually because the authors have found that manual washing is most effective. If ELISA washer is used the number of wash cycles must be increased.
25. Concentrations of oligonucleotide probes and antibody, hybridization temperature, and incubation times correspond to those used in the authors' laboratory. However, it may be necessary to optimize each of these parameters, with those given in the protocol serving as a good starting point. For oligonucleotide probes, the authors have found 1 pmol of each as a universally suitable concentration.
26. This mixture can be prepared in advance and stored frozen at –20°C.
27. Denaturation and hybridization can also be carried out in heat-resistant microtiter plates on corresponding dry heat blocks or thermal cycling machines. This

increases the capacity of reactions that can be analyzed and allows easy transfer of samples after hybridization with a multichannel pipet.

28. The aqueous phase can be transferred together with the mineral oil. The oil does not interfere with binding if you carry out binding on a microplate shaker.
29. It may take a few minutes to dissolve the tablet. Therefore, make sure the PNPP has dissolved completely and is mixed homogeneously before adding the substrate solution to the well.
30. In case a low signal-to-background ratio is encountered in the analysis, the following hints may help to solve problems.
    a. A high background is the result of nonspecific binding of individual reaction components (digoxigenin-labeled probe or the antibody) to the solid phase. First, try to increase the time for blocking the solid phase. Nonspecific binding of oligonucleotide probes can also be reduced by the addition of up to 1 μg single-stranded DNA (e.g., salmon sperm DNA or random oligonucleotides) to the hybridization reaction. Finally, try different sera. Some are simply not suitable for blocking.
    b. A low specific signal can occur if (in sequential order) the hybrid is not formed, if the binding of the hybrid or of the antibody is insufficient, or by inactivation of one of the functional components. Begin with the last step to localize and solve the problem.
    c. Insufficient specific binding of the hybrid can result from incomplete biotin labeling of the probe (use only probes that are purified by high-performance liquid chromatography or by polyacrylamide gel electrophoresis) or from a too high concentration of biotin-labeled probe (the number of binding sites is limited and excess free biotin-labeled probe will outcompete the hybrid). Low specific antibody binding can be the result of incomplete digoxigenin labeling of the probe *(see above)* or a too low concentration of the digoxigenin-labeled probe. Finally, it should be noted that some sera interfere with antibody binding and must simply be replaced.
    d. Insufficient formation of the hybrid is the least likely of all possible reasons for low signal-to background ratio. It is the result of incomplete denaturation (control the temperature and allow sufficient time for denaturation) or of competition by side products from the amplification process (check on an agarose gel).

References

1. Stromberg, K., Hurley, N. E., Davis, N. L., Rueckert, R. R., and Fleissner, E. (1974) Structural studies of avian myeloblastosis virus: comparison of polypeptides in virion and core component by dodecyl sulfate-polyacrylamide gel electrophoresis. *J. Virol.* **13,** 513–528.
2. Panet, A., Baltimore, D., and Hanafusa, T. (1975) Quantitation of avian RNA tumor virus reverse transcriptase by radioimmunoassay. *J. Virol.* **16,** 146–152.
3. Krakower, J. M., Barbacid, M., and Aaronson, S. A. (1977) Radioimmunoassay for mammalian type C viral reverse transcriptase. *J. Virol.* **22,** 331–339.

4. Coffin, J. M. (1996). Retroviridae: The viruses and their replication, in *Fields Virology* 3rd ed. (Fields, B. N., Knipe, D. M., Howley, P. M., et al., eds.), Lippincott-Raven, Philadelphia, PA, pp. 1767–1847.
5. Schüpbach, J. and Böni, J. (1993) Verfahren zum Nachweis reverser Transcriptase (Process for detecting reverse transcriptase). 118 pp, 25 figs., PCT International Office Publication Nr. WO 93/23560.
6. Silver, J., Maudru, T., Fujita, K., and Repaske, R. (1993) An RT-PCR assay for the enzyme activity of reverse transcriptase capable of detecting single virions. *Nucleic Acids Res.* **21,** 3593,3594.
7. Heneine, W., Yamamoto, S., Switzer, W. M., Spira, T. J., and Folks, T. M. (1995) Detection of reverse transcriptase by a highly sensitive assay in sera from persons infected with human immunodeficiency virus type 1. *J. Inf. Dis.* **171,** 1210–1216.
8. Pyra, H., Böni, J., and Schüpbach, J. (1994) Ultrasensitive retrovirus detection by a reverse transcriptase assay based on product enhancement. *Proc. Natl. Acad. Sci. USA* **91,** 1544–1548.
9. Böni, J., Pyra, H., and Schüpbach, J. (1996) Sensitive detection and quantification of particle-associated reverse transcriptase in plasma of HIV-1 infected individuals by the product-enhanced reverse transcriptase assay. *J. Med. Virol.* **49,** 23–28.
10. Weissmahr, R. N., Schüpbach, J., and Böni, J. (1997) Reverse transcriptase activity in chicken embryo fibroblast culture supernatants is associated with particles containing EAV-0 (endogenous avian retrovirus) RNA. *J. Virol.* **71,** 3005–3012.
11. Conrad, B., Weissmahr, R. N., Böni, J., Arcari, R., Schüpbach, J., and Mach, B. (1997) A human endogenous retroviral superantigen as candidate autoimmune-gene in type 1 diabetes. *Cell* **90,** 303–313.
12. Schüpbach, J., Pyra, H., Jendis, J., Tomasik, Z., and Böni, J. (1996) Isolation of an in vitro transmissible agent with reverse transcriptase activity from a blood donor with a borderline-positive HIV-1 serology for more than five years. *Clin. Diagn. Virol.* **5,** 197–203.
13. Griffiths, D. J., Venables, P. J. W., Weiss, R. A., and Boyd, M. D. (1997) A novel exogenous retrovirus sequence identified in humans. *J. Virol.* **71,** 2866–2872.
14. Böni, J., Opravil, M., Tomasik, Z., Rothen, M., Bisset, L., Grob, P. J., Lüthy, R., and Schüpbach, J. (1997) Simple monitoring of antiretroviral therapy with a signal-amplification–boosted human immunodeficiency virus type 1 p24 antigen assay with heat-denatured plasma. *AIDS* **11,** F47–F52.
15. Böni, J., Stalder, J., Reigel, F., and Schüpbach, J. (1996) Detection of reverse transcriptase activity in live attenuated virus vaccines. *Clin. Diagn. Virol.* **5,** 43–53.
16. Alaeus, A., Lidman, K., Sönnerborg, A., and Albert, J. (1997) Subtype-specific problems with quantification of plasma HIV-1 RNA. *AIDS* **11,** 859–865.
17. Kwok, S. and Higuchi, R. (1989) Avoiding false positives with PCR. *Nature* **339,** 237,238.

25

Identifying and Characterizing HIV Protease Inhibitors

Eric S. Furfine

1. Introduction

HIV protease catalyzes the hydrolysis of specific peptide bonds of viral polyproteins, thus processing these polyproteins into their active components. These protein processing reactions are requisite for viral replication. Therefore, the HIV protease is an ideal target for the chemotherapeutic treatment of HIV disease *(1–3)*. HIV protease is an aspartyl protease, and the aspartyl protease inhibitor, pepstatin, was one of the first identified inhibitors of HIV protease. More potent inhibitors have been designed and synthesized since, in fact, four protease inhibitors—saquinavir (Ro-31,8959), ritonavir (ABT-538), indinavir (L-735,524), and Nelfinavir (AG1343)—are effective in clinical trials to treat HIV disease *(4–6)* and recently were approved by the Food and Drug Administration for the chemotherapeutic treatment of HIV infections. Other protease inhibitors in clinical trials are VX-478 (141W94) and ABT-378. Notwithstanding these early successes, it is difficult to comply with these drug's dosing regiments. Furthermore, viral resistance to individual inhibitors and cross-resistance to multiple inhibitors occur in vivo *(7,8)*. Therefore, a medical need still exists for new HIV protease inhibitors with different resistance profiles.

Although many of the HIV protease substrates in vivo are large molecular weight polyproteins, HIV protease is capable of efficiently hydrolyzing some polypeptide substrates as small as hexapeptides. Fluorescence-based substrates, such as the one described herein *(9)*, were thus designed to take advantage of this substrate specificity. Fluorescence-based assays are among the most commonly utilized assays for HIV protease, and in many cases, these assays utilize fluorescence energy transfer techniques (**Fig. 1**). In this example of fluorescence energy transfer, the p-NO_2-phenylalanine has fluorescence at a wave-

From: *Methods in Molecular Medicine, vol. 24: Antiviral Methods and Protocols*
Edited by: D. Kinchington and R. F. Schinazi © Humana Press Inc., Totowa, NJ

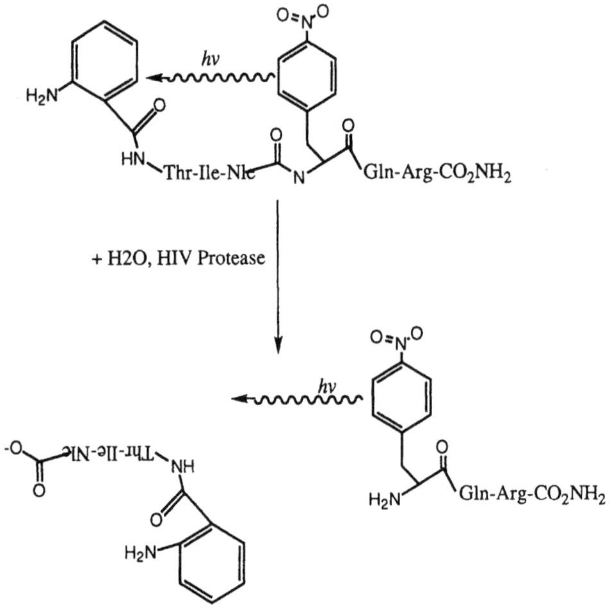

Fig. 1. Fluorescence-based assay of HIV protease: the fluorescence energy transfer technique. Nle is norleucine. The top squiggly line indicates that fluorescent light emmitted by the nitorphenylalanine is absorbed by the aminobenzoyl group. The bottom squiggly line indicates that the light no longer is absorbed by the aminobenzoyl group because it has rotated away and has begun to dissociate.

length where a nearby quenching group (2-amino benzoyl) can absorb the emitted light. Because the 2-amino benzoyl moiety and the p-NO_2-phenyl moiety are on the same molecule, and in relatively close proximity, the fluorescence of the p-NO_2-phenyl moiety is drastically quenched by the 2-amino benzoyl moiety. When the substrate in hydrolyzed, the 2-amino benzoyl group is no longer in close proximity, as it can diffuse away, and the fluorescence of the p-NO_2-phenyl moiety is not quenched significantly. For example, with this substrate, observe the five- to sixfold increase in fluorescence is observed on substrate hydrolysis.

There are other examples of HIV protease substrates that utilize the fluorescence energy transfer technique. Perhaps the strongest characteristic of these assays is that they provide a continuous readout of enzyme activity. Another advantage is their sensitivity (they use small concentrations of enzyme). The disadvantage of these assays is that they are susceptible to interference by some compounds (inhibition artifacts) because of inner and outer filter effects (*see* **Notes 8–10**). Other assays, for example, those based on radioactivity or high-performance liquid chromatography (HPLC) analysis of products are tedious to run, but are less susceptible to interference or inhibition artifacts.

The fluorescence-based assay described herein is used to screen large libraries of compounds, in 96-well format, for the ability to inhibit HIV protease and to accurately determine the affinity of identified inhibitors for the enzyme. Much of the discussion in this section will be widely applicable to fluorescence-based assays and enzyme assays in general. Because numerous potent inhibitors of HIV protease have been identified, part of this procedure outlines the analysis required to deal with these potent compounds. Like any enzyme assay, preparing this assay for routine use can be divided into three parts: (1) determination of an appropriate enzyme concentration for assay, (2) determination of the substrate concentration dependence (K_m and V_{max}), and (3) determination of inhibitor concentration dependence (IC_{50} and K_i values). Parts one and two do not need to be repeated every time inhibitor assays are run—only once to check new batches of enzyme or to "troubleshoot" any problems with the assay.

2. Materials

2.1. Equipment

1. PerSeptive Biosystems (Framingham, MA) 96-well fluorescence plate reader with a 320 ± 20 nm excitation filter (made by reversing the respective emission filter) and a 420 ± 20 nm emission filter (or any other equivalent fluorescence plate reader and filters).
2. 12-channel pipeters (5–40 µL and 40–250 µL ranges or similar).
3. 96-well, polypropylene round-bottomed plates (Costar 3794).
4. 96-well, flat-bottomed fluorescence reader plates (PerSeptive Biosystems CFCPN9650).
5. Reservoirs for multichannel pipetting of buffers and so forth (Costar, Cambridge, MA).

2.2. Software

1. Microsoft Excel or Sigma Plot (Jandel Scientific, Corte Madera, CA) or any database software that allows curve fitting.

2.3. Materials

1. Stock substrate solution of 10 m*M* 2-aminobenzoyl-Thr-Ile-Nle-Phe(NO_2)-Gln-Arg-NH_2 (commercially available custom peptide synthesis), 5 mg in dimethyl sulfoxide (DMSO) 500 µL.
2. MES (0.5 *M*, pH 5.5) is prepared by dissolving 49.5 g MES (Sigma, St. Louis, MO) and 5 g NaOH in 400 mL water. The pH is adjusted to 5.5 with concentrated NaOH (5 *M* or greater) and the volume brought to 500 mL with water. The final solution is filtered through sterile 0.22 µm filters for storage.
3. Enzyme stock solution can be purchased from Bachem Bioscience (Torrance, CA) or prepared as described (*see* **ref. *10***). The author's stock solutions typically contained 100 m*M* sodium MES, pH 6.5, 10% glycerol, 5% ethylene glycol, and 50 m*M* dithiothreitol (DTT); and were stable for more than 1 yr at –70°C. Stock

concentration is 6 μ*M* active sites (≥0.12 mg/mL protein). (Determination of active site concentration is described in **Subheading 3.**) Any stock solution >0.5 μ*M* active sites provided in the commercially available buffer should be fine.

4. Enzyme working solution is prepared by diluting the stock solution of enzyme (6 μ*M*) 1:600 into cold (on an ice bath) enzyme dilution buffer (100 m*M* MES at pH 5.5, 400 m*M* NaCl, 0.2% PEG-8000, prepared analogously to assay buffer). The working solution is stored on ice and should be used within 10 min of dilution of the stock.
5. Assay buffer with substrate contains 2-aminobenzoyl-Thr-Ile-Nle-Phe(NO_2)-Gln-Arg-NH_2 (10 μ*M*) in 100 m*M* MES at pH 5.5, 400 m*M* NaCl, 0.2% PEG-8000, and 2.5% DMSO. To make the solution, 50 μL of 10 m*M* substrate stock is diluted into 1.2 mL of DMSO. To the diluted substrate is added 10 mL of 0.5 *M* MES, 10 mL of 4 *M* NaCl, 250 μL of 40% PEG-8000, and the volume is increased to 50 mL with filtered (0.22 μm) water. The solution is typically good for several days if stored at room temperature.
6. Inhibitor solutions (in DMSO).

3. Method

3.1. Determining a Working Enzyme Solution

1. Set up key parameters of the fluorescence plate reader: time to read plate = 3 min; 12 readings of the plate, gain = 90, reads/well = 42. Other fluorometers may have other parameters or different scales. The key is that an instrument must be set such that (1) 200 μL of a 10 μ*M*, substrate must give a measurable signal above background, (2) the machine must be able to also detect fluorescence five- to sixfold above this level without saturating the detection technology, and (3) the machine must completely read the plate at these settings within 3 min.
2. At least 4 mL of assay buffer with substrate is placed into a reservoir (to be used later).
3. Enzyme dilution buffer (10 μL) is pipeted into wells A1–A12 of a flat-bottomed, 96-well fluorescence plate. Enzyme stock solution (10 μL if ≤ 0.2 mg/mL protein) is diluted into well A1, and then 10 μL from well A1 is threefold serially diluted through well A12.
4. Using a 12-channel pipeter, 190 μL of buffer is transferred simultaneously to each of wells A1–A12.
5. The plate is then placed in the fluorescence plate reader and data collection is initiated. Twelve readings are collected (one every 3 min) over a total of approx 33 min.
6. For an appropriate enzyme concentration, the fluorescence increase should be linear with time (over the 33 min of the assay) and no more than 20% of the substrate should be utilized (*see* **Subheading 3.4.** for additional details). Typically, if the listed filters are used on the noted fluorometer, there is a five- to sixfold increase in fluorescence when the substrate is completely hydrolyzed to products. The test for a given system is to add a large amount of enzyme to a substrate solution to completely hydrolyze it. Then, using equal volumes and concentrations of components, measure the fluorescence of hydrolyzed substrate

($F[p]$)) of buffer alone ($F[b]$) and of substrate ($F[s]$). $[F(p) - F(b)]/[F(s) - F(b)] = Q$, where Q is the fluorescence delta extinction coefficient, which should approximate five. If Q is not ≥ 4 in the system, enough enzyme may not have been added, or suffiecient time may not have elapsed to complete hydrolysis, or better filters for the instrument or a different instrument may be needed. To test the percent of substrate hydrolyzed, measure the change in fluorescence over the reaction time (dF). $100 \cdot (dF/Q)$ = the percent of substrate hydrolysis.

3.2. Determination of K_m for Substrate

1. Set up plate reader (*see* **Subheading 3.1.**).
2. To a polypropylene COSTAR plate, wells A1–H1, add 12.5 µL of 800, 700, 600, 500, 400, 300, 200, and 100 µ*M* fluorescent substrate in DMSO. Repeat procedure for wells A2–H2. These stock substrate concentrations are diluted 1:20 in the assay.
3. At least 4 mL of enzyme dilution buffer (which serves as the assay buffer here) is placed into a reservoir. Then, using 8 tips on a 12-channel pipeter, 240 µL of buffer is transferred simultaneously to each of wells A1–H1 and mixed by pipetting up and down, and then A2–H2 and mixed.
4. Enzyme working solution (10 µL, as determined *above* or as specified by the "reagents and solutions") is pipeted into wells A1–H1 and A2–H2 of a flat-bottomed, 96-well fluorescence plate. Using 8 tips on a 12-channel pipeter, 190 µL of substrate solutions in the polypropylene plate are transferred simultaneously to the corresponding well of the fluorescence plate with enzyme.
5. The plate is then placed in the fluorescence plate reader and data collection is initiated. Twelve readings are collected (one every 3 min) over a total of approx 33 min.
6. The rates of product formation (fluorescence/s) are plotted vs final substrate concentration and fitted to the Michaelis Menten equation, as described in **Subheading 3.4.**

3.3. Screening Inhibitors

1. Set up plate reader (*see* **Subheading 3.1.**).
2. To a polypropylene plate, wells A1–H1, add 200 µL of any eight inhibitor solutions at 2 m*M* in DMSO. To the remaining wells of the plate, add 140 µL of DMSO. Serially dilute 70 µL of the 400 µ*M* inhibitor solutions threefold (using eight tips on a 12-channel pipeter), leaving the last column (A12–H12) as DMSO alone (these wells will serve as "no inhibitor" controls). This plate is a reservoir of stock inhibitor dilution solutions that can be used multiple times if stored frozen. Using a 2 m*M* stock solution of inhibitor gives a 50 µ*M* in the assay as highest concentration of inhibitor. One may want to start with lower stock concentrations if you are screening a series in which molecules with similar structures have known activity. Furthermore, one may want to use twofold dilutions instead of threefold dilutions to cover the appropriate range more carefully. A last scenario is testing potent inhibitors, such as 141W94; one may want to start with a high stock concentration of 40–60 n*M* (2–3 n*M* final concentration) and

serial dilute by 1.5-fold. Finally, replicates of any given compound typically are not tested because there are already 12 data points for each titration curve using this method.

3. Transfer 5.5 µL from all wells of the polypropylene plate with DMSO solutions to a fresh polypropylene plate. Fill a reservoir with at least 25 mL of assay buffer with substrate. To all the wells of the new plate, add 215 µL of assay buffer with substrate and mix. This procedure dilutes the inhibitors 1:40.
4. Fill a reservoir with 2 mL of enzyme working solution. Then, using a 12-channel pipetter, add 10 µL to all wells of a flat-bottomed, 96-well fluorescence plate. Using a 12-channel pipeter, 190 µL of substrate/inhibitor solutions in the polypropylene plate are transferred simultaneously to the corresponding well of the fluorescence plate with enzyme.
5. The plate is then placed in the fluorescence plate reader and data collection is initiated. Twelve readings are collected (one every 3 min) over a total of approx 33 min.
6. The rates of product formation (fluorescence/s) are plotted vs final inhibitor concentration and fitted to the appropriate equation, as described in **Subheading 4.7.**

3.4. Data Analysis

3.4.1. Rates of Substrate Hydrolysis

1. The first step to analyze the data from any part of the basic protocol is to transfer the data from the fluorometer to an appropriate software, such as Excel. Usually the manufacturer of the fluorometer can help with this process. Sometimes the instrument comes with software to complete the analysis described in **step 2**. Ultimately, what is wanted is a series of fluorescence values from all given wells plotted vs time.
2. Using the selected software, fit the parameters of a line (fluorescence = slope·t + intercept). The slope that best fits the data is proportional to the rate of substrate hydrolysis in that well. The value obtained for the slope will have units of fluorescence/time (e.g., fluorescence U/s). It is the author's experience that fluorescence increases linearly with time for approx 30 min if not more than 20% of the substrate is hydrolyzed over that time course (*see* **step 6** of **Subheading 3.1.**). However, if fluorescence is not linear for the whole time course, one must pick a range of time points to fit where fluorescence increase is linear with time. All analyses discussed herein require the use of initial rates, which are defined as the range of data where product formation is linear with time.
3. Fluorescence values are converted into molar units by using the Q value determined in **step 6** of the **Subheading 3**. In our case, the Q value has units of fluorescence U/10 µM of substrate converted to product. This conversion is important for determining kcat values (turnover number for the enzyme) from V_{max} values, but is not necessary to determine K_m, IC_{50}, or K_i values.

3.4.2. Selecting a Working Enzyme Concentration

1. Fit data to obtain the rates of substrate hydrolysis (**Subheading 3.4.1.**).
2. Select the concentration of enzyme that resulted in <20% of the substrate hydrolyzed over the time course of the assay (this is usually a requirement to keep

product formation linear with time at any substrate concentration above or below the K_m value). Typically, at least 10% of the substrate must be hydrolyzed to give a sufficient signal (rate of hydrolysis) to accurately measure inhibition of this signal. Remember to determine the kinetic parameters for inhibitors (IC_{50} or K_i values). One must be able to accurately measure rates of hydrolysis significantly less than the control (uninhibited) rate of substrate hydrolysis. For example, it is best to be able to accurately measure rates that are 10% or less of the control (uninhibited) rate.

3.4.3. Determining the Kinetic Constants (e.g., K_m) for the Fluorescent Substrate

1. Determine the rates of product formation (fluorescence/s) at each substrate concentration. If done as described in **Subheading 3.**, the experiment will have been done in duplicate.
2. Plot the rates of product formation vs [substrate] and fit **Eq. 1** (the Michaelis Menten equation) to the data:

$$V = V_{max} \cdot [S/(S + K_m)] \tag{1}$$

Where V is the rate of substrate hydrolysis at a given substrate concentration (S), V_{max} is the maximal rate of substrate hydrolysis (a constant), and K_m (another constant) is the concentration of substrate that gives one-half the maximal rate of hydrolysis. Under the present conditions of the assay, the K_m value for this substrate is 16 μM.

3.4.4. Characterizing Inhibiton of HIV Protease

1. Rates of substrate hydrolysis (**Subheading 3.3.1.**) are plotted vs concentration of inhibitors. Typically, the average of the eight control (uninhibited) rates in each fit is used (data from column 12 of a full microtiter plate). The uninhibited velocity is a limiting value, and it is useful to have several values averaged to define it. This value is particularly important when using **Eq. 4** in which the uninhibited rate is used to normalize all values (*see* **step 4**).
2. Some concentrations of inhibitors reduce the rate of product formation so little that there is a slight negative drift of fluorescence that results in a small negative slope (rate). It is best to eliminate negative rates from the fit, or set them equal to zero.
3. **Eq. 2** is fit to each data set, where V is the rate of substrate hydrolysis, $[I]$ is the concentration of inhibitor, V_0 is the uninhibited rate of hydrolysis (a constant in this case), and IC_{50} (another constant) is the concentration of inhibitor that results in one-half the uninhibited rate.

$$V = V_0 \cdot IC_{50}/([I] + IC_{50}) \tag{2}$$

K_i values were calculated from IC_{50} values (**Eq. 3**). Data from the inhibition of HIV protease by pepstatin illustrate typical results (**Fig. 2A**).

$$K_i = IC_{50}/\{1 + [S]/K_m\} \tag{3}$$

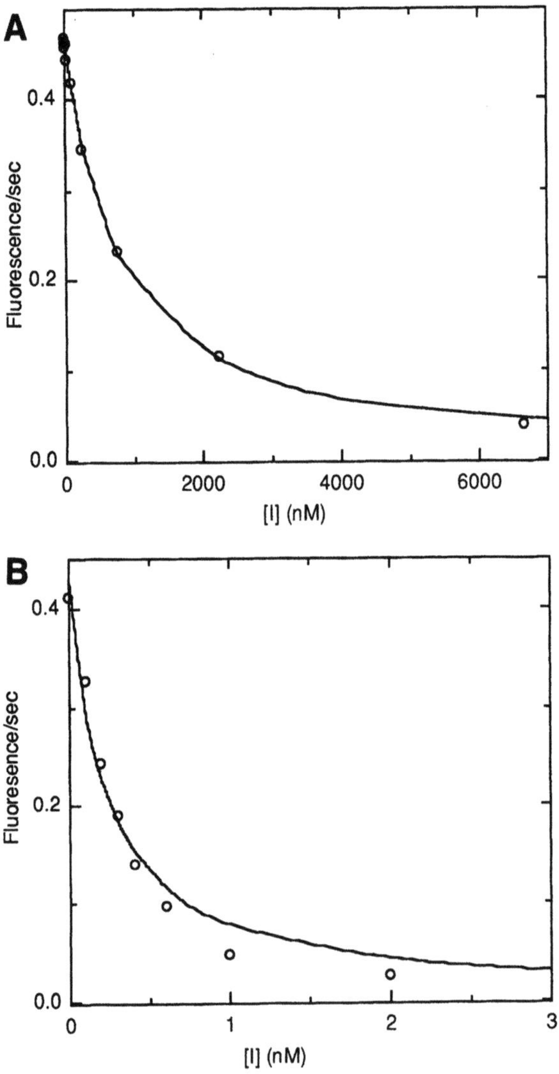

Fig. 2. Inhibition of HIV protease with pepstatin and 141W94. **(A)** The solid line is the fit of **Eq. 2** to the data with an IC_{50} value of 700 ± 20. **(B)** The solid line is the fit of **Eq. 2** to the data with an IC_{50} value of 0.22 ± 0.003.

4. Sometimes inhibitors are extremely potent and have IC_{50} values that are similar to or smaller than the enzyme concentration in the assay (0.5–1 n*M* in our case). In these cases, it is not possible to use **Eq. 2** to fit the data effectively (*see* **Notes 14–17**). Instead, **Eq. 4** is used to fit the data, where *F* is the fraction of enzyme bound to inhibitor [F =1 – (V_{inh}/V_0), where V_{inh} is the steady-state velocity in the presence of inhibitor and V_0 is the velocity of uninhibited enzyme], IC_{50} is the concentration of inhibitor that binds 50% of the enzyme if the enzyme concentra-

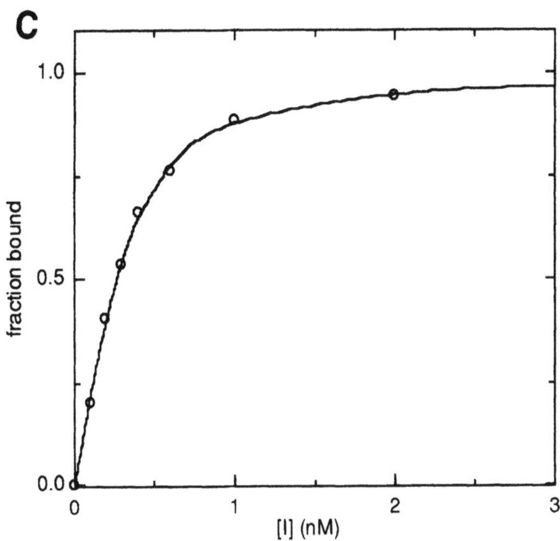

Fig. 2 *(continued)*. Inhibition of HIV protease with pepstatin and 141W94. **(C)** The solid line is the fit of **Eq. 4** to the data with $IC_{50} = 0.096 \pm 0.007$ n*M* and $[E] = 0.34 \pm 0.002$ n*M*.

tion could be much less than the IC_{50}, $[E]$ is the total active site concentration of enzyme, and $[I]$ is the total concentration of inhibitor.

$$F = \frac{[I] + [E] + IC_{50} - \{([I] + [E] + IC_{50})^2 - 4 \cdot [I] \cdot [E]\}^{1/2}}{2[E]} \quad (4)$$

5. Example results of a tight-binding inhibitor (141W94) are shown in **Fig. 2B, C**. Once again, K_i values were calculated from IC_{50} values using **Eq. 3**. Note that the fit of **Eq. 4** to the data results in an estimate of the enzyme active site concentration. This is the most useful way to determine active enzyme concentration (as opposed to protein concentrations, *see* **Subheading 4.**).

4. Notes

4.1. Low Substrate Concentration

1. Low substrate concentrations are defined relative to the K_m for the substrate. In this case, low substrate concentrations would be <16 μ*M*, or less than the K_m. At low substrate concentrations, most of the enzyme is not bound up by substrate at any point in the assay.
2. Typically, the author likes to operate screens for inhibitors using low substrate concentrations because most of the enzyme is "free" or unbound. This means that one is close to observing a direct interaction of enzyme and inhibitor, rather than a competition between substrate and inhibitor for the enzyme. With less competition with substrate, one is more likely to discover a lead molecule (one can identify weaker inhibitors as starting leads).

3. Low substrate concentrations also help to evaluate tight-binding inhibitors. Tight-binding inhibitors work at lower concentrations and take longer times (sometimes minutes) to reach steady-state. Using low substrate concentrations minimizes the time to reach steady-state. The concepts of slow-, tight-binding inhibitors are reviewed ***(11)***.
4. This fluorogenic substrate has an apparent solubility limit of approx 30–40 μ*M*, yet another reason to keep the substrate concentration low. Solutions of 10 μ*M* substrate in assay buffer can be stored at room temperature for a week or more, but cooling the solution or raising the substrate concentration much will likely result in precipitation over time.

4.2. Inhibitor Screening Strategies

5. When trying to identify a lead inhibitor for an enzyme, typically a diverse chemical library is screened for enzyme inhibition at a single enzyme concentration. Subsequently, any "active" molecules are analyzed for potency (and prioritized) by monitoring the concentration dependence of the inhibition.
6. Often, one is studying an enzyme with known inhibitors and inhibitor "scaffolds." A scaffold is a core part of the molecule that binds an enzyme or receptor. Additions and modifications of the scaffold change the binding properties and biological activity of the scaffold. In this case, very few molecules tested will be inactive (since analog inhibitors are based on an "active" scaffold). Therefore, it is more time efficient to examine the concentration dependence in the initial assay rather than first to screen for activity and then "titrate." The method described in **Subheading 3.3.** details a method to determine the concentration dependence of an inhibitor. The data obtained from this method can is sufficient to estimate the affinities of moderate- and tight-binding inhibitors.
7. A simple modification of the assay in **Subheading 3.3.** allows the screening of diverse chemical libraries at a single inhibitor concentration. The only change is that all wells of the plate that were to contain dilutions of 8 given inhibitors now contain 84 inhibitors at one fixed concentration.

4.3. Fluorescence Quenching and Inhibition Artifacts

8. One disadvantage of this assay, and any fluorescence-based assay, is that some compounds quench the fluorescence of the substrate and appear to inhibit the enzyme activity even though they are not binding the enzyme. Quenching the substrate fluorescence can occur two ways: (1) as inner filter effects and (2) as outer filter effects. Inner filter effects occur when the compound absorbs in the same wavelength range that the substrate does. If the compound absorbs much of the light, then there is no light to be absorbed by the substrate, and then the substrate fluorescence is quenched. An outer filter effect occurs when the compound absorbs light at the wavelength of the substrate fluorescence. In this case, the compound absorbs the fluorescent light that does not reach the detector, and the substrate fluorescence is quenched.
9. Both inner and outer filter effects are monitored simply be observing the fluorescence of the substrate (without enzyme!) in the presence and absence of com-

pound. If the substrate fluorescence is quenched by the compound, then there is an inner or outer filter effect. When there is have an inner or outer filter effect, it is possible (perhaps likely) that the compound does not bind the enzyme. *All compounds that appear to inhibit the enzyme in this assay should be tested for inner and outer filter effects.*

10. It is possible to minimze or sometimes eliminate inner and outer filter effects by lowering the compound concentration until the substrate fluorescence is not quenched (this may or may not be practical). Alternatively, an assay that is not fluorescence based (e.g., HPLC-based detection) does not have inner and outer filter effects.

4.4. Enzyme Dissociation

11. HIV protease is a homodimer of 10 kDa subunits. The active site is formed across the interface of the two subunits. Therefore, the dimeric structure is required for activity and monomer subunits are inactive.
12. The enzyme dissociates to some degree during an assay, depending on the final conditions *(12)*. Observation of nonlinear kinetics (decay of enzyme activity over the time course) in the uninhibited enzyme assays may be the result of enzyme dissociation.
13. The dissociation of the dimer to inactive monomers is what limits the concentration of enzyme used in the assay. Typically, dissociation can be limited by increasing salt concentrations (e.g., NaCl 400–000 m*M*), increasing enzyme concentration, lower pHs (4.0–5.5), PEG-8000 (0.1–0.3%), and/or BSA (1 mg/mL).

4.5. Tight-Binding Inhibitors and Active Site Concentrations

14. When inhibitors have binding constants (K_i or IC_{50} values) that are similar to or smaller than the enzyme active site concentration, the kinetic data must be fit by the quadratic equation (**Eq. 4**). **Eq. 4** is used because the assumptions that were made to derive the standard hyperbolic equation (**Eq. 2**) are violated by potent inhibitors. For example, **Eq. 2** assumes that the enzyme concentration is much smaller than the inhibitor concentration, such that the amount of *E-I* complex does not significantly effect total [*I*]. If the IC_{50} value is 0.5 n*M*, then one would need to measure kinetic data near 0.5 n*M*, which is roughly equivalent to [*E*] in the author's assay. This requirement clearly violates the [*I*] >>> [*E*] assumption. Furthermore, if an IC_{50} value were 0.1 n*M* (or less), most inhibitor molecules added to a reaction containing 1 n*M* enzyme would be bound to enzyme because the [*E*] is higher than the IC_{50} value. Thus, the inhibitor would "titrate" active sites.
15. **Eq. 4** is derived based on an exact solution to the binding equation for *E* and *I*. Thus, the fit of **Eq. 4** to inhibition data results in an estimate of both [*E*] and IC_{50} value. The kinetics of tight-binding inhibitors are presented in more detail in **ref.** ***12***.
16. How does one know when to use **Eq. 4**? In general, in the absence of any other information, the best method to determine whether **Eq. 4** should be used is to compare the fit of **Eq. 4** to the fit of **Eq. 2**. If **Eq. 2** does not result in a good fit of the data, e.g., big errors in the IC_{50} value (>40%) or if the fitted curve does not go through many of the data points, try **Eq. 4**. Furthermore, if it is appropriate to use

Table 1
Typical Results of Tight-Binding and Weaker Inhibitors

Compound	K_i (nM)
Pepstatin	500 ± 20
141W94	0.066 ± 0.006
Indinavir	0.24 ± 0.06
Saquinavir	0.033 ± 0.005
Ritonavir	0.012 ± 0.003
AG 1343	0.31 ± 0.06

Eq. 4, the fit of **Eq. 2** will usually result in an IC_{50} value at least five- to 10-fold larger than that from **Eq. 4** and the IC_{50} value of **Eq. 2** will often approximate $[E]$ from **Eq. 4** (within two- to threefold). However, if the fit of **Eq. 4** results in $[E] <<<$ IC_{50} value, then **Eq. 4** is not to be used. Examples of "borderline cases" usually result in IC_{50} values from either fit being similar (within two- to threefold).

17. Protein concentrations do not necessarily accurately estimate active sites, even when proteins are pure based on sodium dodecyl sulfate-polyacrylamide gel electrophoresis. Typically, protein concentrations yield upper estimates of active site concentrations. The best method to determine active sites is based on an activity, such as inhibitor binding. Therefore, tight-binding inhibitors are often the best method to determine the active site concentration of an enzyme. As a general rule, the best estimates of active site concentration come when the maximal enzyme concentration used in the assay is at least five- to 10-fold greater than the inhibitor IC_{50} value.

4.6. Other Conditions and Variations

18. This assay works well over a variety of pH values (4.0–6.5) with a variety of buffers, including MES, citrate, and acetate. It is also possible to vary the salt concentration.
19. In recent times, HIV protease with mutations that confer resistance to protease inhibitors have been examined ***(10)***. This assay works for these mutant proteases as well. However, typically these mutant proteases have reduced catalytic efficiency with this substrate and require higher (10-fold or more) enzyme concentrations to see activity.

4.7. Data Analysis and Typical Results

20. The procedures include the equations used and some recommended software to fit the equations to the data. While this set of procedures is not the only way to analyze the data, it has been found to be the most useful and flexible. For example, there are software programs available for fitting enzyme kinetic data; however; the generic software mentioned in **Subheading 2.** works well.
21. **Table 1** shows some typical results (K_i values) of tight-binding and weaker inhibitors.

References

1. Huff, J. R. (1991) HIV protease: A novel chemotherapeutic target for AIDS. *J. Med. Chem.* **34,** 2305–2314.
2. Norbeck, D. W. and Kempf, D. J., (1991) in *Annual Reports in Medicinal Chemistry* (Bristol, J. A., ed.), Academic, San Diego, pp. 141–150.
3. Dark, P. L. and Huff, J. R. (1994) HIV protease as an inhibitor target of the treatment of AIDS. *Adv. Pharmacol.* **25,** 399–454.
4. Jacobsen, H., Brun-Vezinet, F., Duncan, I., Hanggi, M., Ott, M., Vella, S., Weber, J., and Mous, J. (1994) Genotypic characterizations of HIV-1 from patients aftger prolonged treatment withproteinase inhibitor saquinavir, in *III International Workshop on HIV Drug-Resistance,* **3,** p. 16.
5. Ho, D. D., Neumann, A. V., Perelson, A. S., Chen, W., Leonard, J. M., and Markowitz, M. (1995) Rapid turnover of plama virions and CD4 lymphocytes in HIV-1 infection. *Nature* **373,** 123–126.
6. Wei, X., Ghosh, S. K., Taylor, M., E., Johnson, V. A., Emini, E. A., Deutsch, P., Lifson, J. D., Bonhoeffer, S., Nowak, M. A., Hahn, B. H., Saag, M. S., and Shaw, G. M. (1995) Viral dynamics in human immunodeficiency virus type-1 infection. *Nature* **373,** 117–122.
7. Richman, D. D. (1995) Protease uninhibited. *Nature* **374,** 494.
8. Condra, J. H., Schleif, W. A., Blahy, O. M., Gabryelski, L. J., Graham D. J., Quintero, J. C., Rhodes, A., Robbins, H. L., Roth, E., Shivaprakash, M., Titus, D., Yang, T., Teppler, H., Squires, K. E., Deutsch, P. J., and Emini, E. A. (1995) In vivo emergence of HIV-1 variants resistant to multiple protease inhibitors. *Nature* **374,** 569–571.
9. Toth, M. V. and Marshall, G. R. (1990) A Simple continuous fluorometric assay for HIV protease. *Int. J. Peptide Protein Res.* **36,** 544–550.
10. Maschera, B., Darby, G., Palú, G., Wright, L. L., Tisdale, M., Myers, R., Blair, E. D., and Furfine, E. S. (1996) Human immunodeficiency virus: Mutations in the protease that confer resistance to saquinavir increase the dissociation rate constant of the protease-saquinavir complex. *J. Biol. Chem.* **271,** 33,231–33,235.
11. Morrison, J. F. and Walsh, C. T. (1988) The behavior and significance of slow-binding enzyme inhibitors. *Adv. Enz.* **61,** 201–301.
12. Jordan, S. P., Zugau, J., Darke, P. L., and Kuo, L. C. (1992) Activity and dimerization of human immunodeficiency virus protease as a function of solvent composition and enzyme concentration. *J. Biol. Chem.* **267,** 20,028–20,032.

26

Retroviral Integrase

A Novel Target in Antiviral Drug Development and Basic In Vitro Assays with the Purified Enzyme

Abhijit Mazumder, Nouri Neamati, Sanjay Sunder, Joshua Owen, and Yves Pommier

1. Introduction

Two critical events are the signature of the life cycle of retroviruses *(1)*. The first is reverse transcription, whereby the single-stranded RNA genome of the retrovirus is copied into double-stranded DNA. The second of these events is integration, whereby this viral DNA is inserted into a chromosome of the host cell, establishing what is known as the proviral state. The proviral state is required for efficient replication of retroviruses. This crucial second event is catalyzed by the integrase enzyme. Retroviruses encode the integrase at the 3' end of the *pol* gene. Integrase is generated by the retroviral protease as a proteolytic cleavage product of the *gag-pol* fusion protein precursor, and is contained in the virus particle. During viral infection, integrase catalyzes the excision of the last two nucleotides from each 3' end of the linear viral DNA, leaving the terminal dinucleotide CA-3P-OH at these recessed 3' ends. This activity is referred to as the 3'-processing or dinucleotide cleavage. After transport to the nucleus as a nucleoprotein complex ("preintegration complex"), integrase catalyzes a DNA strand transfer reaction (3'-end joining) involving the nucleophilic attack of these ends on a host chromosome. Completion of the integration process requires removal of the two unpaired nucleotides at the 5' ends of the viral DNA and gap repair reactions that are thought to be accomplished by cellular enzymes. For recent reviews, *see* Andrake and Skalka *(2)* and Rice et al. *(3)*.

Mutation analyses of the integrase gene have demonstrated that integration is essential for productive viral infection. Therefore, integration is among the

From: *Methods in Molecular Medicine, vol. 24: Antiviral Methods and Protocols*
Edited by: D. Kinchington and R. F. Schinazi © Humana Press Inc., Totowa, NJ

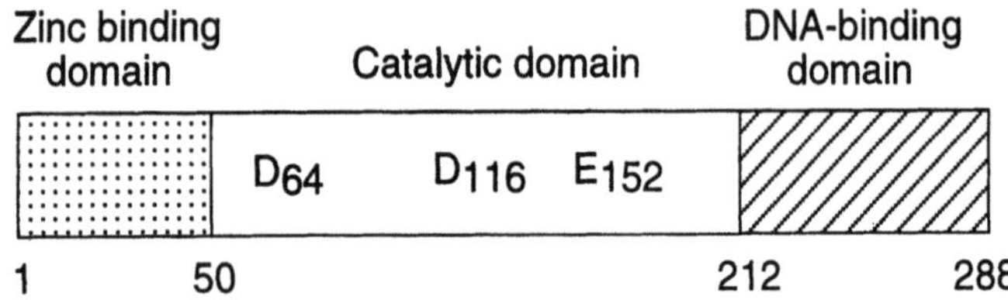

Fig. 1. The three domains of HIV-1 integrase. The central core domain contains three conserved acidic residues common to all retroviral integrases (DD[35]E motif *[2,3]*).

enzymatic steps in the replication cycle of HIV that can be targeted for chemotherapeutic intervention. The activities of various compounds as inhibitors of HIV integrase ***(4–10)*** and HIV-1 preintegration complexes ***(11)*** have been reported. The authors' laboratory has used and developed in vitro assays to derive biochemical information about the integrase ***(12–15)*** and applied this knowledge to the design and development of integrase inhibitors.

1.2. Assays

Figure 1 is a schematic representation of the three domains of HIV-1 integrase. The assays routinely used to measure the effects of inhibitors on the catalytic activities of HIV-1 integrase are depicted in **Fig. 2**.

1.2.1. Dual Assays to Measure Both 3'-Processing and Strand Transfer

A dual assay (**Fig. 2A**) can be used to measure both catalytic activities of integrase *(16,17)*. The 3'-processing reaction (**step 1**) liberates a GT dinucleotide, resulting in the generation of a 19-mer oligonucleotide from a 21-mer substrate. The strand transfer (3'-end joining) reaction (**step 2**) results in the insertion of one 3'-processed oligonucleotide into another target DNA, yielding higher molecular weight species that migrate slower than the 21-mer substrate. There are also species that migrate faster than the 21-mer substrate. These bands represent the "mirror image" of the integration products (i.e., the smaller species produced near the 5'-end). However, quantitation is more convenient on the larger species.

1.2.2. The Strand Transfer Assay

A strand transfer assay can also be performed to determine whether the strand transfer reaction is truly being inhibited or whether the inhibition of the 3'-processing reaction causes the decrease in the subsequent strand transfer

Fig. 2. *(continued on opposite page)* Catalytic activities of HIV-1 integrase. The asterisk denotes the location of the ^{32}P radiolabel. The length of the strands are denoted by the numbers above each strand. In the schematic of the expected results, left lane is DNA alone and right lane is DNA plus integrase. 3'-P, 3'-processing; ST, strand trans-

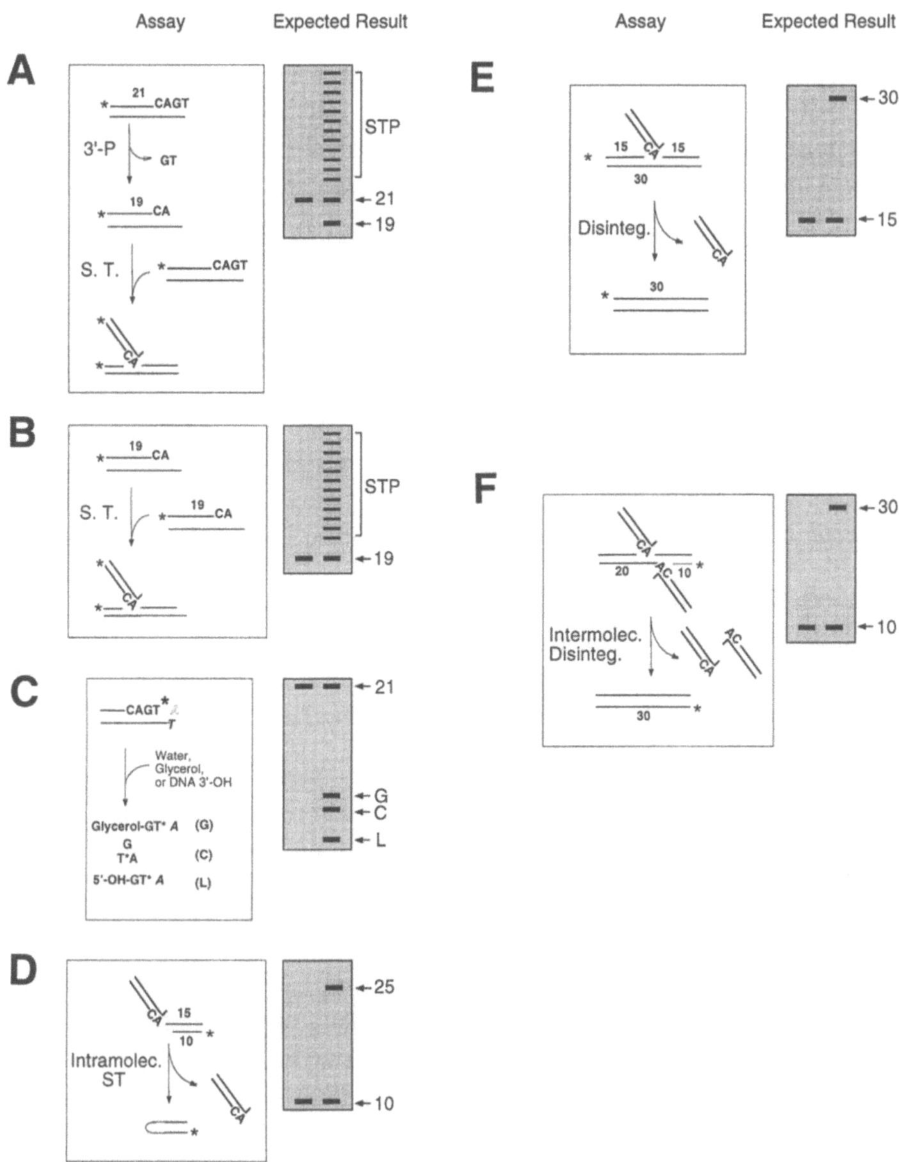

fer (3'-end joining); STP, strand transfer products. **(A)** Dual assay for 3'-processing and strand transfer using a blunt-ended 21-mer; **(B)** assay for strand transfer using a "precleaved" 19-mer; **(C)** assay for 3'-processing using DNA substrate labeled at the 3'-end to determine choice of nucleophile; **(D)** assay for intramolecular strand transfer using a gapped DNA substrate; **(E)** intramolecular disintegration using a branched DNA substrate having a Y structure; **(F)** intermolecular disintegration using a branched DNA substrate having an X structure.

products. The strand transfer (3'-end joining) step by itself can be measured using a "precleaved" substrate containing a recessed 3' end (**Fig. 2B**). If inhibition of strand transfer using this preprocessed substrate is observed in the same concentration range as that seen with the blunt-ended, duplex oligonucleotide substrate (**Fig. 2A**), the compound can be described as inhibiting both steps of the integration reaction: 3'-processing and strand transfer.

1.2.3. The Choice of Nucleophile in Phosphodiester Cleavage

Inhibition of 3'-processing can be further analyzed using DNA substrates labeled at the 3'-end. The choice of nucleophile in the 3'-processing reaction *(18,19)* can be measured using a substrate DNA that has been radiolabeled (and extended by one base pair *[13]* for convenience of radiolabeling) at the 3'-end (**Fig. 2C**). The extents of glycerolysis, circular nucleotide formation, and hydrolysis can then be assayed. If a compound inhibits glycerolysis, hydrolysis, and circular nucleotide formation to the same extent, it can be described as exerting a global inhibition in the 3'-processing reaction (glycerol, water, or the hydroxyl group of the viral DNA terminus).

1.2.4. Hairpin Formation

An intramolecular strand transfer reaction, resulting in the formation of a hairpin structure *(12)*, can be assayed using a gapped DNA substrate (**Fig. 2D**). All four of these assays require the full-length integrase.

1.2.5. Disintegration Reactions

The binding site of active compounds can be investigated using either of two assays that can be performed with deletion mutants of HIV-1 integrase. Intramolecular (**Fig. 2E**) *(20–22)* or intermolecular (**Fig. 2F**) disintegration reactions *(12,23,24)* can be used with full-length IN^{I-288}, IN^{1-212}, IN^{50-288}, or IN^{50-212}.

1.2.6. DNA Binding Assays

The two assays used to assess the effects of inhibitors on integrase are shown in **Fig. 3**. When a linear DNA substrate is used, the full-length IN^{1-288}, IN^{1-212}, or IN^{50-288} can be assayed. A photocrosslinking procedure (**Fig. 2A**) uses short wavelength ultraviolet light to induce free radicals that will crosslink the integrase to the DNA *(25,26)*. A recently developed chemical crosslinking traps a Schiff base formed between an appropriately positioned ε-amino group of a lysine on the enzyme and an enzymatically introduced aldehydic abasic site via reduction with sodium borohydride *(15)*.

2. Materials

2.1. Enzymes and Equipment

1. Oligonucleotide substrates: AE117, 5'-ACTGCTAGAGATTTTCCACAC-3'; AE118, 5'-GTGTGGAAAATCTCTAGCAGT-3'; AE1'57, 5'-GAAAGCGAC

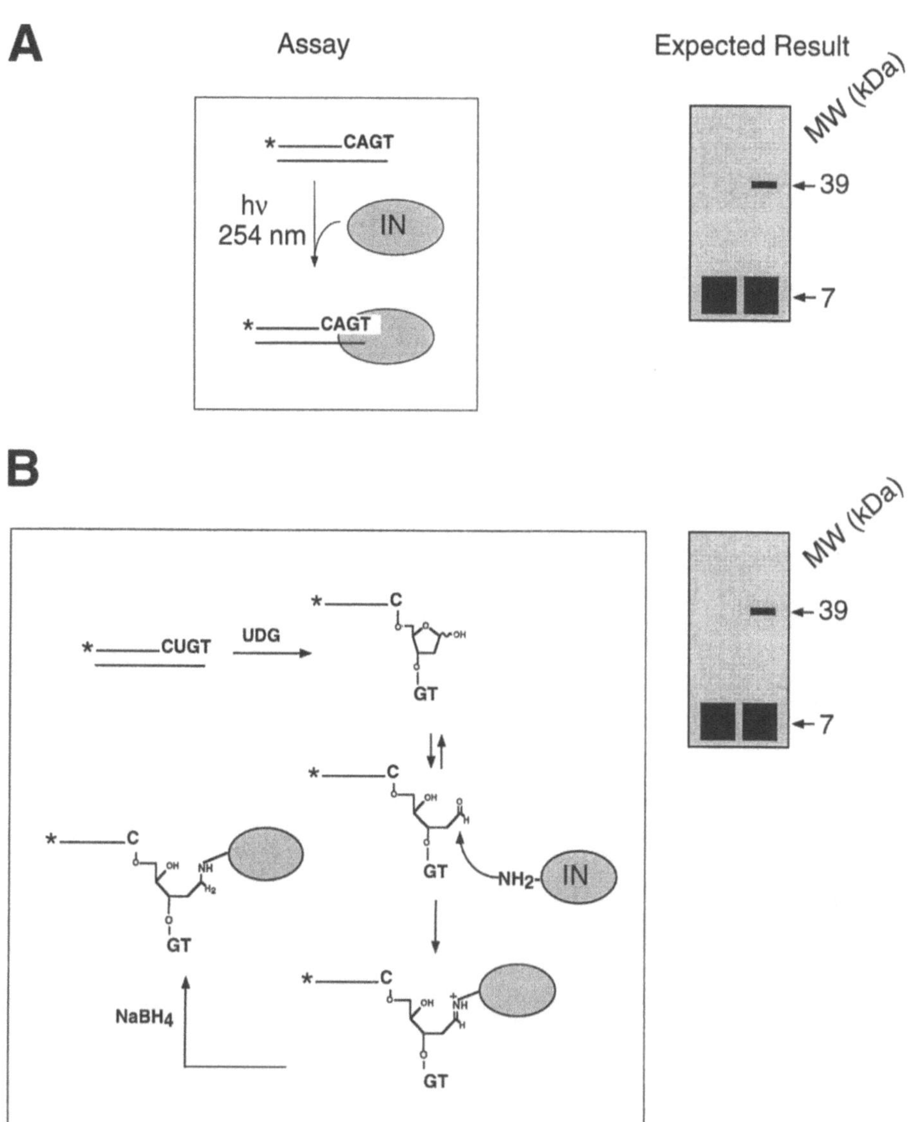

Fig. 3. DNA binding activity of HIV-1 integrase. The asterisk denotes the location of the ^{32}P radiolabel. In the schematic of the expected results, left lane is DNA alone and right lane is DNA plus integrase. **(A)** Photocrosslinking assay for DNA binding; **(B)** chemical crosslinking assay for DNA binding.

CGCGCC-3'; AE146, 5'- GGACGCCATAGCCCCGGCGCGGTCGCTTTC-3'; AE156, 5'-GTGTGGAAAATCTCTAGCAGGGGCTATGGCGTCC-3'; AE118S, 5'-GTGTGGAAAATCTCTAGCA-3'; RM22M, 5'-TACTGCTAGAGATTTTCC

ACAC-3'. The AE117, AE118, and the first 19 nucleotides of AE156 correspond to the U5 end of the HIV-1 long terminal repeat.
2. *Escherichia coli* strain BL21 (DE3, Novagen, Madison, WI).
3. pET-15b plasmid (Novagen) encoding the integrase.
4. Super Broth (Biofluids, Inc., Rockville, MD) or LB Medium (Digene, Beltsville, MD).
5. Rotary shaker set at 37°C.
6. Ampicillin (100 mg/mL stock, Boehringer Mannheim GmbH, Germany).
7. T4 polynucleotide kinase (Gibco-BRL, Gaithersburg, MD).
8. Sodium borohydride (1 *M* stock).
9. Isopropyl β-D-thiogalactopyranoside (IPTG, Boehringer Mannheim).
10. Lysozyme (0.2 mg/mL).
11. Uracil DNA glycosylase (Gibco-BRL).
12. Electrophoresis apparatus and a gel dryer.
13. Terminal transferase (Boehringer Mannheim).
14. γ-[^{32}P]-ATP (Dupont-NEN).
15. α-[^{32}P]-cordycepin triphosphate (Dupont-NEN).
16. Spectrophotometer.
17. Chelating Sepharose column FF (Pharmacia, Biotech, Sweden).
18. G-25 Sephadex quick-spin column (Boehringer Mannheim).
19. Homogenizer.
20. Nickel chelating column.
21. Ultraviolet (UV) transilluminator (254 nm wavelength).
22. Phosphorimager (Molecular Dynamics, Sunnyvale, CA).
23. Microcentrifuge and ultracentrifuge.

2.2. Solutions and Buffers

1. Dialysis/enzyme buffer: 25 m*M* HEPES pH 7.5, 2 m*M* ethylenediaminetetra-acetic acid (EDTA), 10 m*M* dithiothreitol (DTT), 1 *M* NaCl, 10% glycerol, water (total vol = 1 L).
2. Denaturing 20% polyacrylamide gel solution: 0.09 *M* Tris-borate, pH 8.3, 2 m*M* EDTA, 20% acrylamide, 8 *M* urea.
3. DNA cocktail (for 31 reaction tubes): 125 m*M* 3-[*N*-morpholino]propanesulfonic acid (MOPS) (100 µL), 100% glycerol (50 µL), H_2O (63 µL), DNA (20 µL).
4. INT cocktail (for 30 reaction tubes): 100 m*M* $MnCl_2$ (3.6 µL), 1 mg/mL bovine serum albumin (BSA) (48 µL), 100 m*M* 2-mercaptoethanol (48 µL), H_2O (63 µL), and 10 µ*M* integrase (15 µL).
5. Loading dye solution: 98% deionized formamide, 10 m*M* EDTA, 0.025% xylene cyanol, 0.025% bromophenol blue.
6. Lysis buffer: 20 m*M* Tris-HCl, pH 8.0, 0.1 m*M* EDTA, 2 m*M* 2-mercaptoethanol, 0.5 *M* NaCl, 5 m*M* imidazole, 0.2 mg/mL lysozyme.
7. Sodium dodecyl sulfate-polyacrylamide gel electrophoresis (SDS-PAGE) buffer: 100 m*M* Tris-HCl, pH 6.8, 4% 2-mercaptoethanol, 4% SDS, 0.2% bromophenol blue, 20% glycerol.
8. TNM buffer: 20 m*M* Tris-HCl, pH 8.0, 2 *M* NaCl, 2 m*M* 2-mercaptoethanol.

3. Methods

3.1. Transformation

HIV-1 integrase can be purified by transformation of *E. coli* strain BL21 (DE3) with a pET-15B plasmid as described ***(16)***.

1. Place 50 μL of *E. coli* solution into two prechilled tubes and keep on ice for 30 min.
2. Add 1 μL of ampicillin-resistant plasmid to one tube and label as integrase. Other tube is a control with no plasmid.
3. Incubate on ice for 1 h.
4. Remove tubes from ice and insert into a water bath at 42°C for exactly 60 s.
5. Immediately place tubes in ice bath and add 900 μL of S.O.C. Medium (or LB Broth) to each tube. Do not cap tightly.
6. Incubate tubes in a rotary shaker at 37°C for 45–60 min.
7. Spread 200–500 μL onto LB agar plates containing 100 μg/mL ampicillin.
8. Let the plates sit at room temperature for 5 min, invert, and incubate the plates overnight at 37°C.

3.2. Inoculation of Cells

1. Inoculate a single colony obtained in **step 8** in **Subheading 3.1.** from plate labeled integrase in 10 mL LB Broth containing ampicillin (10 μL of 100 mg/mL stock)
2. Incubate at 37°C in a rotary shaker.
3. Prepare two 1-L flasks, each with 500 mL of LB Broth. Add 500 μL ampicillin to each flask.
4. Add 5 mL of the cell solution to each flask. Do not cap tightly.
5. Incubate in a rotary shaker at 37°C until an A_{600nm} of 0.8 is reached. This will take 3–5 h.
6. Remove a 0.5-mL sample of the culture for SDS-PAGE. Centrifuge for 1 min in a microcentrifuge. Discard the supernatant and resuspend the cell pellet in 75 μL of SDS-PAGE sample buffer. Store at –20° C.
7. Add IPTG to a final concentration of 0.4 m*M* (0.5 mL of 0.4 *M* IPTG), and incubate for an additional 3 h. Before harvesting cells, save a sample for SDS-PAGE as described in **step 6**.
8. Harvest the cells by centrifugation at 3000*g* for 20 min. Discard the supernatant and store the pellet at –70°C.
9. Resuspend the cell pellet in 10 mL of ice-cold 25 m*M* HEPES, pH 7.5, and 5 m*M* EDTA (1:1 w/v).
10. Centrifuge the cell suspension at 6000*g* for 10 min. Resuspend the cells in 10 mL of lysis buffer and then add lysozyme (0.2 mg/mL).
11. Incubate on ice with occasional stirring until the suspension becomes viscous (approx 30 min).
12. Sonicate in short bursts (10 s) until the lysate is no longer viscous. It is important to sonicate on ice and to carefully monitor the temperature of the lysate between bursts of sonication. Do not let it rise above 8°C.

13. Centrifuge at 40,000*g* for 45 min. Collect and store the supernatant at –20°C, and homogenize the pellet for 30 min in 10 mL of TNM buffer containing 5 m*M* imidazole.
14. Centrifuge again at 40,000*g* for 45 min. Save the supernatant.

3.3. Purification of Integrase

1. Run supernatant(s) on protein gel against known marker to determine integrase band after staining with Coomassie blue. Integrase has a mol wt of 32 kDa and is the prominent protein in the crude lysate.
2. Prepare a 0.5-mL column of Chelating Sepharose FF. Wash the column with 1.5 mL of water, followed with 2.5 mL of 50 m*M* $NiSO_4$, and then with approx 7.5 mL of TNM buffer containing 5 m*M* imidazole.
3. Load the supernatant from **step 14** in **Subheading 3.2.**
4. Wash the column with at least 5 mL of TNM buffer containing 5 m*M* imidazole followed by 5 mL of the same buffer containing 60 m*M* imidazole.
5. Elute with increasing concentrations of imidazole in TNM buffer (50, 300, 450, 600, and 695 m*M*). Repeat two 500-μL washes for each of these five concentrations.
6. Pool the fractions that contain integrase, add EDTA to final concentration of 10 m*M* (10 μL of 500 m*M* EDTA to each 500 μL fraction), and dialyze immediately overnight against dialysis buffer.
7. Determine integrase concentration. HIV-1 integrase has an extinction coefficient of 1.56 at 280 nm.
8. Run fractions on protein gel and stain with Coomassie to determine which one contains integrase.
9. Do an activity assay, described in **Subheading 3.5.**, and store the integrase at –80°C.

3.4. Preparation of Radiolabeled DNA Substrates

To analyze the extents of 3'-processing and strand transfer using 5'-end–labeled substrates, AE118 is 5'-end labeled using T4 PNK and γ-[^{32}P]-ATP (*see* **Note 1**).

1. Prepare a solution containing 10 μL of sterilized distilled water, 7.5 μL of 10X kinase buffer, 5.0 μL of oligonucleotide AE118, 2.5 μL of T4 PNK and 50 μL of γ-[^{32}P]-ATP.
2. Heat the mixture for 45 min at 37°C.
3. Transfer to 85°C heat block and heat for additional 15 min.
4. Add 96 μL of water, 20 μL of 1 *M* NaCl, and 10 μL of oligonucleotide AE117.
5. Heat for 2 min at 85°C.
6. Slow cool in heat block until reaching room temperature.
7. Spin G-25 Sephadex quick spin columns three times to dry.
8. Add 50 μL of DNA solution to each column, spin for 5 min, and collect and store DNA.

3.5. Integrase Reactions

1. Prepare drug dilutions in DMSO.
2. Add 8.6 µL of water to first tube, labeled DNA.
3. Add 7.0 µL of freshly prepared INT cocktail to each of the remaining tubes.
4. Add 1.6 µL of DMSO to each of the integrase controls.
5. Add 1.6 µL of drugs to each appropriate reaction tube.
6. Incubate at 30°C for 30 min.
7. While incubating, prepare DNA Cocktail.
8. After incubation period is complete, add 7.4 µL of "DNA Cocktail" to each reaction tube.
9. Incubate for an additional hour at 30°C.
10. After l h quench with 16 µL of loading dye.
11. Load and run on 20% polyacrylamide gel.
12. Final concentrations: 10% glycerol (w/v), 25 m*M* MOPS pH 7.2, 50 m*M* NaCl, 1 m*M* HEPES, pH 7.5, 50 µ*M* EDTA, 50 µ*M* DTT, 7.5 m*M* $MnCl_2$ or $MgCl_2$ (when specified), 0.1 mg/mL BSA, 10 m*M* 2-mercaptoethanol, 10% DMSO (*see* **Note 2**).

3.6. DNA Binding Assays (UV Crosslinking)

The method used has been described by Yoshinaga et al. *(25)* and Engelman et al. *(26)*.

1. Incubate integrase in INT cocktail with substrate in DNA cocktail as in **Subheading 3.5.** for 5 min at 30°C.
2. Irradiate reactions with a UV transilluminator (254 nm wavelength) from 3 cm above (2.4 mW/cm^2) at room temperature for 10 min.
3. Add an equal volume (16 µL) of 2X SDS-PAGE buffer to each reaction.
4. Heat 20-µL aliquots at 95°C for 3 min.
5. Load on a 12 or 18% SDS-polyacrylamide gel.
5. Run gel at 120 V for 1.5 h.
6. Dry and expose in a PhosphorImager cassette.

3.7. DNA Binding Assays (Schiff Base Formation)

Duplex oligonucleotide substrates containing a single enzymatically generated abasic site are created as follows: Analogs of AE118 are synthesized such that one deoxyuridine replaces each of the wild-type nucleotides in this strand. For example, substrates –1 and –11 *(15)* have the sequences 5'-GTGTGG AAAATCTCTAGCUGT-3' and 5'-GTGTGGAAUATCTCTAGCAGT-3', respectively. Each of these single strands is then radiolabeled and annealed to the complementary strand AE117 as described in **Subheading 3.4.**

1. Remove uracil from duplex oligonucleotides containing deoxyuridine by incubation of 40 mL of end-labeled duplex (500 n*M* stock concentration) with 1 U of uracil DNA glycosylase for 2 h at 30°C.

2. Load on a G-25 Sephadex quick-spin column to remove the unincorporated label and the uracil.
3. The extent of AP site formation is determined by incubation of 0.5 μ*M* of the radiolabeled AP site–containing DNA with 166 m*M* sodium hydroxide for 30 min at 30°C.
4. The extent of cleavage of the oligonucleotide by β- and δ-elimination reactions is quantitated and determined to be 100%, implying that all the uracil from the substrate has been excised.
5. Incubate integrase in INT cocktail with the oligonucleotide containing the enzymatically generated abasic site in DNA cocktail (as described in **Subheading 3.5.**) for 2 min at room temperature (*see* **Note 4**).
6. Add freshly prepared solution of sodium borohydride (0.1 *M* final concentration).
7. Incubate for 5 min at 30°C.
8. Add an equal volume (16 μL) of 2X SDS-PAGE buffer to each reaction.
9. Heat 20-μL aliquots at 95°C for 3 min.
10. Load on a 12 or 18% SDS-polyacrylamide gel.
11. Run gel at 120 V for 1.5 h.
12. Dry and expose in a PhosphorImager cassette.

3.8. DNA Electrophoresis, Quantitation, and Data Analysis

1. Quench reactions with an equal volume (16 μL) of loading dye.
2. Run an aliquot (5 μL) on a denaturing 20% polyacrylamide gel.
3. Dry gels, and expose in a Molecular Dynamics Phosphorimager cassette or autoradiography.
4. Analyze using a Molecular Dynamics phosphorimager.
5. Calculate percent inhibition using the following equation:

$$\%I = 100 \times [1 - (D - C)/(N - C)]$$

   where C, N, and D are the fractions of DNA substrate converted to product for DNA alone (C), DNA plus integrase (N), and integrase plus drug (D).
6. Determine IC_{50} by plotting the log of drug concentration vs percent inhibition, and determine the concentration that produces 50% inhibition.

4. Notes

1. To analyze the extent of strand transfer using the "precleaved" substrate, AE118S is 5'-end labeled, annealed to AE117, and column purified as above. To analyze the choice of nucleophile for the 3'-processing reaction, AE118 is 3'-end labeled using α-[^{32}P]-cordycepin triphosphate and terminal transferase ***(18,19)***. The transferase is heat-inactivated and RM22M is added to the same final concentration. The mixture is then heated at 95°C, allowed to cool slowly to room temperature, and run on a G-25 spin column as in **Subheading 3.4.** To determine the extent of 30-mer target strand generation during disintegration ***(20)***, AE,157 is 5'-end labeled, annealed to AE156, AE146, and AE117, and column purified as in **Subheading 3.4.**

2. When magnesium is used as the divalent metal ion, polyethylene glycol is substituted for BSA at a final concentration of 5% to increase activity ***(28)***. Preincubation for 30 min of the enzyme with inhibitor is performed to optimize the inhibitory activity in the 3'-processing reaction ***(29)***. Disintegration reactions ***(20)*** are performed as above with a Y oligonucleotide (i.e., the branched substrate in which the U5 end is "integrated" into target DNA).
3. For inhibition of DNA binding experiments, integrase is preincubated with the inhibitor for 30 min at 30°C in INT cocktail prior to the subsequent addition of the radiolabeled viral DNA substrate in DNA cocktail.
4. For inhibition of DNA binding experiments, integrase in INT cocktail is preincubated with the inhibitor for 30 min at 30°C prior to the subsequent addition of the radiolabeled viral DNA substrate in DNA cocktail. Incubation is continued for an additional 5 min prior to the addition of borohydride.

References

1. Varmus, H. E. and Brown, P. O. (1989) in *Mobile DNA* (Berg, D. and Howe, M., eds.), Am. Soc. Microbiol., Washington, DC, pp. 53–108.
2. Andrake, M. D. and Skalka, A. M. (1996) *J. Biol. Chem.* **271,** 19,633–19,636.
3. Rice, P., Craigie, R., and Davies, D. R. (1996) *Curr. Opin. Struct. Biol.* **6,** 76–83.
4. Cushman, M., Golebiewski, W. M., Pommier, Y., Mazumder, A., Reymen, D., De Clerq, E., Graham, L., and Rice, W. G. (1995) *J. Med. Chem.* **38,** 443–452.
5. LaFemina, R. L., Graham, P. L., LeGrow, K., Hastings, J. C., Wolfe, A., Young, S. D., Emini, E. A., and Hazuda, D. J. (1995) *Antimicrob. Agents Chemother.* **39,** 320–324.
6. Fesen, M. R., Kohn, K. W., Leteurtre, F., and Pommier, Y. (1993) *Proc. Natl. Acad. Sci. USA* **90,** 2399–2403.
7. Robinson, W. E., Jr., Reinecke, M. G., Abdel-Malek., S., Jia, Q., and Chow, S. A. (1996) *Proc. Natl. Acad. Sci. USA* **93,** 6326–6331.
8. Bouziane, M., Cherny, D. I., Mouscadet, J. F., and Auclair, C. (1996) *J. Biol. Chem.* **271,** 10,359–10,364.
9. Mazumder, A., Wang, S., Neamati, N., Nicklaus, M., Sunder, S., Chen, J., Milne, G. W. A., Rice, W. G., Burke, T. R. J., and Pommier, Y. (1996) *J. Med. Chem.* **39,** 2472–2481.
10. Mazumder, A., Neamati, N., Ojwang, J. O., Sunder, S., Rando, R. F., and Pommier, Y. (1996) *Biochemistry* **35,** 13,762–13,771.
11. Farnet, C. M., Wang, B., Lipford, J. R., and Bushmarn, F. D. (1996) *Proc. Natl. Acad. Sci. USA* **93,** 9742–9747.
12. Mazumder, A., Engelman, A., Craigie, R., Fesen, M., and Pommier, Y. (1994) *Nucleic Acids Res.* **22,** 1037–1043.
13. Mazumder, A., Gupta, M., and Pommier, Y. (1994) *Nucleic Acids Res.* **22,** 4441–4448.
14. Mazumder, A., and Pommier, Y. (1995) *Nucleic Acids Res.* **23,** 2865–2871.
15. Mazumder, A., Neamati, N., Pilon, A., Sunder, S., and Pommier, Y. (1996) *J. Biol. Chem.* **271,** 27,330–27,338.
16. Craigie, R., Fujiwara, T., and Bushman, F. (1990) *Cell* **62,** 829–837.

17. Katz, R. A., Merkel, G., Kulkosky, J., Leis, J., and Skalka, A. M. (1990) *Cell* **63,** 87–95.
18. Engelman, A., Mizuuchi, K., and Craigie, R. (1991) *Cell* **67,** 1211–1221.
19. Vink, C., Yeheskiely, E., van der Marel, G. A., van Boom, J. H., and Plasterk, R. H. (1991) *Nucleic Acids Res.* **19,** 6691–6698.
20. Chow, S. A., Vincent, K. A., Ellison, V., and Brown, P. O. (1992) *Science* **255,** 723–726.
21. Sherman, P. A., Dickson, M. L., and Fyfe, J. A. (1992) *J. Virol.* **66,** 3593–3601.
22. Bushman, F. D., Engelman, A., Palmer, I., Wingfield, P., and Craigie, R. (1993) *Proc. Natl. Acad. Sci. USA* **90,** 3428–3432.
23. Chow, S. A. and Brown, P. O. (1994) *J. Virol.* **68,** 7869–7878.
24. van Den Ent, F. M. I., Vink, C., and Plasterk, R. H. A. (1994) *J. Virol.* **68,** 7825–7832.
25. Yoshinaga, T., Kimura-Ohtani, Y., and Fujiwara, T. (1994) *J. Virol.* **68,** 5690–5697.
26. Engelman, A., Hickman, A. B., and Craigie, R. (1994) *J. Virol.* **68,** 5911–5917.
27. Jenkins, T. M., Engelman, A., Ghirlando, R., and Craigie, R. (1996) *J. Biol. Chem.* **271,** 7712–7718.
28. Engelman, A. and Craigie, R. (1995) *J. Virol.* **69,** 5908–5911.
29. Fesen, M., Pommier, Y., Leteurtre, F., Hiroguchi, S., Yung, J., and Kohn, K. W. (1994) *Biochem. Pharmacol.* **48,** 595–608.

IV

Human Papilloma Virus

27

Papillomavirus DNA Replication

Maureen C. Ferran and Alison A. McBride

1. Introduction

Papillomavirus genomes replicate and are maintained as stable extrachromosomal plasmid DNA (episomes) in many cell lines (reviewed in **ref.** ***1***). This process requires the viral E1 and E2 proteins and the origin of replication ***(2,3)***. The minimal origin of replication consists of an E1 binding site, an E2 binding site, and an AT rich region that probably facilitates origin unwinding (*see* **Fig. 1**). The E1 protein is an ATP-dependent helicase that specifically binds to and unwinds the origin ***(4–6)***. The E2 protein is the major transcriptional transactivator of the virus but it is also required for viral DNA replication. The E2 protein probably plays more of an auxiliary role in DNA replication; it has been shown to cooperatively bind to the origin with the E1 protein ***(7–11)***, to alleviate repression of replication by nucleosomes ***(12)***, and to interact with cellular replication proteins (RPA) ***(13)***.

To date, the most successful antiviral targets have been directed against viral-specific enzymes. Therefore, the ATPase and helicase activities of the E1 protein are attractive targets. Papillomavirus DNA replication may also be inhibited by compounds that interfere with the ability of E1 to bind DNA or to interact with the E2 protein. This chapter will describe a method to assay for specific E1 DNA binding and cooperative origin binding with the E2 protein and a method to transiently assay papillomavirus DNA replication. The methods described are for bovine papillomavirus type 1 (BPV-1), which has been the molecular prototype of the papillomaviruses. However, the methods can easily be adapted to assay for human papillomavirus replication.

1.1. E1 DNA Binding and E1-E2 Cooperative DNA Binding Assay

In this assay, E1 protein (and E2 protein) is incubated with a mixture of ^{32}P-labeled DNA fragments, one of which contains the viral replication origin

From: *Methods in Molecular Medicine, vol. 24: Antiviral Methods and Protocols*
Edited by: D. Kinchington and R. F. Schinazi © Humana Press Inc., Totowa, NJ

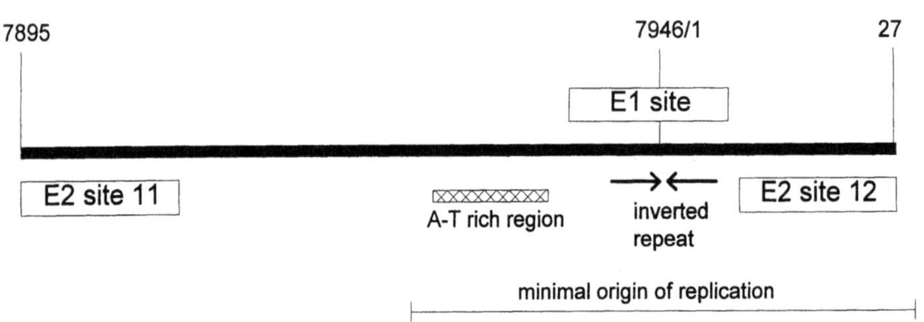

Fig. 1. Diagram of the BPV-1 replication origin.

(which includes an E1 binding site flanked by two E2 binding sites). The resulting DNA-protein complexes are immunoprecipitated with an E1-specific antibody, and E1-bound DNA is analyzed by gel electrophoresis. This method involves the following steps and is outlined in **Fig. 2**: preparation of the origin-containing DNA probe; synthesis of E1 and E2 proteins by in vitro translation; DNA-protein immunoprecipitation assay; and analysis of the DNA products (options 1 and 2).

1.2. Replication Assay

In this method, papillomavirus DNA is transfected into cells and DNA replication is assayed at various times after infection. Low molecular weight extrachromosomal DNA is isolated and analyzed by Southern blotting. Unreplicated input DNA and replicated DNA can be distinguished by their susceptibility to the restriction enzymes *Dpn*I and *Mbo*I. Nonreplicated plasmid DNA that has been isolated from dam+ bacteria is methylated at the N^6 position of the adenine residues in the sequence GATC and is susceptible to cleavage by *Dpn*I and resistant to *Mbo*I cleavage. Conversely, DNA replicated in eukaryotic cells has lost this methylation and can be cleaved by *Mbo*I but not by *Dpn*I. The method is outlined in **Fig. 3** and has been adapted from that of Ustav and Stenlund *(2)*. This assay involves the following steps: preparation of the BPV-1 replicon; electroporation of eukaryotic cells with viral DNA; extraction of low molecular weight DNA; preparation of a viral DNA probe; and analysis of the DNA products by Southern blotting.

2. Materials

2.1. E1-E2 Cooperative DNA Binding Assay

2.1.1. Preparation of Labeled DNA Fragments

1. *Bam*HI, *Hin*dIII, *Afl*III restriction enzymes, and buffers.
2. DNA polymerase I large (Klenow) fragment (2 U/μL) (*see* **Note 1**).

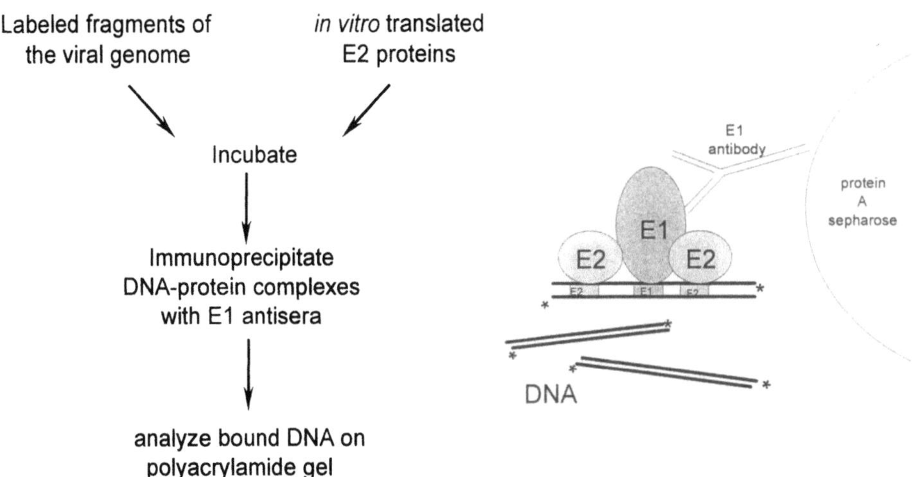

Fig. 2. Outline of the E1-E2 cooperative binding assay.

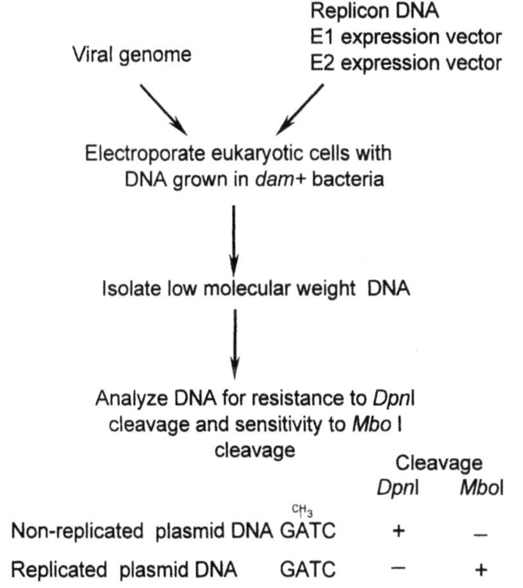

Fig. 3. Outline of the transient replication assay.

3. Origin-containing plasmid, such as pKS ori (**Fig. 4**).
4. 10X Klenow buffer: 100 m*M* Tris-HCl, pH 7.5, 100 m*M* $MgCl_2$, 10 m*M* DTT.
5. 10 m*M* dATP, 10 m*M* dGTP, 10 m*M* TTP.
6. ^{32}P-dCTP (>3000 Ci/mmol).
7. 0.5 *M* Ethylenediaminetetra-acetic acid (EDTA).

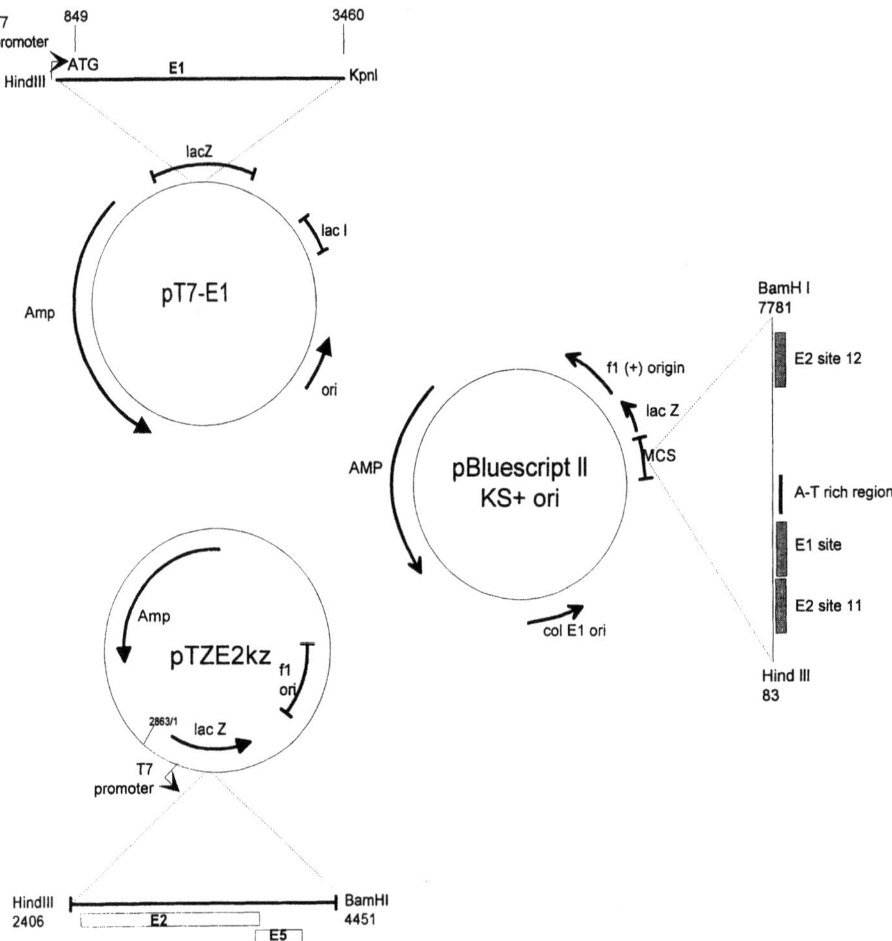

Fig. 4. Diagrams of the E1 and E2 expression plasmids used to transcribe and translate viral gene products and diagram of the plasmid containing the BPV-1 replication origin.

8. ProbeQuant G-50 Micro columns (Pharmacia Biotech, Piscataway, NJ).
9. TE buffer: 10 m*M* Tris-HCl, pH 8.0, 1 m*M* EDTA.

2.1.2. Agarose Gel Electrophoresis

1. Agarose.
2. 10X TBE: 1.0 *M* Tris, 0.9 *M* boric acid, 0.01 *M* EDTA.
3. Ethidium bromide (10 mg/mL).
4. Sucrose loading buffer: 40% sucrose (w/v), 0.25% (w/v) bromophenol blue.
5. Horizontal gel electrophoresis apparatus.
6. UV light box and photography equipment.
7. DNA molecular weight markers.

2.1.3. Polyacrylamide Gel Electrophoresis for Analysis of Labeled DNA Probe and Analysis of E1- and E2-Bound DNA (Option 2)

1. Sucrose loading buffer: 40% sucrose (w/v), 0.25% (w/v) bromophenol blue. Store aliquots at –20°C.
2. 10X TBE: 1.0 *M* Tris, 0.9 *M* boric acid, 0.01 *M* EDTA.
3. 30% Acrylamide:bis-acrylamide (29:1).
4. 10% Ammonium persulfate (fresh).
5. Tetramethylethylenediamine (TEMED).
6. Vertical gel electrophoresis apparatus.
7. Plastic cling film (e.g., Saran Wrap).
8. 3MM paper.
9. Gel fixative (10% methanol; 7.5% acetic acid) for Option 2.
10. Gel dryer.
11. Autoradiography film and cassettes.

2.1.4. In Vitro Translation of E1 and E2 Proteins

1. Plasmids pT7E1 and pT7E2 (*see* **Fig. 4**).
2. TNT™ T7 coupled transcription/translation kit (Promega, Madison, WI).
3. RNasin (Promega).
4. ^{35}S-Methionine (1000 Ci/mmol, 10 mCi/mL; *see* **Note 2**).

2.1.5. Analysis of E1 and E2 Proteins and for Analysis of E1 and E2 DNA-Protein Complexes (Option 1)

1. Standard Laemelli sodium dodecyl sulfate-polyacrylamide gel electrophoresis (SDS-PAGE) equipment and reagents.
2. 1X and 2X SDS-sample buffer: 1X: 50 m*M* Tris-HCl, pH 6.8, 2% SDS, 10% glycerol, 0.001% bromophenol blue, 100 m*M* dithiothreitol (DTT) (add fresh).
3. Gel fixative: 10% acetic acid, 40% methanol.
4. ENLIGHTNING (DuPont, Wilmington, DE).
5. 3MM paper.
6. Gel dryer.
7. Autoradiography film and cassettes.
8. Phosphorimager (Molecular Dynamics, Sunnyvale, CA) or similar instrument to quantitate proteins.

2.1.6. DNA-Protein Immunoprecipitation Assay

1. 10X binding buffer: 200 m*M* HEPES, pH 7.4, 50 m*M* MgAc, 2 m*M* EDTA, 10 m*M* DTT (add fresh).
2. Buffer C-300: 20 m*M* HEPES, pH 7.9, 25% (v/v) glycerol, 0.3 *M* NaCl,1.5 m*M* $MgCl_2$, 2 m*M* EDTA.
3. NET-100: 50 m*M* HEPES, pH 7.4, 100 m*M* NaCl, 5 m*M* EDTA, 0.1% Triton X-100, 10 m*M* DTT (add fresh).
4. Sheared salmon sperm DNA (10 mg/mL).

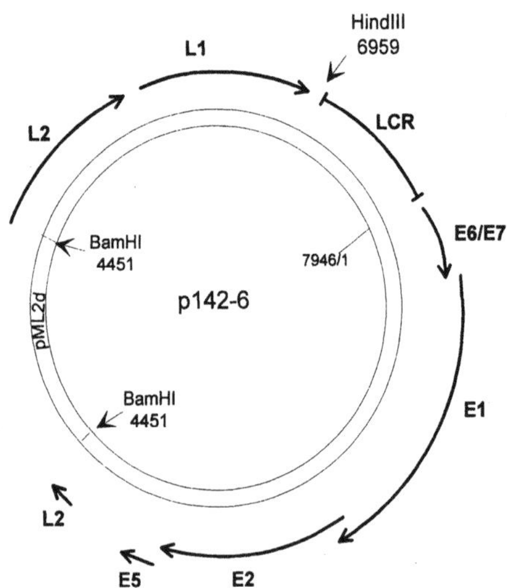

Fig. 5. Diagram of the p142-6 plasmid (BPV-1 genome cloned at the *Bam*HI site in pML2d).

5. E1-specific antiserum (SSQN) (*see* **Note 3**).
6. Protein A-Sepharose CL-4B (Pharmacia), 50% (v/v) slurry in NET-100.
7. 1.7-mL siliconized microfuge tubes (SLICK, PGC Scientific, Gaithersburg, MD).
8. Microfuge tube rotator.
9. Microfuge.
10. Carrier tRNA, 10 mg/mL (Option 1 only).
11. 10% SDS (Option 1 only).
12. "Phenol/chloroform": phenol saturated with TE buffer, chloroform (1:1) (Option 1 only).
13. Ethanol, 95 and 70% (Option 1 only).
14. TE buffer: 10 m*M* Tris-HCl, pH 8.0, 1 m*M* EDTA (Option 1 only).
15. 1X SDS sample buffer: 50 m*M* Tris-HCl, pH 6.8, 2% SDS, 10% glycerol, 0.001% bromophenol blue, 100 m*M* DTT (add fresh), (Option 2 only).

2.2. Replication Assay

2.2.1. Preparation of Viral Replicon

1. Viral DNA, such as p142-6 ***(14)***, cloned into a prokaryotic vector and prepared from bacteria (*see* **Fig. 5**).
2. *Bam*HI restriction enzyme and buffer.
3. "Phenol/chloroform": phenol saturated with TE buffer, chloroform (1:1).
4. "Chloroform": chloroform, isoamyl alcohol (24:1).
5. High concentration T4 DNA ligase (2000 U/µL) (New England Biolabs, Beverly, MA).

6. 10X ligase buffer: 0.5 *M* Tris-HCl, pH 7.6, 100 m*M* $MgCl_2$, 100 m*M* DTT.
7. 10 m*M* adenosine triphosphate (ATP).
8. Ethanol, 95 and 70%.
9. 3 *M* sodium acetate, pH 5.2.
10. 5 *M* ammonium acetate.
11. Sorvall RC5-B or similar floor-model centrifuge.
12. 30 mL COREX tubes or 50-mL Falcon tubes and appropriate swing-out centrifuge rotor.

2.2.2. Agarose Gel Electrophoresis

1. Agarose.
2. 10X TBE: 1.0 *M* Tris, 0.9 *M* boric acid, 0.01 *M* EDTA.
3. Ethidium bromide (10 mg/mL).
4. Sucrose loading buffer: 40% sucrose (w/v), 0.25% (w/v) bromophenol blue.
5. Horizontal gel electrophoresis apparatus.
6. UV light box and photography equipment.
7. Fluorescent ruler.
8. DNA molecular weight markers.

2.2.3. Culture and Electroporation of C127 Cells

1. Routine tissue-culture equipment: CO_2 incubators; laminar flow-hood; tissue culture grade plastics.
2. C127 cells (ATCC CRL 1616, Rockville, MD).
3. Dulbecco's modified Eagle's medium (DMEM) (Life Technologies, Gaithersburg, MD).
4. Fetal bovine serum (FBS).
5. "Trypsin" (0.25% Trypsin, 1 m*M* EDTA in HBSS).
6. DMEM/10% FBS containing 10 m*M* BES, pH 7.2 and 10 m*M* HEPES, pH 7.2.
7. Hemocytometer or Coulter counter.
8. Electroporation cuvet (Bio-Rad [Richmond, CA] or BTX [San Diego, CA], 0.4-mm gap).
9. Electroporation apparatus (Bio-Rad Gene Pulser with Capacitance Extender, BTX ECM 600 or similar instrument).
10. Replicon DNA, 0.1 mg/mL.
11. Carrier DNA, salmon sperm 10 mg/mL.
12. 15-mL centrifuge tubes.
13. Low-speed centrifuge.

2.2.4. Extraction of Low-Mol-Wt DNA

1. Dulbecco's phosphate-buffered saline (D-PBS).
2. Alkaline lysis solution I: 50 m*M* glucose, 25 m*M* Tris-HCl, pH 8.0, 10 m*M* EDTA.
3. Alkaline lysis solution II: 0.2% NaOH, 1% SDS (make fresh).
4. Alkaline lysis solution III: 5 *M* potassium acetate, pH 4.8 (for 500 mL: 300 mL 5 *M* potassium acetate, 57.5 mL glacial acetic acid, 142.5 mL dH_2O).

5. Cell scrapers.
6. Microfuge and microfuge tubes.
7. Isopropanol.
8. Digestion buffer: 20 m*M* Tris-HCl, pH 8.0, 100 m*M* NaCl, 10 m*M* EDTA, 0.2% SDS; 200 µg/mL proteinase K (add fresh).
9. "Phenol/chloroform": phenol saturated with TE buffer, chloroform (1:1).
10. "Chloroform": chloroform, isoamyl alcohol (24:1, v/v).
11. 3 *M* sodium acetate, pH 5.2.
12. Ethanol, 95% and 70%.
13. TE buffer: 10 m*M* Tris-HCl, pH 8.0; 1 m*M* EDTA.
14. RNase A (10 mg/mL).

2.2.5. Preparation of Probe

1. Viral DNA cloned into a prokaryotic vector, p142-6 ***(14)***.
2. *Bam*HI.
3. Random Prime DNA Labeling kit (Boehringer Manheim, Indianapolis, IN).
4. α^{32}P-dCTP (>3000 Ci/mmol).
5. 0.5 *M* EDTA.
6. G50 spin columns (ProbeQuant G-50 Micro columns, Pharmacia Biotech).

2.2.6. Digestion of Low-Mol-Wt DNA and Detection of Papillomavirus DNA by Southern Blotting

1. *Dpn*I, *Mbo*I, and *Hin*dIII restriction enzymes and buffers.
2. Materials for agarose gel electrophoresis as in **Subheading 2.2.2.**
3. 0.25 *M* HCl.
4. Denaturing solution: 0.5 *M* NaCl/0.5 *M* NaOH.
5. Neutralizing solution: 0.5 *M* NaCl/0.5 *M* Tris-HCl, pH 7.5.
6. 20X SSC: 3 *M* NaCl, 0.3 *M* sodium citrate, pH 7.0.
7. Magnagraph Nylon Transfer Membrane (Micron Separations, Westboro, MA), Nytran (Schleicher & Schuell, Keene, NH) or similar membrane.
8. 3MM paper.
9. Plastic cling film (e.g., Saran Wrap).
10. Blot pads or paper towels.
11. UV-stratalinker (Stratagene, La Jolla, CA).
12. 50X Denhardt's: 1% Ficoll (type 400), 1% polyvinylpyrrolidone (PVP), 1% BSA (Fraction V). Store at –20°C.
13. 20% SDS.
14. 10 mg/mL sheared salmon sperm DNA.
15. Wash buffer: 0.1% SDS/0.1X SSC.
16. Hybridization oven containers or blot bags and heat sealer.
17. Hybridization oven, heated water bath, or air shaker.
18. Plastic box to set up blot and wash blot.
19. Autoradiography film and cassettes.

3. Methods

3.1. E1-E2 Cooperative DNA Binding Assay

3.1.1. Preparation of ^{32}P-Labeled DNA Fragments

1. Digest 20 µg pKS ori+ plasmid DNA with *Bam*HI, *Hin*dIII, and *Afl*III (*see* **Fig. 4** and **Note 4**). This will provide a stock of digested probe DNA for several experiments. The final reaction volume should equal 200 µL, and, therefore, the DNA concentration is 0.1 µg/mL.
2. Analyze 5 µL (0.5 mg) of digested DNA on a 1% agarose/1X TBE gel using standard methods. DNA can be stored at –20°C. After digestion there should be three bands: a 250-bp band containing the origin, a 400-bp vector band, and a larger vector band of 2–3 kb.
3. End-label 5 µg digested DNA (enough for 25 binding reactions using 0.2 µg probe per incubation) as follows: 5 µL 10X Klenow buffer (*see* **Note 5**), 50 µL (5 µg) digested DNA, 3 µL 10 m*M* dATP, 3 µL 10 m*M* dGTP, 3 µL 10 m*M* TTP, 20 µL $\alpha^{32}P$-dCTP (>3000 Ci/mmol), and 3 µL (6 U) of Klenow. Adjust the final reaction volume to 100 µL with dH_2O. Incubate at 37°C for 30 min. Stop the reaction by adding of 2 µL of 0.5 *M* EDTA. Adjust probe to 40 ng/µL with dH_2O.
4. Remove unincorporated nucleotides using a spin column, such as ProbeQuant G-50 Micro column, following the manufacturer's directions (*see* **Note 6**).
5. Analyze 1 µL probe on a 5% polyacrylamide/1X TBE gel to ensure that fragments are labeled efficiently. To prepare a 40-mL 5% polyacrylamide gel, use 6.7 mL of 30% stock acrylamide:bis-acrylamide (29:1), 4 mL of 10X TBE, 28.7 mL distilled water. Polymerize acrylamide with 0.6 mL 10% ammonium persulfate and 10 µL TEMED. Dilute 1 µL of probe in 5 µL dH_2O and add 3 µL loading buffer. Load the sample on the gel and electrophorese at 300 V. The gel can be stopped when the bromophenol blue dye has migrated two-thirds of the way down. To detect the probe, remove one glass plate, and wrap the other plate containing the gel with plastic cling film. Place the plate and gel (gel side down) on a piece of X-ray film (*see* **Note 7**). Expose for approx 15 min and develop the film.

3.1.2. Preparation of Proteins

1. Use Promega's TNT T7 kit to translate E1 and E2 proteins, according to the manufacturer's directions (**Note 8**). For the E1/E2 cooperative binding assay, approx 25 µL of each protein is required per reaction. In addition, enough unprogrammed (blank) lysate should be translated for use as controls and to dilute the E1 and E2 proteins to equal concentrations. For each 50 µL reaction the components are mixed gently on ice in the following order: 25 µL TNT lysate; 2 µL reaction buffer; 1 µL RNA polymerase; 1 µL amino acids minus methionine; 4 µL ^{35}S-methionine (1000 Ci/mmol, 10 mCi/mL); 1 µL RNasin; X µL DNA (1 µg); 15-X µL H_2O. The reaction is incubated at 30°C for 90 min.
2. Analyze each translation reaction on a 12% SDS-polyacrylamide gel. Mix 1 µL translation reaction with 10 µL 1X SDS sample buffer and heat to 100°C before

loading on gel. Minigels work well for this analysis, and electrophoresis can be completed within 1–2 h. The gel is fixed in methanol/acetic acid for 1 h with several changes of fixative to remove unincorporated ^{35}S-methionine. The ^{35}S signal is enhanced by soaking the gel in ENLIGHTNING for 20 min. The gel is dried onto 3MM paper using standard methods.
3. Analyze gel on Phosphorimager. Expose dried gel to screen for 3 h to overnight. Quantitate proteins and adjust concentration of each with unprogrammed lysate so that they all have equal concentrations of E1 or E2 protein (*see* **Note 9**).
4. Store proteins at –70°C.

3.1.3. E1 DNA Binding and E1-E2 Cooperative DNA Binding Assay

1. Mix the following at room temperature in siliconized microfuge tubes (volumes are per reaction): 10 µL 10X binding buffer, 25 µL buffer C-300 (*see* **Note 10**), 9 µL dH_2O, 1 µL sheared salmon sperm DNA (10 mg/mL), 25 µL TNT E1 protein, and 25 µL TNT™ E2 protein (*see* **Note 11**).
2. Spin out insoluble protein in microfuge at 18°C for 10 min.
3. Aliquot 5 µL probe DNA (0.2 µg) to a new set of siliconized microfuge tubes.
4. Transfer the supernatant from **step 2** to the new tube containing the probe. Mix well but do not vortex. Incubate at room temperature for 1–4 h.
5. Meanwhile, wash protein A sepharose (100 µL per sample) three times with NET-100 and suspend in original volume of NET-100. Bind 5 µL affinity-purified E1-specific antiserum (SSQN) to 100 µL of washed protein A sepharose for each incubation reaction. Rotate at 4°C for 1 h.
6. Wash antibody/sepharose three times with NET-100 and suspend in original volume using NET-100.
7. Add 100 µL antibody/protein A sepharose to each binding reaction and rotate in a tumble-mixer (to keep sepharose from settling) at room temperature for 1 h.
8. Wash sepharose three times with NET-100: pellet sepharose in microfuge for 5 s, aspirate buffer, and add 1 mL fresh NET-100. Mix by inverting tubes several times (do not vortex). Work quickly at this stage in batches of no more than six tubes.

3.1.4. Analysis of DNA Products

3.1.4.1. Option 1

In this option, the DNA is extracted from the complexes with SDS and phenol/chloroform and ethanol-precipitated before being analyzed on a polyacrylamide gel. Option 2 is quicker and probably less prone to losses.

1. Add 300 µL NET-100 to sepharose pellet. Mix well and remove 30 µL slurry to examine proteins (add an equal volume of 2X SDS-sample buffer and analyze by SDS-PAGE).
2. Add SDS to the remaining 270 µL slurry to a final concentration of 1%. Add 10 µg carrier tRNA per tube. Shake at room temperature for 20 min.

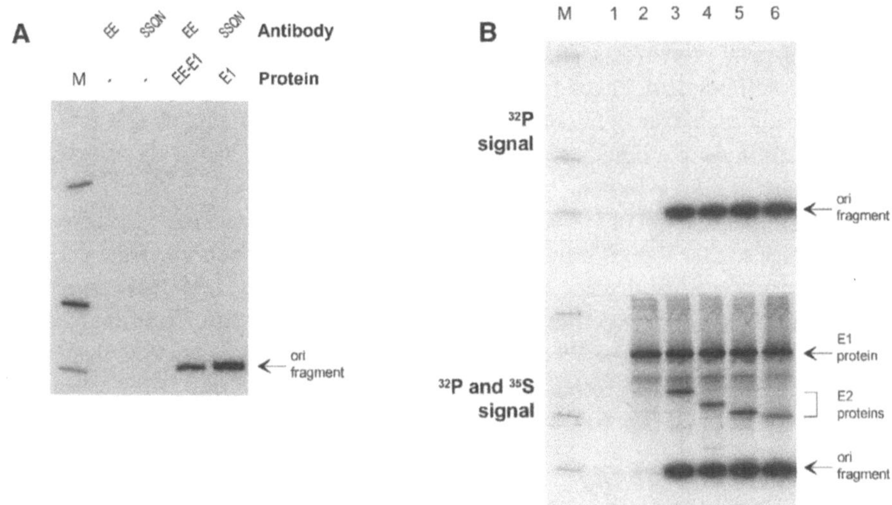

Fig. 6. **(A)** E1 binding assay. Lane M contains the input ^{32}P-labeled DNA fragments from pKS+ ori. These fragments were incubated with 100 µL TNT lysate containing either no E1 protein (–), EE-E1 protein (E1 with an EE epitope fused at the N-terminus), or wild-type E1. DNA-protein complexes were immunoprecipitated with either E1-specific antiserum (SSQN) or EE-specific antibody. E1-bound DNA was extracted and analyzed by gel electrophoresis (option 1). **(B)** E1-E2 cooperative binding assay. Lane M contains the input ^{32}P-labeled DNA fragments from pKS+ ori. These fragments were incubated with 50 µL control TNT lysate (lane 1), 25 µL E1 lysate and 25 µL control lysate (lane 2) and 25 µL E1 lysate and 25 µL control lysates (lanes 3–6). Lane 3 contains wild-type E2 protein and lanes 4–6 contain E2 proteins with deletions in the "hinge" region ***(15)***. DNA-protein complexes were immunoprecipitated with E1-specific antiserum (SSQN), and E1-bound DNA was extracted and analyzed by gel electrophoresis (option 2).

3. Extract DNA with phenol chloroform. Remove aqueous phase (avoid interface) and add to 1 mL ethanol. Samples can be stored overnight at –20°C at this stage, if necessary.
4. Pellet DNA in microfuge for 10 min. Wash pellet with 70% ethanol. Carefully aspirate off all traces of ethanol and air dry pellet.
5. Dissolve pellet in 20 µL TE buffer. Add 5 µL sucrose loading buffer (use frozen aliquots).
6. Load samples on 5% polyacrylamide gel (29:1, made as in **Subheading 3.1.1., step 5** for probe). As a marker, run a 1:200 dilution of probe on each gel. Dilute 1 µL probe in 199 µL TE buffer. Mix 5 µL diluted probe, 10 µg (1 µL) tRNA, 10 µL H_2O, and 5 µL sample buffer.
7. Electrophorese gel at 250 V until bromophenol blue dye is close to the bottom.
8. Fix gel in methanol/acetic acid for 1 h, dry onto 3MM paper and expose to autoradiograph film (*see* **Fig. 6** and **Note 12**).

3.1.4.2. Option 2

1. Resuspend protein A sepharose pellet in 100 µL 1X SDS-PAGE sample buffer. Mix well but do not heat. Shake at room temperature for 15 min.
2. Spin out sepharose in microfuge and transfer the supernatant to a new tube. Load 50 µL of sample onto a 12% SDS-polyacrylamide gel. Run 1 ng of probe as a marker in sample buffer.
3. Electrophorese gel at 100 V until dye runs through the stacking gel. Increase the voltage to 200 V until bromophenol blue is close to the bottom of the gel.
4. Fix gel in methanol/acetic acid (do not enhance) and dry onto 3MM paper.
5. Expose the gel to two films in an autoradiography cassette. The film closest to the gel will contain the ^{35}S and ^{32}P signals and is useful for checking that the size and quantity of the proteins are as expected. The second film will have only the ^{32}P DNA signal (*see* **Fig. 6**).

3.2. Replication Assay

3.2.1. Recircularization of BPV-1 Replicon

1. Cleave 10–200 µg cloned viral genome (or other replicon DNA) with appropriate enzyme to remove vector sequences. *Bam*HI removes the pML2d vector from p142-6 (**Note 13**).
2. Check 0.5 µg digested DNA by agarose gel electrophoresis to ensure that digestion is complete.
3. Remove the restriction enzyme by extracting once with "phenol/chloroform" and once with "chloroform." Add sodium acetate, pH 5.2 to a final concentration of 0.3 *M*. Add 2.5 vol of 95% ethanol and centrifuge for 10 min in a microfuge. Aspirate ethanol and wash pellet with 70% ethanol. Air-dry pellet.
4. Suspend DNA in TE (assume approx 80% recovery).
5. Ligate DNA at 5 µg/mL overnight at 16°C. Use 2 mL 10X ligase buffer, 2 mL 10 m*M* ATP, and 5 µL high-concentration T4 DNA ligase for a 20-mL ligation (100 µg DNA).
6. Extract DNA by phenol/chloroform extraction. Add sodium acetate, pH 5.2 to a final concentration of 0.3 *M*. Add 2.5 vol of 95% ethanol and centrifuge for 10 min at 6500*g*. Because of the large volumes, it is necessary to use 30-mL Corex tubes or disposable 50-mL tubes (Falcon). A large pellet should be visible as the ATP will precipitate and act as carrier.
7. Suspend pellet in 200 µL TE buffer. Add 200 µL 5 *M* ammonium acetate. Precipitate DNA with 1 mL 95% ethanol (ATP should not precipitate in ammonium acetate). Centrifuge in microfuge for 10 min at room temperature. Wash pellet in 95% ethanol (not 70%). Air-dry pellet.
8. Dissolve pellet in TE at 0.1 mg/mL (assume 80% recovery) and check on recovery by agarose gel electrophoresis.

3.2.2. Electroporation of C127 Cells for Transient Replication Assay

1. C127 cells are cultured in DMEM media supplemented with 10% FBS and grown in a 10% CO_2 incubator. C127 cells should be subconfluent and actively growing

at the time of transfection. These assays use a large number of cells. There are approx 0.5×10^7 C127 cells in a large (175-cm^2) subconfluent flask (**Note 15**).

2. Trypsinize cells and count using a hemocytometer or Coulter counter. Collect cells by centrifugation at 100*g* for 5 min. Resuspend cells at a density of 1.0×10^7/mL for C127 cells in DMEM/10% FBS/10 m*M* BES, pH 7.2/10 m*M* HEPES, pH 7.2. Store cells at room temperature until ready to use.
3. Add the DNA to be electroporated (0.1–1 µg) to a disposable electroporation cuvette (with 0.4-mm gap). Add salmon sperm carrier DNA to a total of 50 µg and dH_2O to a total of 20 mL.
4. Add 250 µL cell suspension to each cuvet. Mix gently and proceed with the electroporation. The settings for electroporation with the Bio-Rad Gene Pulser are as follows: 960 µF; 220 V. The settings using the BTX ECM 600 are as follows: 1200 µF; Resistance Timer R5; 220 V (**Note 15**).
5. After electroporation, the cell/DNA mix is left at room temperature for 10–15 min.
6. While the cells are standing at room temperature, aliquot 10 mL DMEM/10% FBS into 15 mL centrifuge tubes. After incubation, remove the cell/DNA mix from the cuvette with a 1-mL pipet and layer it on top of the DMEM/10% FBS. Spin at 100*g* for 5 min. Dead cells and denatured serum should stay on the top and live cells should pellet.
7. Aspirate media and resuspend C127 cells pellet in 6 mL complete media. Plate 1 mL cells per 10-cm dish and add 9 mL complete media.
8. Cells can be harvested at different time intervals. Normally, we collect samples at 3 and 5 d posttransfection. BPV-1 will transform C127 cells and so, if desired, a plate can be kept for 2–3 wk to measure transformation efficiency (**Note 17**).

3.2.3. Extraction of Low-Mol-Wt Extrachromosomal DNA

1. Wash culture plates in PBS. Carefully aspirate any excess liquid and sit plate on ice.
2. Add 600 µL of a 1:2 mixture of alkaline lysis plasmid prep solutions I and II (8.8 mL H_2O; 1 mL 10% SDS; 5 mL solution I; 0.2 mL 10 *N* NaOH). Tilt plate back and forth to distribute liquid over entire plate. Cells should lyse. Incubate on ice for 5 min.
3. Add 300 µL solution III to each plate. This will precipitate proteins and chromosomal DNA. Scrape lysate into a microcentrifuge tube, mix well by inverting the tube several times (do not vortex), and incubate on ice for 10 min.
4. Spin lysate at 4°C for 5 min. Add supernatant to 0.6 vol of isopropanol. Mix well. Samples can be stored at –20°C at this stage.
5. Collect nucleic acids by centrifugation in a microfuge for 10 min at 4°C. Dissolve pellet in 200 µL HIRT digestion buffer. Incubate at 37°C for 30 min and then at 50°C for 30 min.
6. Extract samples with an equal volume of "phenol/chloroform" and then with an equal volume of "chloroform."
7. Add 20 µL 3 *M* sodium acetate, pH 5.2. Add 600 µL 95% ethanol to precipitate nucleic acids.
8. Collect nucleic acids by centrifugation in a microfuge for 10 min at 4°C. Dissolve pellet in 200 µL TE. Add 20 µL 3 *M* sodium acetate and reprecipitate with 600 µL ethanol.

9. Collect nucleic acids by centrifugation, wash pellet in 70% ethanol, and air-dry.
10. Dissolve pellet in 50 µL TE containing 20 µg/mL RNase A. Incubate at 68°C for 20 min.
11. Digest 25 µL of the DNA sample with *Dpn*I and an enzyme to linearize the genome (*Hin*dIII), and the remaining 25 µL of DNA with *Mbo*I and an enzyme to linearize the genome (*Hin*dIII). Digest for several hours with an excess of restriction enzyme to ensure that cleavage is complete.

3.2.4. Preparation of ^{32}P-Labeled DNA Probe

1. Digest viral genome with a restriction enzyme that will linearize the DNA (*Bam*HI or *Hin*dIII).
2. Label 50 ng probe using the random prime method according to the manufacturer's directions.
3. Separate unincorporated nucleotides from labeled DNA using a ProbeQuant G-50 Micro column.

3.2.5. Southern Blot

1. Prepare a 0.8% agarose gel in 1X TBE. Ethidium bromide can be added to the gel (10 µL of 10 mg/mL solution/100 mL gel) and to the buffer (100 µL/L of buffer) or gels can be stained after electrophoresis. Do not include ethidium bromide in gel when separating uncut supercoiled DNA as it can affect the migration.
2. Agarose gels (100 mL; 11 × 14 cm^2) can be electrophoresed overnight at 8 mA or in several hours at 40 mA. After electrophoresis, photograph gel with a fluorescent ruler alongside the marker lane. The replicon is not usually observed with ethidium bromide staining, but cellular mitochondrial DNA and a low level of cellular genomic DNA are usually present.
3. Optional step (but necessary for uncut supercoiled DNA). Depurinate DNA by soaking gel in 1 L of 0.25 *M* HCl for 15 min.
4. Denature DNA by soaking gel in 1 L of 0.5 *M* NaCl/0.5 *M* NaOH for 1 h.
5. Soak gel in 1 L of 0.5 *M* NaCl/0.5 *M* Tris-HCl, pH 7.5 for 1 h to neutralize DNA.
6. Transfer DNA to a nylon membrane as shown in **Fig. 7**. In a dish of 10X SSC, place a piece of 3MM paper over a platform so that the ends of the paper dip into the buffer and act as wicks. Place the gel on the platform and roll out any bubbles with a pipet. Add a sheet of nylon membrane (prewetted in dH_2O) and then two sheets of prewetted 3MM paper. Roll out any bubbles between the gel, membrane, and 3MM paper with a pipet. Next add two dry sheets of 3MM paper and a stack of paper towels or blot pads. Add a 500 g weight to the top. Gels are usually transferred overnight, but 4 h is probably sufficient.
7. Remove the blot pads and lift off the 3MM paper and membrane. Keep the membrane on the 3MM paper as this helps to prevent it from drying out. Crosslink DNA to the membrane using the UV-stratalinker. Use the "auto crosslink" program that delivers 120 mJ.
8. Place the nylon membrane in a blot bag or hybridization tube with 50 mL prehybridization mix (3X SSC, 2% SDS, 5X Denhardt's, 0.2 mg/mL sheared

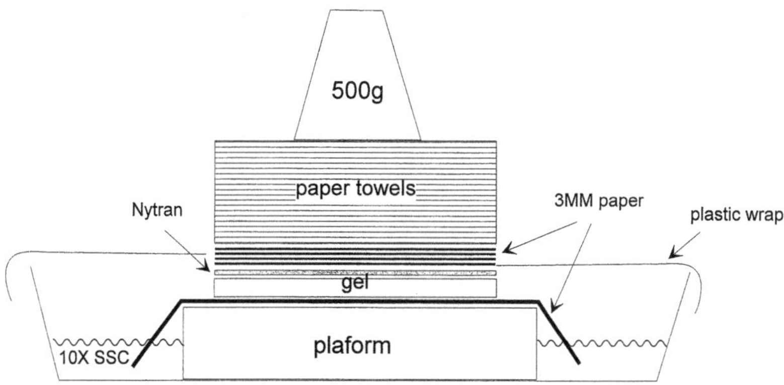

Fig. 7. Southern blotting. DNA fragments that have been separated by gel electrophoresis are transferred to nylon membrane, such as Nytran, as shown in the diagram and as described in the text.

carrier DNA; *see* **Note 18**). Heat salmon sperm DNA to 100°C for 10 min before adding to the solution. Incubate in hybridization oven, water bath, or air shaker at 65°C. Prehybridization times can range from 1 h to overnight.

9. Add 50 ng ^{32}P-labeled DNA probe to carrier DNA and heat to 100°C for 10 min. Add to 10 mL hybridization mix (3X SSC, 2% SDS, 5X Denhardt's, 0.2 mg/mL sheared carrier DNA). Remove prehybridization solution and replace with hybridization solution containing probe. Incubate in hybridization oven or shaker overnight at 65°C.
10. Preheat wash buffer (0.1% SDS/0.1X SSC) to 65°C. Remove filter from bag and place in plastic box. If using hybridization tubes, carry out initial washes in tube and then transfer to plastic box. Rinse twice with approx 500 mL wash buffer. Wash blot three times for 30 min in 1 L of wash buffer. Wash in shaker, water bath or hybridization oven at 65°C.
11. Air-dry blot. Mount on a piece of 3MM paper and cover with plastic film. Expose to autoradiography film (*see* **Fig. 8**).

4. Notes

4.1. E1 Binding and E1-E2 Cooperative DNA Binding Assay

1. Some sources of Klenow do not label all DNA fragment equally, particularly if the terminal nucleotide is to be labeled. Boehringer Mannheim's Klenow enzyme gives consistently good results.
2. We use Amersham's (Arlington Heights, IL) Redivue ^{35}S-methionine, which can be stored at 4°C.
3. The SSQN antiserum recognizes an epitope at the N-terminus of BPV-1 E1 (residues 90–110). The assay also works well when a synthetic epitope is fused to the N-terminus of the El protein and an antibody that recognizes the epitope is used

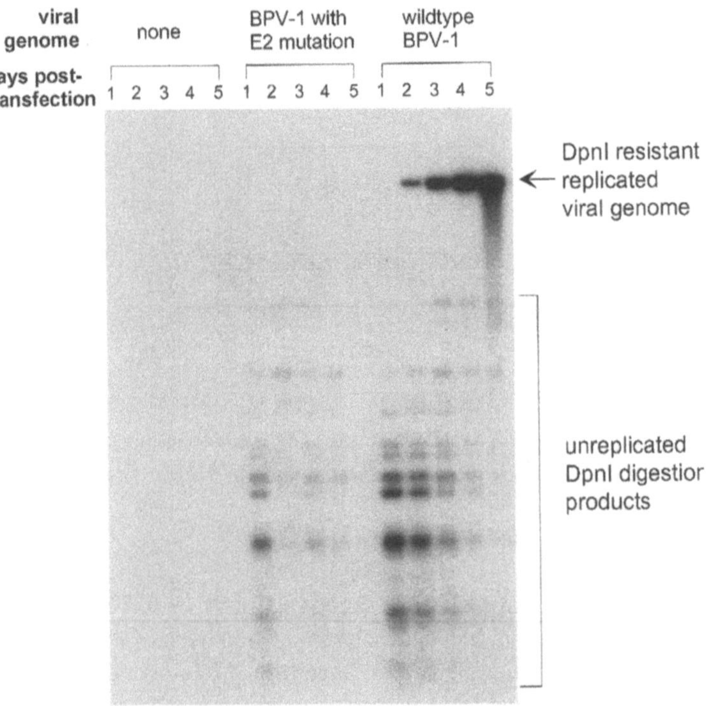

Fig. 8. Replication assay. Recircularized viral genomes were transfected into C127 cells by electroporation. and low molecular weight DNA was isolated every day for 5 d posttransfection. The DNA was cleaved by *Hin*dIII and *Dpn*I, and replicated viral genomes were detected by Southern blot analysis as described in the text.

to precipitate E1 complexes (the authors use an EE epitope ***(16)***. Antibodies that bind to the C-terminal two-thirds of E1 may interfere with E1 DNA binding and/ or interaction with the E2 protein.

4. Any plasmid that contains the replication origin can be used as a probe (even the entire viral genome). Select a restriction enzyme that will generate a range of fragment sizes that can easily be identified. The labeling method and ^{32}P-labeled nucleotide to be used will depend on the type and sequence of the DNA fragment end.
5. Only 5 µL of 10X buffer is added because the 50 µL digested DNA is already in buffer.
6. Use TE buffer for the ProbeQuant G-50 columns rather than the STE buffer recommended by the manufacturer.
7. If using individually wrapped double-sided autoradiography film (such as Xomat AR), the film can be exposed to the gel while it is still in its paper envelope. The envelope can then be taken to the darkroom for film development.
8. The E2 protein can be synthesized by first transcribing RNA from the E2 plasmid and then translating this RNA in an in vitro translation system. However, the

authors have found that the E1 protein can only be efficiently translated using the coupled transcription and translation TNT system (Promega). This may be owing to secondary structure in the E1 RNA that inhibits translation.

9. When quantitating in vitro translated proteins based on ^{35}S incorporation, the number of methionines in each protein must be taken into account.
10. The final salt concentration of the binding reaction has been estimated to be 150 m*M* NaCl. TNT lysates are assumed to be 150 m*M* NaCl, and so if a different volume of TNT lysate is added to the reaction, the volume of buffer C-300 must be adjusted accordingly.
11. In most cases, 25 µL E1 protein and 25 µL E2 protein give good cooperative binding. If the addition of E2 does not greatly enhance E1 binding, then it may be necessary to decrease the volume of E1 protein so that it is limiting. To assay for E1 binding in the absence of E2, it is better to increase the volume of the E1 lysate to 50–100 µL (*see* **Fig. 6A**).
12. 5% Polyacrylamide gels are quite fragile. Instead of placing the gel directly onto the 3MM paper for drying, pick up the gel in a bundle with both hands and lay it upside down on the plastic wrap. Smooth it out flat and then lay a damp piece of 3MM on top.

4.2. Replication Assay

13. It is not absolutely necessary to remove the prokaryotic vector sequences from the replicon before use, but the replicon will replicate more efficiently if they are removed. Some investigators linearize the replicon but do not religate it. The replicon will be ligated within the transfected cell but it will often have deletions at the site of linearization.
14. Instead of using the viral genome as a replicon (which will also express the E1 and E2 proteins), it is possible to cotransfect a plasmid containing the origin together with separate expression vectors for the E1 and E2 proteins. Under these circumstances, it is better to generate by polymerase chain reaction a specific probe (of approx 200 nucleotides) that spans the origin region. The amplified fragment can be labeled by the random primer method as described in **Subheading 3.2.4.**
15. If separate E1 and E2 expression plasmids and replicons are being used in the replication assay (as described in **Note 14**), it is better to use Chinese hamster ovary (CHO) cells. The level of replication signal is much higher using these cells compared with C127 cells, perhaps because they have a much higher transfection efficiency. The authors have not tried the BPV-1 genome in CHO cells. Replication assays using human papillomaviruses have been successful in a number of cell types, such as SCC-13, COS-7, NIH-3T3, and 293 cells ***(17–19)***.
16. The electroporation procedure is the same for C127 and CHO cells except as follows: CHO cells are cultured in F12 media supplemented with 10% FBS and grown in a 5% CO_2 incubator; a 175-cm^2 70% confluent flask contains approx 2×10^7 CHO cells; CHO cells should be suspended at 2.0×10^7/mL for electroporation; CHO cells are electroporated at 250 V; after electroporation, CHO cells are divided into 10, 10-cm plates.

17. When using separate E1 and E2 expression plasmids and replicons, it is better to harvest DNA at shorter times after infection (2 and 4 d) because the viral genomes have a plasmid maintenance function that maintains them at a stable copy number compared to the expression vectors, which will be lost after several cell divisions.
18. Do not mix 20X SSC and SDS together directly or a precipitate will form.

References

1. Howley, P. M. (1995) *Papillomavirinae*: the viruses and their replication, in *Virology* (Fields, B. N., Knipe, D. M., and Howley, P. M., eds.), Lippincott-Raven, Philadelphia, pp. 2045–2076.
2. Ustav, M. and Stenlund, A. (1991) Transient replication of BPV-1 requires two viral polypeptides encoded by the E1 and E2 open reading frames. *EMBO J.* **10,** 449–457.
3. Ustav, M., Ustav, E., Szymanski, P., and Stenlund, A. (1991) Identification of the origin of replication of bovine papillomavirus and characterization of the viral origin recognition factor E1. *EMBO J.* **10,** 4321–4329.
4. Hughes, F. J. and Romanos, M. A. (1993) E1 protein of human papillomavirus is a DNA helicase/ATPase. *Nucleic Acids Res.* **21,** 5817–5823.
5. Jenkins, O., Earnshaw, D., Sarginson, G., Del Vecchio, A., Tsai, J., Kallender, H., Amegadzie, B., and Browne, M. (1996) Characterization of the helicase and ATPase activity of human papillomavirus type 6b E1 protein. *J. Gen. Virol.* **77,** 1805–1809.
6. Yang, L., Mohr, I., Fouts, E., Lim, D. A., Nohaile, M., and Botchan, M. (1993) The E1 protein of bovine papillomavirus 1 is an ATP-dependent DNA helicase. *Proc. Natl. Acad. Sci. USA* **90,** 5086–5090.
7. Blitz, I. L. and Laimins, L. A. (1991) The 68-kilodalton E1 protein of bovine papillomavirus is a DNA binding phosphoprotein which associates with the E2 transcriptional activator in vitro. *J. Virol.* **65,** 649–656.
8. Mohr, I. J., Clark, R., Sun, S., Androphy, E. J., MacPherson, P., and Botchan, M. R. (1990) Targeting the E1 replication protein to the papillomavirus origin of replication by complex formation with the E2 transactivator. *Science* **250,** 1694–1699.
9. Sedman, J. and Stenlund, A. (1995) Co-operative interaction between the initiator E1 and the transcriptional activator E2 is required for replicator specific DNA replication of bovine papillomavirus in vivo and in vitro. *EMBO J.* **14,** 6218–6228.
10. Seo, Y., Muller, F., Lusky, M., Gibbs, E., Kim, H., Phillips, B., and Hurwitz, J. (1993) Bovine papilloma virus (BPV)-encoded E2 protein enhances binding of E1 protein to the BPV replication origin. *Proc. Natl. Acad. Sci. USA* **90,** 2865–2869.
11. Spalholz, B. A., McBride, A. A., Sarafi, T., and Quintero, J. (1993) Binding of bovine papillomavirus E1 to the origin is not sufficient for DNA replication. *Virology* **193,** 201–212.
12. Li, R. and Botchan, M. R. (1994) Acidic transcription factors alleviate nucleosome-mediated repression of DNA replication of bovine papillomavirus type 1. *Proc. Natl. Acad. Sci. USA* **91,** 7051–7055.

13. Li, R. and Botchan, M. R. (1993) The acidic transcriptional activation domains of VP16 and p53 bind the cellular replication protein A and stimulate in vitro BPV-1 DNA replication. *Cell* **73,** 1207–1221.
14. Sarver, N., Byrne, J. C., and Howley, P. M. (1982) Transformation and replication in mouse cells of a bovine papillomavirus—pML2 plasmid vector that can be rescued in bacteria. *Proc. Natl. Acad. Sci. USA* **79,** 7147–7151.
15. Winokur, P. L. and McBride, A. A. (1996) The transactivation and DNA binding domains of the BPV-1 E2 protein have different roles in co-operative origin binding with the E1 protein. *Virology* **221,** 44–53.
16. Grussenmeyer, T., Scheidtmann, K. H., Hutchinson, M. A., Eckart, W., and Walter, G. (1985) Complexes of polyoma virus medium T antigen and cellular proteins. *Proc. Natl. Acad. Sci. USA* **82,** 7952–7954.
17. Chiang, C. M., Ustav, M., Stenlund, A., Ho, T. F., Broker, T. R., and Chow, L. T. (1992) Viral E1 and E2 proteins support replication of homologous and heterologous papillomaviral origins. *Proc. Natl. Acad. Sci. USA* **89,** 5799–5803.
18. Del Vecchio, A. M., Romanczuk, H., Howley, P. M., and Baker, C. C. (1992) Transient replication of human papillomavirus DNAs. *J. Virol.* **66,** 5949–5958.
19. Frattini, M. G. and Laimins, L. A. (1994) The role of the E1 and E2 proteins in the replication of human papillomavirus type 31b. *Virology* **204,** 799–804.

28

Quantitative Immunodetection of Viral Oncoprotein Levels in Human Papillomavirus–Transformed Human Cells

Jeffrey A. Johnson and J. David Gangemi

1. Introduction

Human papillomaviruses (HPV) comprise a genus in the species *Papovaviridae*, which consist of small, naked icosahedral viruses containing circular dsDNA. HPV types 16 and 18 infect squamous epithelium of the genitalia and may infect as many as 45% of the female population in developed countries *(1)*.

HPV-16 encodes a set of early gene oncoproteins (E6 and E7) responsible for cellular immortalization. HPV types 16 and 18 E6 and E7 proteins are known to interact strongly with p53 and retinoblastoma (Rb) tumor suppressor gene products, respectively *(2)*. The association of E6 with p53 marks this tumor suppressor for rapid ubiquitin-mediated proteolysis. Reduced levels of p53 prevent the cell from activating cell cycle arrest and/or induction of apoptosis in genetically mutated cells.

The viral E7 gene product preferentially binds the underphosphorylated, active form of pRb. Hypophosphorylated Rb has the ability to bind DNA and negatively regulate E2F-responsive promoters of genes responsible for driving progression of cell cycling into S-phase and mitosis. E7 is also known to interact with and transactivate several AP-1 transcription factors *(3)*; thus, the coordinated inhibitory and activation properties of this oncoprotein can result in cellular transformation.

Quantitatively assessing oncoproteins in HPV-transformed cells is useful for evaluating viral activity and the potential effectiveness of antiviral therapy *(4)*. The following describes immunodetection methods for assaying levels of human papillomavirus E6 and E7 protein in total protein cell lysates. This pro-

From: *Methods in Molecular Medicine, vol. 24: Antiviral Methods and Protocols*
Edited by: D. Kinchington and R. F. Schinazi © Humana Press Inc., Totowa, NJ

cedure can be utilized to assay any soluble protein, however, its value is better realized in identifying proteins that are more difficult to detect.

2. Materials

1. 100-mm tissue culture dishes and appropriate medium for cell line.
2. 50-mL polypropylene centrifuge tubes.
3. Trypsin-EDTA (for adherent cells) (0.05% trypsin, 0.53 m*M* EDTA·4Na) (Gibco).
4. Tris-buffered saline (TBS) (per liter): Tris base, 2.42 g; NaCl, 8.00 g; H_2O to fill and pH to 7.6 with HCl).
5. Protease inhibitors: aprotinin (10 mg/mL in 0.01 *M* HEPES, pH 8.0), leupeptin (10 mg/mL in water), pepstatin A (1 mg/mL in ethanol), benzamidine (10 m*M* in water), sodium orthovanadate (100 m*M*), paramethylsulfonyl fluoride (PMSF) (10 m*M* in isopropanol) (Sigma).
6. Microcentrifuge (12,000*g* capacity).
7. 1.5-mL microcentrifuge tubes (Eppendorf).
8. Bradford protein assay (Bio-Rad).
9. Bovine serum albumin (BSA) (ELISA grade) (Sigma).
10. Polyoxyethylene-sorbitan monolaurate (Tween-20).
11. Orbital shaker.
12. Natural nitrocellulose membrane (Bio-Rad).
13. Nonfat dry milk (Blotto).
14. Dot-spotting template (dot blotter) (Bio-Rad).
15. 2 mL/well-culture plates (optional).
16. Unlabeled goat antimouse IgG.
17. Anti-HPV-16 E6 mouse monoclonal IgG (Oncogene Research), anti-HPV-16 E6 goat polyclonal IgG (Santa Cruz, Biotech).
18. Anti-HPV-16 E7 mouse monoclonal IgG (Santa Cruz Biotech), anti-HPV-16 E7 goat polyclonal IgG (Santa Cruz, Biotech).
19. Alkaline phosphatase-labeled goat antimouse IgG (Cappel).
20. p-Nitrophenol phosphate (pNPP) SigmaFast tablets with buffer (Sigma).
21. 3 *N* NaOH.
22. Hole puncher, handheld.
23. 96-well flat-bottomed microtiter plates (Corning).
24. ELISA plate reader (Bio-Rad).

3. Methods

3.1. ELISA Assays for HPV E6/E7 Proteins

1. For adherent cultures, trypsinize cells for 5 min and pool plates within each treatment group (4–6 100-mm plates for each group should be sufficient).
2. Harvest cells by centrifugation (7 min at 500*g*).
3. Resuspend cell pellets in cold TBS containing 10 µg/mL aprotinin, leupeptin, and pepstatin, 10 µ*M* benzamidine and 1 m*M* PMSF.

4. Lyse cells on ice by sonication (60 s at 35% power), then transfer lysates to 1.5-mL microcentrifuge tubes.
5. Centrifuge to pellet cell debris for 10 min at 12,000*g* in a microcentrifuge.
6. Determine total protein concentrations of supernatants by Bradford microplate assay (Bio-Rad), or whatever method is available.
7. (Optional) To reduce background signals, incubate supernatants for 3 h at 4%C in 2-mL culture wells that, on the previous day, have been coated with 2 μg/mL of goat antimouse IgG and blocked overnight with 3% BSA/0.5% Tween-20 in buffer. **Note:** All incubations and washes should be made on an orbital shaker (~50 rpm).
8. Incubate natural nitrocellulose membranes in TBS containing 1 μg/mL pAb to E6 or E7 for 30 min at 4°C with shaking.
9. Wash the membranes once with TBS/1% Tween 20.
10. Block nitrocellulose overnight with 5% dry milk (in TBS/0.1% Tween 20) at 4°C with shaking.
11. Apply a layer of parafilm beneath the nitrocellulose membrane and place in a dot-blot apparatus. From each lysate sample, spot 0.5 mg protein/spot onto the nitrocellulose membranes, in triplicate. Be sure to spot groups for each antigen to be detected. Allow to incubate 4 h to overnight at 4°C with shaking.
12. Wash the membranes once with TBS/1% Tween-20.
13. Divide the membrane so that each group can be incubated with a separate primary antibody.
14. Grouped spots are incubated overnight at 4°C with 1 μg/mL of either E6 (Oncogene Research) or E7 (Santa Cruz) mouse monoclonal antibody.
15. Following incubation with primary antibody, wash the membranes with TBS/1% Tween-20 four times for 15 min each.
16. Incubate spotted membranes for 2 h with 0.025 μg/mL alkaline phosphatase-labeled goat antimouse IgG (Cappel).
17. Following incubation with secondary antibody, wash the membranes with TBS/1% Tween-20 four times for 15 min each.
18. Allow the nitrocellulose membranes to briefly dry (~15 min) on clean towels, and then punch out each spot and place into designated wells of a 96-well microtiter plate.
19. React the spots with 100 μL of pNPP substrate (Sigma) until sufficient color development has occurred (30 min–1 h), and then stop the reaction with 50 μL of 3 *N* NaOH.
20. Transfer 100 μL of the supernatants from each well to designated wells into a clean 96-well plate, and read at 405 nm using an available ELISA plate reader.

4. Notes

1. If a sonicator is not available, lysates may be obtained by freeze thawing. For this protocol, lysis buffer (10 m*M* HEPES, pH 7.9, 400 m*M* NaCl, 20% glycerol, 1 m*M* EDTA) is substituted for TBS in **step 3** of **Subheading 3.1.** Additionally, DNase I should be added. Lyse cells by rapid freezing in liquid nitrogen and rapid thaw-

ing in a 50°C water bath. Do this four times and continue procedure at **step 5** of **Subheading 3.1.**

2. Some cell lines have endogenous alkaline phosphatase activity (especially carcinoma lines). In this case, horseradish peroxidase–conjugated goat antimouse IgG can be used (substitute in **step 14** of **Subheading 3.1.**) with appropriate substrate (e.g., 2,2'-azino-di-[3-ethyl-benzthiazoline-6-sulfonic acid] [ABTS]).

References

1. Peto, R. (1986) Introduction: geographic patterns and trends, in *Viral Etiology of Cervical Cancer*, Banbury report 21 (Peto, R. and ZurHausen, H., eds.), Cold Spring Harbor Laboratory, Cold Spring Harbor, NY, pp. 3–15.
2. Vousden, K. H. (1994) Interactions between papillomavirus proteins and tumor suppressor gene products. *Adv. Cancer Res.* **64,** 1–24.
3. Antinore, M. J., Birrer, M. J., Patel, D., Nader, L., and McCance, D. J. (1996) The human papillomavirus type 16 E7 gene product interacts with and trans-activates the AP1 family of transcription factors. *EMBO J.* **15,** 1950–1960.
4. Johnson, J. A. and Gangemi, J. D. (1997) Data presented at the 10th International Conference on Antiviral Research, Atlanta, GA.

V

Influenza Virus

29

Biochemical Methods for the Characterization of Influenza Viruses with Reduced Sensitivity to 4-Guanidino-Neu5Ac2en

Richard C. Bethell, Graham J. Hart, Tony J. Blick, Anjali Sahasrabudhe, and Jennifer L. McKimm-Breschkin

1. Introduction

Viruses that are less sensitive to the influenza neuraminidase (NA)-specific inhibitor 4-guanidino-Neu5Ac2en (zanamavir) *(1)* can be isolated after several passages in MDCK cells in the presence of the inhibitor. Although there are three reports of a mutation in the NA gene at the same conserved site, glu119 *(2–4)*, most of the variants have mutations in the hemagglutinin (HA) gene *(5)*. Many of these mutations appear to lower the affinity of the HA for the cellular receptor, so there is less requirement for significant NA activity for the newly synthesized progeny virus to elute. In this chapter we describe noncell culture-based methods for characterization of both HA and NA variants.

2. Materials

1. 96-well fluorimeter plates, e.g., Optiplate by Packard.
2. 2'-*O*-4-Methylumbelliferyl *N*-acetylneuraminic acid, (MUNANA) (Sigma, St. Louis, MO). 2 m*M* stock solutions should be made up in either 10 m*M* $CaCl_2$ and 100 m*M* sodium acetate buffer, pH 5.5 (IC_{50} determination) or water (slow-binding inhibition determination).
3. 200 m*M* sodium carbonate, pH 9.5.
4. Fluorimeter with microplate attachment, Perkin Elmer model LS50B or similar.
5. Fluorimeter with appropriate temperature-controlled 1-place or motor-driven 4-place cuvet attachment, Perkin Elmer model LS50B or similar.
6. Semimicro quartz fluorescence cuvets with appropriate cuvet adaptors.

From: *Methods in Molecular Medicine, vol. 24: Antiviral Methods and Protocols*
Edited by: D. Kinchington and R. F. Schinazi © Humana Press Inc., Totowa, NJ

7. 500 m*M* 2-[*N*-morpholino]-ethane sulfonic acid (MES), pH 6.5.
8. 20 m*M* $CaCl_2$.
9. Monoclonal antibody (MAb) to native NA, e.g., NC-10 antibody, which binds only to native N9 NA of the NWS/G70C virus, (Rob Webster, St. Jude Children's Research Hospital, Memphis, TN).
10. Polyclonal anti-NA antibody prepared by inoculation of rabbits with pronase-treated purified NA heads ***(6)***.
11. Phosphate-buffered saline (PBS) containing 1% casein, or 1% Tween 20.
12. Sheep antirabbit-HRPO.
13. ABTS, 1 mg/mL in citrate-phosphate buffer, pH 4.5.
14. (Enzyme-linked immunosorbent assay (ELISA) plate reader with 405-nm filter.
15. Monoclonal anti-HA antibody.
16. ELISA plates coated with 20 µg/mL of fetuin.
17. ELISA coating buffer, carbonate/bicarbonate buffer, 0.02 *M*, pH 9.6.
18. 0.5% suspension of chicken erythrocytes.
19. Data analysis software, e.g., Grafit (Erithacus Software Ltd., Staines, Surrey, UK).

3. Methods

3.1. Enzyme Inhibitor, IC_{50} Determination

3.1.1. Determination of Enzyme Activity by MUNANA Assay

NA activity is initially determined over a range of virus dilutions. To determine virus titers for which the enzyme activity is linear, this is generally in the range of 0.5–2 HA units.

1. Prepare dilutions of a drug-free virus stock in PBS. Mix 50 µL of virus and 50 µL of MUNANA mix in 96-well fluorimeter plates.
2. Incubate at 37°C for 1 h.
3. Stop reactions with 260 µL sodium carbonate.
4. Quantify fluorescence in a fluorimeter, e.g., Perkin Elmer, with an excitation wavelength of 365 nm and a slit width of 2.5 nm, and an emission wavelength of 450 nm with a slit width of 20 nm.
5. Plot fluorescence units (FU) vs virus dilution. Select two dilutions of virus for which the activity is in the linear portion of the curve.

3.1.2. Determination of Enzyme Inhibition by MUNANA Assay

1. Mix 25 µL of (2X) virus dilution determined from the enzyme assay and 25 µL of half $\log_{10}$ dilutions of 4-guanidino-Neu5Ac2en, ranging from 1 to 0.0001 µ*M*.
2. Incubate for 30 min at room temperature.
3. Add 50 µL of MUNANA in buffer, and incubate at 37°C for 1 h.
4. Stop reactions and quantify as above.
5. Plot $\log_{10}$ (drug concentration) vs percent inhibition. If the two dilutions of virus are in the linear range the curves should overlay each other and the IC_{50} values should be similar.

3.2. Determination of Slow-Binding Inhibition of NA

4-Guanidino-Neu5Ac2en is a slow-binding inhibitor of wild-type neuraminidases *(8)* (for a complete explanation of slow-binding inhibition *see* **ref. *9***). In contrast, 4-guanidino-Neu5Ac2en no longer binds slowly to those mutant neuraminidases from viruses with reduced sensitivity that have thus far been characterized; in such cases 4-guanidino-Neu5Ac2en is a rapid-binding "classical" competitive inhibitor of the enzyme. Consequently, comparison of K_i values (for rapid-binding inhibition of neuraminidase) or K_d values (for slow-binding inhibition of neuraminidase) is the most appropriate biochemical measure of the loss of sensitivity of the viral neuraminidase to inhibition by this compound when comparing the properties of neuraminidases from resistant viruses with those of the comparator wild-type strain.

3.2.1. Determination of Enzyme Dilution

1. Prepare dilutions of virus in PBS. Combine 60 µL MES solution, 48 µL $CaCl_2$ solution, 3 µL MUNANA solution, and water in the fluorescence cuvets.
2. Add virus to give a final volume of 0.6 mL in the cuvet.
3. Monitor fluorescence (excitation wavelength 365 nm, emission wavelength 450 nm) continuously for 1 h.
4. Construct plots of fluorescence against time.
5. Select a virus dilution giving rise to rates of fluorescence increase that are are linear for the duration of the assay.

3.2.2. Determination of K_m for MUNANA

1. Combine 60 µL MES solution, 48 µL $CaCl_2$ solution, MUNANA solution (final concentration range 10–150 µ*M*), and water in the fluorescence cuvets.
2. Add the appropriate dilution of virus to give a final volume of 0.6 mL in the cuvet.
3. Monitor fluorescence (excitation wavelength 365 nm, emission wavelength 450 nm) continuously for 1 h.
4. From plots of fluorescence against time, derive an initial rate (v) of fluorescence increase (FU/s).
5. Derive K_m for MUNANA from Lineweaver-Burk (1/v vs 1/[MUNANA]) or other suitable plot.

3.2.3. Determination of K_i (Rapid-Binding Inhibition) or K_d (Slow-Binding Inhibition) for 4-Guanidino-Neu5Ac2en

1. Prepare dilutions of virus in PBS. Combine 60 µL MES solution, 48 µL $CaCl_2$ solution, MUNANA solution (final concentration $5 \times K_m$), 4-guanidino-Neu5Ac2en (concentration range should give final rates of fluorescence increase that are 2–20-fold lower than the rate in an inhibitor-free control reaction), and water in the fluorescence cuvets.
2. Add virus to give a final volume of 0.6 mL in the cuvet.

3. Monitor fluorescence (excitation wavelength 365 nm, emission wavelength 450 nm) continuously for 1 h.
4. Construct plots of fluorescence against time.
5. If the plots of fluorescence against time are linear, 4-guanidino-Neu5Ac2en is a rapid-binding inhibitor of the neuraminidase. In this case derive initial rates (v) of fluorescence increase (FU/s) for each inhibitor concentration and the uninhibited control reaction. The K_i value can be calculated from a plot of 1/v vs [4-guanidino-Neu5Ac2en] by the method of Dixon *(10)*, using the K_m value for MUNANA obtained in **Subheading 3.2.2.**
6. If, unlike the data from the uninhibited control reaction, the plots of fluorescence against time are curved rather than linear, 4-guanidino-Neu5Ac2en is a slow-binding inhibitor of the neuraminidase. The data obtained at each inhibitor concentration should be fitted to the equation:

$$F = A + v_s.t + (v_o - v_s).\ (1 - e^{-k.t})\ /\ k \tag{1}$$

in which *F* represents the measured fluorescence, *t* represents time, and the values of the other parameters are obtained from the data-fitting routine at each inhibitor concentration.
7. Plots of *k* vs [4-guanidino-Neu5Ac2en] should be linear. The K_d value is given by the relationship:

$$K_d = {}^{Int}/_{Sl}.(1 + [MUNANA]\ /\ K_m) \tag{2}$$

where *Int* is the intercept obtained from the linear fit and *Sl* is the slope obtained from the linear fit.

3.3. Thermal Stability of Mutant NA and HA Proteins

Because of the destabilizing effect of the mutations on the structure of the mutant proteins, the NA mutant and some of the HA mutants display a marked thermolability. The NA mutant loses both enzyme activity as well as reactivity to the NC-10 mAb, which only recognizes the native NA *(7)*. The HA mutants lose the ability to bind to the receptor on red blood cells, resulting in a decrease in the hemagglutination titer, or to the sialic acids on fetuin in a fetuin-based ELISA assay.

3.3.1. Stability of NA Enzyme Activity

1. Prepare a dilution of virus that has approx 50 FU of activity after a 1 h incubation.
2. Incubate triplicate aliquots in water baths at 0, 37, 45, 55, and 60°C for 1 h.
3. Assay activity in the MUNANA assay as described above for 1 h at 37°C.
4. Calculate residual activity as a percentage of original activity at 0°C. Plot percent activity vs temperature and compare inactivation of mutant to parent virus NA.

3.3.2. Stability of NA Protein in an ELISA

1. Coat ELISA plates overnight with 10 µg/mL of protein A purified anti-NA MAb (e.g., NC-10 for G7oC N9 NA) in carbonate coating buffer, pH 9.6.

2. Block with PBS-Tween 20 for 30–60 min at room temperature.
3. Add dilutions of virus in PBS-casein and bind for 1 h at room temperature.
4. Wash in PBS-Tween 20, add polyclonal rabbit anti-NA sera in PBS-casein, and incubate 1 h at room temperature.
5. Wash, and add sheep antirabbit-HRPO conjugate.
6. Develop with ABTS.
7. Determine a suitable dilution that is in the linear range of absorbance.
8. Prepare aliquots of this dilution and incubate at the same temperatures as for the enzyme activity assays described in **Subheading 3.3.1.**
9. Calculate the binding of heat-treated viruses compared to virus held at 0°C.

3.4. Hemagglutinin ELISA

1. Coat ELISA plates overnight with 20 µg/mL of fetuin in coating buffer *(2)*. Block in PBS-Tween 20 for 1 h.
2. Serially dilute virus stocks in PBS and incubate 4 h to overnight at 4°C.
3. Wash in PBS-Tween 20.
4. Add monoclonal anti-HA in PBS-casein.
5. Wash and add antimouse-HRPO in PBS-casein.
6. Develop with ABTS and read in ELISA plate reader at 405 nm.
7. Select a dilution of the virus stock in the linear range of absorbance.
8. Prepare aliquots of this dilution and incubate replicates at the same temperatures as for the enzyme activity assays.
9. Calculate the binding of heat-treated viruses compared to virus held at 0°C.

3.5. Hemagglutination Elution

Some mutant viruses elute from chicken erythrocytes in the presence of drug. This may be the result of either a weakly binding HA, or a resistant NA that is still active in the presence of the drug. This assay is also useful in the absence of drug when the parent HA binds fairly strongly and elutes poorly. Variants are readily characterized by their ability to elute more rapidly than the parent virus.

1. Serially dilute virus in 50 µL of PBS, then add 50 µL of chicken erythrocytes.
2. Incubate for 45 min at 4°C in U-bottom microtiter plates. Determine dilution of virus containing 4 HA units. Photocopy the plate as a record of the titer.
3. Shift the plate to 37°C to determine how rapidly both the parent and variant viruses elute.
4. Preincubate 4 HA units with serial twofold dilutions of 4-guanidino-Neu5Ac2en for 30 min at room temperature starting from 10 µg/mL. Keep one well for the elution control of virus with PBS.
5. Add erythrocytes and incubate for a further 45 min at 4°C.
6. Photocopy plates for a record of the titer, then incubate at 37°C to allow elution of the virus.
7. Photocopy plates again and record the concentration of drug at which virus still elutes.

3.6. Quantifying NA "Specific Activity" by ELISA

Relative NA specific activity can be quantified using a combination of the NC-10 MAb-based ELISA for quantifying the relative amount of native protein and comparing this to the enzyme activity for the same dilutions in a MUNANA-based enzyme assay. Either purified NA prepared by pronase treatment of virus or whole virus can be used in both assays.

3.6.1. Purification of NA (6)

1. Inoculate 10-d-old embryonated eggs with the virus at approx 10–100 pfu/egg.
2. Harvest allantoic fluid after 48 h incubation.
3. Pellet the virus directly from the allantoic fluid and resuspend in 0.5% of the initial volume.
4. Pronase treat the virus for 2 h at 37°C, spin down cores at 100,000*g*, and save the first NA-containing supernatant.
5. Resuspend cores in PBS in half of the original volume.
6. Pronase cores again for 2 h at 37°C and spin them down.
7. Pool two NA-containing supernatants.
8. Extract with an equal volume of chloroform to remove lipids.
9. Concentrate approx 10-fold and purify NA over a Superose 12 column. NA tetramers elute immediately after the void volume.
10. Concentrate to between 1/100 and 1/1000 the original volume of allantoic fluid by ultrafiltration.
11. Protein concentration is estimated by an A_{280} value of 1.0, corresponding to approx 0.5 mg/mL NA.

3.6.2. NA Quantification

1. Titrate the relative amounts of NA protein for the parent and variant NA samples using the MAb-based ELISA described in **Subheading 3.3.2.**
2. Using the same dilutions titrate the NA enzyme activity in a MUNANA assay.
3. Plot the ELISA absorbance values for each dilution of the NA samples. On the same graph plot the NA enzyme activity for the same dilutions. The relative specific activity of the parent and the potential mutant can be determined by comparing the enzyme activities for the same absorbance values in the linear portion of the curves.

4. Notes

1. Since the NA enzyme is more sensitive to the inhibitor in an enzyme inhibition assay than in cell culture, virus stocks must be drug-free for accurate determination of enzyme activity and drug sensitivity. Thus, if virus stocks are grown in the presence of drug, they need to be dialysed overnight with 3–4 changes of buffer to remove bound 4-guanidino-Neu5Ac2en. This also includes the picking of plaques from an agarose overlay containing high concentrations of drug. Suf-

ficient drug can be carried over into the amplified culture to significantly inhibit enzyme activity.

2. The monoclonal NC-10 antibody only recognizes the native conformation of the NA from NWS/G70C (N9) virus; hence, the calculation of NA specific activity is based on activity of only native NA. If a polyclonal antibody is used to capture the NA the activity will be based on total NA protein, not just native NA. In the case of our NA mutant this was critical, since the NA is unstable and activity calculations are grossly different if one calculates activity of total vs native NA protein.
3. Inactivation of the HA can also be followed by the HA titer before and after heat treatments. However, it is more difficult to accurately determine a difference of half a well in an agglutination assay, whereas half the absorbance in an ELISA assay is accurately determined.
4. Virus for HA ELISA is incubated on the fetuin plates at 4°C to decrease NA cleavage of fetuin. Straight PBS is used in the initial incubation because the casein interferes with virus binding to the fetuin.
5. Although the A_{280} gives an approximate value for the total amount of NA protein, this does not necessarily represent native protein. Binding to an MAb recognizing only the native NA is the only way of determining the relative amount of native NA protein.

References

1. von Itzstein, M., Wu, W. Y., Kok, G. B., Pegg, M. S., Dyason, J. C., Phan, T. V., Smythe, M. L., White, H. F., Oliver, S. W., Colman, P. M., Varghese, J. N., Ryan, D. M., Woods, J. M., Bethell, R. C., Hotham, V. J., Cameron, J. M., and Penn, C. R. (1993) Rational design of potent sialidase-based inhibitors of influenza virus replication. *Nature* **363,** 418–423.
2. Blick, T. J., Tiong, T., Sahasrabudhe, A., Varghese, J. N., Colman, P. M., Hart, G. J., Bethell, R. C., and McKimm-Breschkin, J. L. (1995) Generation and characterization of an influenza virus neuraminidase variant with decreased sensitivity to the neuraminidase-specific inhibitor 4-guanidino-Neu5Ac2en. *Virology* **214,** 475–484.
3. Gubareva, L. V., Bethell, R. C., Hart, G. J., Murti, K. G., Penn, C. R., and Webster, R. G. (1996) Characterization of mutants of influenza A virus selected with the neuraminidase inhibitor 4-guanidino-Neu5Ac2en. *J. Virol.* **70,** 1818–1827.
4. Staschke, K. A., Colacino, J. M., Baxter, A. J., Air, G. M., Bansal, A., Hornback, W. J., Munroe, J. E., and Laver, W. G. (1995) Molecular basis for resistance of influenza viruses to 4-guanidino-Neu5Ac2en. *Virology* **214,** 642–646.
5. McKimm-Breschkin, J. L., Sahasrabudhe, A. V., Tiong, T., Marshall, D., Hart, G. J., Bethell, R. C., and Penn, C. R. (1996) Generation and characterization of variants of the NWS/G70C influenza virus after in vitro passage in 4-amino-Neu5Ac2en and 4-guanidino-Neu5Ac2en. *Antimicrob. Agents Chemother.* **40,** 40–46.
6. McKimm-Breschkin, J. L., Caldwell, J. B., Guthrie, R. E., and Kortt, A. A. (1991) A new method for the purification of the influenza A virus neuraminidase. *J. Virol Methods* **32,** 121–124.

7. McKimm-Breschkin, J. L., Blick, T. J., McDonald, M., and Colman, P. M. (1996) Mutation in the influenza virus neuraminidase gene resulting in decreased sensitivity to the neuraminidase inhibitor 4-guanidino-Neu5Ac2en leads to instability of the enzyme. *Virology* **225,** 240–242.
8. Hart, G. J. and Bethell, R. C. (1995) 2,3-Didehydro-2,4-dideoxy-4-guanidino-N-acetylneuraminic acid (4-guanindino-Neu5Ac2en) is a slow-binding inhibitor of sialidase from both influenza A and influenza B virus. *Biochem. Mol. Biol. Int.* **36,** 695–703.
9. Morrison, J. F. and Walsh, C. T. (1988) The behaviour and significance of slow-binding enzyme inhibitors. *Adv. Enzymol. Relat. Areas Mol. Biol.* **61,** 201–301.
10. Dixon, M. (1953) The determination of enzyme inhibitor constants. *Biochem. J.* **55,** 170, 171.

30

Virological Methods for the Generation and Characterization of Influenza Viruses with Reduced Sensitivity to 4-Guanidino-Neu5Ac2en

Jennifer L. McKimm-Breschkin, Anjali Sahasrabudhe, Tony J. Blick, Amanda J. Jowett, and Richard C. Bethell

1. Introduction

The compound 4-guanidino-Neu5Ac2en (zanamivir) has been described as a selective inhibitor of the influenza virus neuraminidase (NA) *(1)*. Viruses that are less sensitive to this inhibitor can be isolated after several passages in MDCK cells in the presence of the inhibitor. Variants isolated so far have had mutations predominantly in the hemagglutinin (HA) gene *(2)*. Many of these mutations appear to lower the affinity of the HA for the cellular receptor, so that there is less requirement for significant NA activity for the newly synthesized progeny virus to elute. There are three reports of a mutation in the NA gene, all at the same conserved site, glu 119 *(3–5)*. In this chapter, the authors describe methods for the isolation of the mutants, and for their characterization in cell culture based assays.

2. Materials

1. MDCK cells.
2. 4-guanidino-Neu5Ac2en, 4-amino-Neu5Ac2en, Neu5Ac2en.
3. Growth medium, Dulbecco's Modified Eagles Medium/Hams F12, supplemented with 10% fetal calf serum and glutamine, penicillin, streptomycin, and fungizone.
4. Maintenance medium, Minimal Eagles Medium and Liebovitz L15, 1:1, without serum, but with glutamine, penicillin, streptomycin, and fungizone. For virus culture add 0.1% TPCK-treated trypsin (Worthington) at 2 μL/mL.
5. PBS.
6. Indubiose agarose.

From: *Methods in Molecular Medicine, vol. 24: Antiviral Methods and Protocols*
Edited by: D. Kinchington and R. F. Schinazi © Humana Press Inc., Totowa, NJ

7. Assay medium, DCCM-1 (defined cell culture medium—Biological Industries) supplemented with glutamine, penicillin, streptomycin, 0.001% DEAE Dextran, TPCK-treated trypsin, and 0.5% indubiose agarose.
8. 5% gluteraldehyde in water.
9. 10% carbol fuchsin in water.
10. Anti-NA antibody to virus used, e.g., monoclonal NC-10 to the N9 NA of the NWS/G70C virus we have used, (Rob Webster, St. Jude Children's Medical Research Centre, Memphis, TN), or polyclonal anti-NA sera.
11. 1% formalin in normal saline, 0.15 *M*.
12. 0.05% neutral red in water.
13. Antinucleoprotein antibody, (monoclonal HB65 ATCC or polyclonal).
14. Microscope slides, and diamond pen or knife.
15. Nail polish.
16. Antisheep or antimouse antibody conjugated with FITC.
17. Fluorescent microscope.

3. Methods

3.1. Liquid Culture of Influenza

1. Seed MDCK cells in a 6-well cluster dish; use when confluent.
2. Prepare virus dilution at approx 0.1 plaque forming unit (PFU)/cell.
3. Remove growth medium, wash twice with prewarmed phosphate-buffered saline (PBS), and inoculate each well with the diluted influenza virus.
4. After adsorption, add 4 mL of maintenance medium containing drug at the 50% inhibitory concentration (IC_{50}) to four wells.
5. Add maintenance medium to the other two wells as controls.
6. After 2 d growth, scrape cells in each well into the medium.
7. Inoculate the resulting virus onto confluent MDCK cells in a 6-well cluster dish as in **step 3**.
8. After adsorption, add 4 mL of maintenance medium containing drug at $2 \times IC_{50}$ to four wells.
9. Add maintenance medium to the control wells.
10. Repeat **step 6**.
11. Continue to passage viruses as above and/or plaque-purify the viruses by plaque picking (*see* **Subheading 3.2.**).

3.2. Plaque Picking

1. Seed MDCK cells in a 6-well cluster dish, use when confluent.
2. Prepare six serial log_{10} dilutions of each virus.
3. Remove growth medium, wash twice with prewarmed PBS, and inoculate each dilution of virus into one well of the dish. Set up three plates for each virus.
4. After adsorption, add assay medium containing drug at approx $5 \times IC_{50}$ for plate one, $10 \times IC_{50}$ for plate two.
5. Add assay medium to plate three.
6 After 3 d growth, examine each plate for influenza plaques.

7. Pick any plaques present on plates one and two using a sterile pipet tip. Place agarose/plaque plug into maintenance medium.
8. Add glutaraldehyde to plate three for 2 h, remove agarose overlay, and add carbol fuchsin to each well for 30 min. Wash off stain and count plaques to determine the titer of each virus.
9. Repeat plaque picking using virus produced from **step 7**.
10. Repeat again to produce a plaque-purified virus stock ready for characterization.

3.3. Limiting Dilution Passaging of Virus

A limiting dilution method of passaging is preferable to blind passaging because virus that grows with the latter method may not be owing to the emergence of resistant variants, but owing to the virus swamping the amount of drug used.

1. Seed MDCK cells in a 24-well cluster dish, use when confluent.
2. Prepare four serial $\log_{10}$ dilutions of virus to be passaged, e.g., 10^{-2} to10^{-5}.
3. Remove growth medium, wash with PBS, and inoculate five wells across dish with each dilution of virus.
4. After adsorption, remove inoculum and add 1 mL of maintenance medium containing drug at approx 2 µg/mL to four wells only.
5. Add maintenance medium to the fifth well for the comparative growth of the diluted virus in the absence of drug.
6. Inoculate serial $\log_{10}$ dilutions of the original stock in the sixth well, for detection of spontaneous mutations owing to passaging.
7. After 3 d, observe cells for evidence of cytopathic effect (CPE).
8. Screen for virus growth by removing 50 µL of supernatant and testing for virus antigen in a slot-blot immunoassay, e.g., using an anti-NA antibody.
9. Virus from the most dilute sample showing growth is used for the next passage. This applies to both virus grown in drug and the control passage virus.
10. Once the virus appears to be growing to higher titers, increase the drug concentration in the subsequent passage by twofold.
11. Passaged virus can be plaqued under concentrations of drug known to inhibit the plaque size of the parent virus. Larger plaques can be picked as potential resistant variants.
12. Sensitivity of passaged virus to drug is then determined in a plaque inhibition assay, in a microtiter CPE inhibition assay in liquid culture, or in a yield reduction assay.

3.4. Plaque Reduction Assay

1. Seed MDCK cells in 60-mm, tissue culture Petri dishes, or 6-well cluster dishes.
2. After cells are confluent, remove growth medium, wash cells with PBS, and add approx 100 PFU of virus to each dish.
3. Adsorb virus for 1 h, remove the inoculum, and overlay cells with agarose containing $\log_{10}$ dilutions of 4-guanidino-Neu5Ac2en ranging from 0.0003 to 3.0 µg/mL, 4-amino-Neu5Ac2en ranging from 0.01 to 100 µg/mL or Neu5Ac2en ranging from 0.01 to 100 µg/mL.

4. After 4 d at 37°C, fix plaques with formalin for a minimum of 4 h to allow formalin to penetrate through the agarose.
5. Remove agarose and stain plaques with neutral red.
6. Determine sensitivity by the relative decrease in both size and number of plaques.
7. HA mutants are characteristically equally crossresistant to Neu5Ac2en and the 4-amino derivative in the plaque assay.

3.5. $TCID_{50}$ Determination of Drug Sensitivity

The drug sensitivity in liquid culture is determined using approx 100 $TCID_{50}$ of virus. The infectivity of the virus stock therefore needs to be initially determined in a $TCID_{50}$ assay.

3.5.1. $TCID_{50}$ Infectivity Assay

1. Seed MDCK cells in growth medium in 96-well plates and grow to confluency.
2. After overnight incubation, remove growth medium and add 100 µL of maintenance medium to each well.
3. Serially dilute both the control virus and the potential variant virus in quadruplicate, across the 96-well plate in half log_{10} or twofold dilutions. Depending on estimated titer of stock, start dilutions between 10^{-3} and 10^{-5}.
4. After 4 d, fix cells with formalin-saline for a min. of 1 h.
5. Flick off supernatants and then stain monolayers with neutral red for a minimum of 1 h.
6. End point is the last dilution showing virus CPE. A dilution of virus containing approx 100 $TCID_{50}$ is used in the subsequent drug sensitivity assay.

3.5.2. CPE Inhibition Assay for Drug Sensitivity

1. Seed MDCK cells in growth medium in 96-well plates and grow to confluency.
2. Remove growth medium and add maintenance medium.
3. Dilute drug across plate in half log_{10} dilutions starting from 30 µg/mL.
4. Add 100 $TCID_{50}$ of either the control or variant virus to each well. Use quadruplicates for each virus at each drug concentration. Add virus without drug to four wells as controls for cpe.
5. Incubate cultures for 4 d, after which fix and stain as for the infectivity assay.
6. Drug sensitivity is determined as the last dilution of drug inhibiting the development of virus CPE.
7. Sensitivity of the variant is compared to the sensitivity of the parent control virus.

3.5.3. Yield Reduction Assay

Sensitivity in liquid culture can also be assessed in a yield reduction assay. This can also be useful for some variant viruses that may not cause distinct CPE in a $TCID_{50}$ assay.

1. Seed MDCK cells in growth medium in a 24-well cluster dish.
2. When almost confluent, remove medium and add virus at 0.1 PFU/cell in 100 µL.

3. Adsorb for 1 h at room temperature and remove inoculum.
4. To duplicate wells, add log_{10} dilutions of drug in 1 mL of maintenance medium from 30 to 0.003 μg/mL. Leave one pair of wells without drug for the control.
5. Incubate for 24 h.
6. Remove supernatants.
7. Assay virus yields either by a $TCID_{50}$ assay or by a plaque assay.
8. Compare yields of parent and variant virus for each drug dilution and compare these to the control yields without drug.

3.6. Resistance Reversion

To determine the stability of the resistance phenotype, variant virus is serially passaged by limiting dilution, in the absence of drug.

1. Inoculate serial log_{10} dilutions of virus across six wells in a 24-well cluster dish.
2. Grow three rows in the absence of drug. Add drug to each dilution of virus in the fourth row, to determine the relative drug sensitivity.
3. Observe virus growth after 3 d in culture, and quantitate by a slot blot immunoassay using an anti-NA antibody.
4. Select virus from the most dilute well showing growth, for the subsequent passage.
5. Test virus for the resistant phenotype in an enzyme inhibition assay, or in a plaque assay, either when the virus appears more sensitive or after 10 passages.
6. If the variant is now sensitive, the mutated gene needs to be sequenced to determine whether there has been a back mutation(s) to the original amino acid(s), or whether there has been a complementary mutation suppressing the original one(s).

3.7. Adsorption Assay

Many of the influenza mutants that demonstrate in vitro resistance to 4-guanidino-Neu5Ac2en have mutations in the HA gene, rather than in the NA gene. These mutant HAs appear to have a reduced affinity for the cellular receptor, which means that they have less requirement for NA activity for the elution of newly synthesized progeny. However, it also means that their binding to the cellular receptor at the adsorption phase may be less efficient. Efficiency of adsorption can be followed by allowing the virus only limited time to attach before removal, and assessing the numbers of cells infected, by staining for synthesis of the viral nucleoprotein 5–6 h postinfection. The adsorption step is carried out on ice to synchronize the infection and to ensure that virus can only adsorb to, but not be internalized by, the cells.

1. Cut microscope slides into quarters using a diamond pen, and sterilize in a beaker containing 70% ethanol.
2. Remove slides and place several in a Petri dish, or a large 100-mm, square sterile plastic dish. These do not need to be tissue culture treated, because the cells only need to grow on the slides. Allow to air-dry in a biohazard cabinet.

3. Seed MDCK cells into Petri dishes, using approx 20% more volume and cells than would be normally used for that size dish.
4. When cells are just confluent, wash slides in cold PBS and remove to individual dishes.
5. Cool dishes on ice, in a cold room. Inoculate with 50–100 μL of virus, at an multiplicity of infection of approx 5.
6. Adsorb on ice, removing inoculum and washing cells with PBS after 10, 20, 40, and 60 min.
7. For control of maximum adsorption, allow virus to adsorb for 60 min on ice, followed by 60 min at 37°C before removal.
8. Add maintenance medium containing 0.5% fetal calf serum, this maintains the cell integrity better than without the serum.
9. After 6 h at 37°C, fix slides in acetone, air-dry, and store at –20°C.
10. Divide each slide into two halves by painting a line of nail polish across slide. For staining balance slides on two wooden skewers in a dish containing a damp paper towel. Add 50 μL of diluted antinucleoprotein antibody to one-half only of each slide. Cover dish and incubate at room temperature for 30–60 min.
11. Wash slides by immersing in a small container of PBS, and blot dry by dabbing edge on paper towel.
12. Add antispecies antibody conjugated with fluoresceine isothiocyanate, to whole slide, and incubate at room temperature in humidified container for 30–60 min.
13. Wash in PBS, followed by a brief wash in distilled water, and air-dry. View with fluorescent microscope.
14. Compare numbers of cells infected under maximum adsorption conditions, to limited adsorption period. Compare variants to parent control virus.
15. A decrease in adsorption efficiency is indicative of an HA mutation.

4. Notes

1. If too high an inoculum of virus is used in the $TCID_{50}$ drug sensitivity assay, the viruses are not particularly sensitive.
2. Picking of large plaques under higher concentrations of drug has yielded only HA mutants. The NA mutants isolated so far produce smaller plaques than the parent virus without drug in the overlay, although they do continue to plaque under concentrations of drug that are inhibitory to the parent virus.
3. To try to avoid selection of weakly binding HA variants, the passaged virus can be adsorbed for only 10–15 min before being washed off with warmed PBS *(3)*.

References

1. von Itzstein, M., Wu, W. Y., Kok, G. B., Pegg, M. S., Dyason, J. C., Phan, T. V., Smythe, M. L., White, H. F., Oliver, S. W., Colman, P. M., Varghese, J. N., Ryan, D. M., Woods, J. M., Bethell, R. C., Hotham, V. J., Cameron, J. M., and Penn, C. R. (1993) Rational design of potent sialidase-based inhibitors of influenza virus replication. *Nature* **363,** 418–423.
2. McKimm-Breschkin, J. L., Blick, T. J., Sahasrabudhe, A. V., Tiong, T., Marshall, D., Hart, G. J., Bethell, R. C., and Penn, C. R. (1996) Generation and character-

ization of variants of the NWS/G70C influenza virus after in vitro passage in 4-amino-Neu5Ac2en and 4-guanidino-Neu5Ac2en. *Antimicrob. Agents Chemother.* **40,** 40–46.

3. Blick, T. J., Tiong, T., Sahasrabudhe, A., Varghese, J. N., Colman, P. M., Hart, G. J., Bethell, R. C., and McKimm-Breschkin, J. L. (1995) Generation and characterization of an influenza virus neuraminidase variant with decreased sensitivity to the neuraminidase-specific inhibitor 4-guanidino-Neu5Ac2en. *Virology* **214,** 475–484.
4. Gubareva, L. V., Bethell, R. C., Hart, G. J., Murti, K. G., Penn, C. R., and Webster, R. G. (1996) Characterization of mutants of influenza A virus selected with the neuraminidase inhibitor 4-guanidino-Neu5Ac2en. *J. Virol.* **70,** 1818–1827.
5. Staschke, K. A., Colacino, J. M., Baxter, A. J., Air, G. M., Bansal, A., Hornback, W. J., Munroe, J. E., and Laver, W. G. (1995) Molecular basis for resistance of influenza viruses to 4-guanidino-Neu5Ac2en. *Virology* **214,** 642–646.

Index

W

X

Y

Z

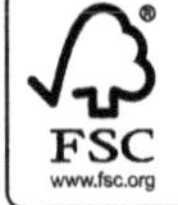

MIX
Papier aus verantwortungsvollen Quellen
Paper from responsible sources
FSC® C105338

If you have any concerns about our products,
you can contact us on
ProductSafety@springernature.com

In case Publisher is established outside the EU,
the EU authorized representative is:
Springer Nature Customer Service Center GmbH
Europaplatz 3, 69115 Heidelberg, Germany

Printed by Libri Plureos GmbH
in Hamburg, Germany